# Biomarkers in Neurodegenerative Diseases 2.0

# Biomarkers in Neurodegenerative Diseases 2.0

Editor

**Arnab Ghosh**

MDPI • Basel • Beijing • Wuhan • Barcelona • Belgrade • Manchester • Tokyo • Cluj • Tianjin

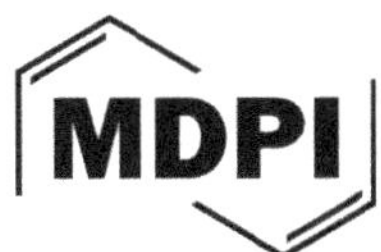

*Editor*
Arnab Ghosh
Cleveland State University
USA

*Editorial Office*
MDPI
St. Alban-Anlage 66
4052 Basel, Switzerland

This is a reprint of articles from the Special Issue published online in the open access journal *Biomedicines* (ISSN 2227-9059) (available at: https://www.mdpi.com/journal/biomedicines/special_issues/biomarkers_neurodegenerative_2).

For citation purposes, cite each article independently as indicated on the article page online and as indicated below:

| LastName, A.A.; LastName, B.B.; LastName, C.C. Article Title. *Journal Name* **Year**, *Volume Number*, Page Range. |
|---|

**ISBN 978-3-0365-5731-1 (Hbk)**
**ISBN 978-3-0365-5732-8 (PDF)**

# Contents

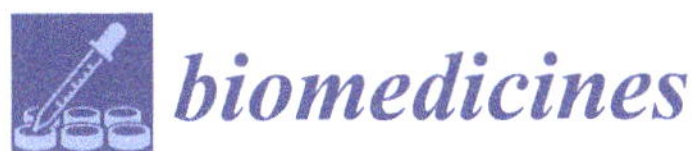 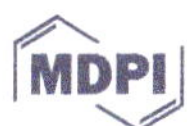

*Review*

# Mechanistic Insights into Alzheimer's Disease Unveiled through the Investigation of Disturbances in Central Metabolites and Metabolic Pathways

**Raúl González-Domínguez [1,2,*], Álvaro González-Domínguez [3], Ana Sayago [1,2], Juan Diego González-Sanz [4], Alfonso María Lechuga-Sancho [3,5,6] and Ángeles Fernández-Recamales [1,2]**

1 AgriFood Laboratory, Faculty of Experimental Sciences, University of Huelva, 21007 Huelva, Spain; ana.sayago@dqcm.uhu.es (A.S.); recamale@dqcm.uhu.es (Á.F.-R.)
2 International Campus of Excellence CeiA3, University of Huelva, 21007 Huelva, Spain
3 Inflammation, Nutrition, Metabolism and Oxidative Stress Study Group (INMOX), Biomedical Research and Innovation Institute of Cádiz (INiBICA), Research Unit, Puerta del Mar University Hospital, 11009 Cádiz, Spain; alvaro.gonzalez@inibica.es (Á.G.-D.); alfonso.lechuga@uca.es (A.M.L.-S.)
4 Department of Nursing, COIDESO Research Center, University of Huelva, 21007 Huelva, Spain; juan.gonzalez@denf.uhu.es
5 Pediatric Endocrinology, Department of Pediatrics, Puerta del Mar University Hospital, 11009 Cádiz, Spain
6 Area of Pediatrics, Department of Child and Mother Health and Radiology, Medical School, University of Cádiz, 11002 Cádiz, Spain
* Correspondence: raul.gonzalez@dqcm.uhu.es; Tel.: +34-959-219-975

**Citation:** González-Domínguez, R.; González-Domínguez, Á.; Sayago, A.; González-Sanz, J.D.; Lechuga-Sancho, A.M.; Fernández-Recamales, Á. Mechanistic Insights into Alzheimer's Disease Unveiled through the Investigation of Disturbances in Central Metabolites and Metabolic Pathways. *Biomedicines* **2021**, *9*, 298. https://doi.org/10.3390/biomedicines9030298

Academic Editor: Arnab Ghosh

Received: 2 February 2021
Accepted: 12 March 2021
Published: 14 March 2021



**Abstract:** Hydrophilic metabolites are closely involved in multiple primary metabolic pathways and, consequently, play an essential role in the onset and progression of multifactorial human disorders, such as Alzheimer's disease. This review article provides a comprehensive revision of the literature published on the use of mass spectrometry-based metabolomics platforms for approaching the central metabolome in Alzheimer's disease research, including direct mass spectrometry, gas chromatography-mass spectrometry, hydrophilic interaction liquid chromatography-mass spectrometry, and capillary electrophoresis-mass spectrometry. Overall, mounting evidence points to profound disturbances that affect a multitude of central metabolic pathways, such as the energy-related metabolism, the urea cycle, the homeostasis of amino acids, fatty acids and nucleotides, neurotransmission, and others.

**Keywords:** central metabolites; Alzheimer's disease; mass spectrometry; central metabolic pathways

## 1. Alzheimer's Disease and Metabolomics: The Challenge of Hydrophilic Metabolites

Alzheimer's disease (AD) is nowadays a major health problem due to the dramatic population aging worldwide. As this neurodegenerative disorder presents great variability of complex clinical symptoms and a long pre-symptomatic period, the underlying etiological factors remain a tangled meshwork to be unraveled. In this respect, mounting evidence points to a multifactorial and systemic crosstalk of heterogeneous pathological mechanisms, encompassing the well-known proteopathies associated with the deposition of β-amyloid plaques and the hyper-phosphorylation of tau protein, but also other cellular perturbations related to oxidative stress and inflammation, energy-related disturbances, altered neurotransmission, and metal homeostasis, among others [1–3]. Considering this multifaceted nature, numerous authors have extensively explored the potential of metabolomics for holistically elucidating the characteristic molecular alterations behind the onset and progression of AD [4,5]. In this vein, nuclear magnetic resonance (NMR) and reversed-phase liquid chromatography coupled to mass spectrometry (RPLC-MS) are currently the gold standard techniques in metabolomics, and most of the literature published on AD research is based on their application to brain, cerebrospinal fluid (CSF), blood, and other biological matrices. However, it is recognized that the low sensitivity and low spectral resolution of NMR considerably reduce its coverage, thus impeding comprehensive metabolomics analysis [6]. On the other hand, although great efforts have been made to develop large-scale RPLC-MS metabolomics approaches [7], this analytical platform is usually limited to the determination of low and medium polarity metabolites, such as lipids (i.e., lipidomics) [8], aromatic amino acids and their microbiota derivatives [9], some nutrients and food-related metabolites (i.e., nutrimetabolomics) [10,11], and a few other metabolite classes. Accordingly, the efficient profiling of hydrophilic metabolites is still a methodological challenge. Hydrophilic metabolites comprise multiple chemical classes, including sugars, most amino acids and derivatives, biogenic amines, organic acids, and many others, which are in turn involved in a multitude of central metabolic pathways, such as the energy-related metabolism (e.g., glycolysis, tricarboxylic (TCA) cycle), the urea cycle, the one-carbon metabolism, and others. Therefore, orthogonal analytical tools are crucial to approach this essential piece of the human metabolome puzzle, namely direct mass spectrometry (DMS), gas chromatography-mass spectrometry (GC-MS), hydrophilic interaction liquid chromatography-mass spectrometry (HILIC-MS), and capillary electrophoresis-mass spectrometry (CE-MS).

DMS fingerprinting, based on the direct introduction of the sample extracts into the mass spectrometer, shows great utility for high-throughput and comprehensive metabolomics analysis thanks to the lack of a chromatographic or electrophoretic separation prior to MS detection, which inherently bias the method coverage [12]. However, this screening tool suffers from considerable ion suppression and the impossibility of resolving isomeric metabolites, which make the use of complementary approaches mandatory. Among MS-based hyphenated methods, GC-MS has been widely employed in metabolomics because of its reproducibility, chromatographic resolution, sensitivity, and selectivity [13]. This technique usually requires the application of a derivatization process before the analysis for increasing the volatility and thermal stability of metabolites, thus enabling the profiling of numerous low molecular weight central metabolites, such as amino acids, sugars, organic and fatty acids, amines, and many other primary metabolites. To avoid this derivatization step, which may represent an important source of variability and bias, the use of HILIC-MS is significantly increasing over the last years to analyze hydrophilic metabolites [14]. Complementarily, the coupling CE-MS provides orthogonal separation performance to LC and GC approaches for the analysis of highly polar and ionic metabolites [15]. Nonetheless, HILIC and CE present serious reproducibility-related limitations (e.g., drifts in retention/migration times along sequence runs) and reduced sensitivity compared with the most robust RPLC-MS and GC-MS platforms, which consequently hinder their application in large-scale metabolomics. Although much less employed in metabolomics, other RPLC-based alternatives for approaching polar metabolites include the use of ion-pair agents or derivatization to reduce the polarity of hydrophilic metabolites. However, ion pairing may provoke ion suppression during MS analysis, contamination of the MS ion source, and column instability, whereas common derivatization protocols (e.g., dansylation) are time-consuming and considerably reduce the method coverage toward specific metabolites classes that are sensitive to the derivatizing reagent. As a complementary approach, the use of imaging mass spectrometry is gaining great importance for in situ metabolomics analysis to map the molecular mechanisms underlying neurodegenerative disorders [16]. These techniques can complement traditional MS platforms relying on the investigation of postmortem and peripheral biofluid samples, thus facilitating the association between metabolomics and histological data. However, the application of these tools in AD research is still scarce and mainly limited to the lipidome [16]. Therefore, considering the inherent limitations of each one of all the platforms usually employed in metabolomics, more and more authors have emphasized the benefit of combining complementary techniques to obtain comprehensive metabolomics coverage [17].

The next sections of this review article provide an overview of the literature published over the last years aimed to explore the AD-characteristic disturbances in central metabolites and associated metabolic pathways through the application of the MS-based metabolomics platforms that are described above, as summarized in Table 1. The literature search was conducted in three online databases (Scopus, Web of Science, PubMed), using the search terms "Alzheimer", "metabolomics", "mass spectrometry", "gas chromatography", "hydrophilic interaction liquid chromatography", "capillary electrophoresis", and "direct infusion". Studies not focused on the hydrophilic metabolome were discarded.

**Table 1.** Summary of hydrophilic-oriented metabolomics studies on Alzheimer's disease.

| Study Population | Analytical Platform | Biological Sample | Key Results (Altered Pathways) | Ref. |
|---|---|---|---|---|
| AD (N = 22)/healthy controls (N = 18) | DMS | serum | Energy metabolism (glucose, carnitine, creatine), fatty acid metabolism (free fatty acids, eicosanoids), neurotransmission (dopamine), phospholipid homeostasis | [18] |
| AD (N = 22)/healthy controls (N = 18) | DMS | serum | Phospholipid homeostasis | [19] |
| AD (N = 22)/healthy controls (N = 18) | DMS | serum | Nitrogen metabolism (guanidine, arginine, putrescine), fatty acid metabolism (eicosanoids), neurotransmission (kynurenine), phospholipid homeostasis | [20] |
| AD (N = 19)/healthy controls (N = 17) | DMS + RPLC-MS | serum | Phospholipid homeostasis | [21] |
| AD (N = 30)/healthy controls (N = 30) | DMS (APPI) | serum | Energy metabolism (creatine, malic acid), fatty acid metabolism (free fatty acids, fatty acid amides), neurotransmission (dopamine, serotonin, picolinic acid), phospholipid and sphingolipid homeostasis | [22] |
| APP × PS1 (N = 30)/WT (N = 30) | DMS (ESI+APPI) | serum | Energy metabolism (glucose, carnitine, creatine), fatty acid metabolism (free fatty acids, eicosanoids), nitrogen metabolism (urea), amino acid metabolism, lipid homeostasis | [23] |
| APP × PS1 (N = 10)/WT (N = 10) | DMS | urine | Unidentified discriminant signals | [24] |
| APP × PS1 (N = 30)/WT (N =30) | DMS | hippocampus, cortex, cerebellum, olfactory bulb | Energy metabolism (pyruvic acid), fatty acid metabolism (free fatty acids, acyl-carnitines, eicosanoids), nucleotide metabolism, nitrogen metabolism (urea, N-acetylspermidine), amino acid metabolism, neurotransmission (dopamine), phospholipid homeostasis | [25] |
| APP × PS1 (N = 30)/WT (N = 30) | DMS | liver, kidney, spleen, thymus | Energy metabolism (glycolysis, TCA, creatine), fatty acid metabolism (free fatty acids, acyl-carnitines, eicosanoids), nucleotide metabolism, nitrogen metabolism (urea, polyamines), amino acid metabolism, lipid homeostasis | [26] |
| APP × PS1 × IL4-KO (N = 7)/APP × PS1 (N = 7)/WT (N = 7) | DMS | serum | Fatty acid metabolism (eicosanoids), nitrogen metabolism (urea, citrulline), amino acid metabolism, neurotransmission (dopamine, histamine) | [27] |
| CRND8 (N = 6)/WT (N = 6) | DMS | hippocampus | Energy metabolism (glucose), fatty acid metabolism (eicosanoids, β-oxidation) | [28] |
| CRND8 (N = 6)/WT (N = 6) | DMS | cerebellum | Fatty acid metabolism (eicosanoids), amino acid metabolism, nucleotide metabolism (purines) | [29] |
| AD (N = 9)/healthy controls (N = 9) | GC-MS | hippocampus, entorhinal cortex, middle-temporal gyrus, sensory cortex, motor cortex, cingulate gyrus, cerebellum | Energy metabolism (glycolysis, pentose phosphate, TCA), nucleotide metabolism, nitrogen metabolism (urea), amino acid metabolism | [30] |
| SAMP8 (N = 5, 2 months; N = 6, 7 months; N = 7, 12 months) | GC-MS | hippocampus | Energy metabolism (TCA, lactic acid), nitrogen metabolism (urea), amino acid metabolism, lipid homeostasis | [31] |
| APP × PS1 (N = 12)/WT (N = 11) | GC-MS | hippocampus | Energy metabolism (ketone bodies), amino acid metabolism, sphingolipid homeostasis | [32] |
| TASTPM (N = 16)/WT (N = 5) | GC-MS | whole brain, plasma | Energy metabolism (glycolysis, pentose phosphate), amino acid metabolism, steroid homeostasis | [33] |

**Table 1.** *Cont.*

| Study Population | Analytical Platform | Biological Sample | Key Results (Altered Pathways) | Ref. |
|---|---|---|---|---|
| AD (N = 23)/healthy controls (N = 21) | GC-MS | serum | Energy metabolism (glucose, TCA, lactic acid), fatty acid metabolism (free fatty acids), nucleotide metabolism, nitrogen metabolism (urea, ornithine), amino acid metabolism | [34] |
| AD (N = 24)/MCI (N = 16)/PD (N = 22)/healthy controls (N = 8) | GC-MS | exhaled breath | Phenol (PD) | [35] |
| $APP_{Tg2576}$ (N = 15)/CRND8 (N = 9)/ $APP_{V717I}$ (N = 10)/WT (N = 17 + 9 + 12) | GC-MS | urine | Urinary odorants | [36] |
| AD (N = 47)/MCI (N = 143)/healthy controls (N = 46) | GC-MS + RPLC-MS | serum | Baseline: lipid homeostasis (phospholipids, sphingolipids, sterols) Progression: energy metabolism (2,4-dihydroxybutanoic acid) | [37] |
| AD (N = 57)/MCI (N = 58)/healthy controls (N = 57) | GC-MS + RPLC-MS | plasma | Fatty acid metabolism (free fatty acids), energy metabolism (glycolysis, TCA), one-carbon metabolism, amino acid metabolism, nucleotide metabolism | [38] |
| DS-AD (N = 78)/DS-control (N = 68) | GC-MS + RPLC-MS | plasma | Energy metabolism (anaerobic respiration) | [39] |
| $APP_{Tg2576}$ (N = 3)/PS1 (N = 3)/APP × PS1 (N = 6)/WT (N = 6) | GC-MS + RPLC-MS | hippocampus | Energy metabolism (glycolysis, TCA), nucleotide metabolism, amino acid metabolism, neurotransmission | [40] |
| AD (N = 79)/healthy controls (N = 51) | GC-MS + RPLC-MS | CSF | Neurotransmission (dopamine, noradrenaline, MHPG), cortisol, uridine | [41] |
| AD (N = 40)/healthy controls (N = 38) | GC-MS + RPLC-MS | CSF | Two unidentified discriminant signals | [42] |
| APP × PS1 (N = 30)/WT (N = 30) | GC-MS + RPLC-MS | serum | Energy metabolism (glycolysis, TCA), fatty acid metabolism (free fatty acids, fatty acid amides, acyl-carnitines, eicosanoids), nitrogen metabolism (urea, citrulline), nucleotide metabolism, amino acid metabolism, neurotransmission (serotonin), homeostasis of cholesterol, phospholipids and sphingolipids | [43] |
| APP × PS1 (N = 30)/WT (N = 30) | GC-MS + RPLC-MS | hippocampus, cortex, striatum, cerebellum, olfactory bulb | Energy metabolism (glycolysis, TCA), nitrogen metabolism (urea), amino acid metabolism, neurotransmission (dopamine), phospholipid and sphingolipid homeostasis | [44] |
| APP × PS1 (N = 30)/WT (N = 30) | GC-MS + RPLC-MS | liver, kidney | Energy metabolism (glycolysis, TCA), fatty acid metabolism (free fatty acids, acyl-carnitines), nitrogen metabolism (urea, spermidine), amino acid metabolism, homeostasis of cholesterol, phospholipids and sphingolipids | [45] |
| APP × PS1 (N = 30)/WT (N = 30) | GC-MS + RPLC-MS | spleen, thymus | Energy metabolism (glycolysis, TCA), fatty acid metabolism (free fatty acids, acyl-carnitines), nitrogen metabolism (urea, putrescine), nucleotide metabolism, amino acid metabolism, homeostasis of cholesterol, phospholipids and sphingolipids | [46] |
| AD (N = 15)/healthy controls (N = 15) | HILIC-MS | neocortex | 76 unidentified discriminant signals | [47] |
| AD (N =20)/healthy controls (N = 20) | HILIC-MS | plasma | 54 unidentified discriminant signals | [48] |
| MCI_AD (N = 19)/MCI (N = 16)/healthy controls (N = 37) | HILIC-MS | plasma | Polyamine metabolism, L-arginine metabolism | [49] |
| CRND8 (N = 18/12, 12/18 weeks)/WT (N = 12/12, 12/18 weeks) | HILIC-MS | urine | Aromatic amino acid metabolism, nucleotide metabolism, ascorbate metabolism | [50] |
| AD (N = 15)/MCI (N = 15)/healthy controls (N = 15) | HILIC-MS + RPLC-MS | plasma, CSF | Energy metabolism (glycolysis, TCA), fatty acid metabolism, amino acid metabolism, neurotransmission, lipid homeostasis | [51] |
| AD (N = 21)/MCI_AD (N = 12)/MCI_stable (N = 21)/healthy controls (N = 21) | HILIC-MS + RPLC-MS | CSF | Nucleotide metabolism, amino acid metabolism, neurotransmission | [52] |
| AD (N = 9)/healthy controls (N = 9) | HILIC-MS + RPLC-MS | superior temporal cortex | Amino acid metabolism, neurotransmission | [53] |
| AD (N = 21)/healthy controls (N = 19) | HILIC-MS + RPLC-MS | frontal cortex | Amino acid metabolism, purine metabolism, pantothenate and CoA biosynthesis, phospholipid homeostasis | [54] |
| AD (N = 30)/MCI (N = 30)/healthy controls (N = 30) | HILIC-MS + RPLC-MS | plasma | Sphingolipid metabolism | [55] |

**Table 1.** *Cont.*

| Study Population | Analytical Platform | Biological Sample | Key Results (Altered Pathways) | Ref. |
|---|---|---|---|---|
| AD (N = 23)/MCI_AD (N = 9)/MCI_stable (N = 22)/SCI (N = 19) | CE-MS | CSF | Amino acid metabolism, fatty acid metabolism, one-carbon metabolism | [56] |
| AD (N = 42)/MCI (N = 14)/healthy controls (N = 37) | CE-MS | serum | Amino acid metabolism, fatty acid metabolism, one-carbon metabolism | [57] |
| AD (N = 17)/asymptomatic AD (N = 13)/healthy controls (N = 13) | CE-MS | inferior temporal gyrus, middle frontal gyrus, cerebellum | Nitrogen metabolism (urea, polyamines), one-carbon metabolism, neurotransmission | [58] |
| AD (N = 3)/FTLD (N = 4)/LBD (N = 3)/healthy controls (N = 9) | CE-MS | serum, saliva | Energy metabolism, amino acid metabolism | [59] |
| AD (N = 81)/iNPH (N = 57) | CE-MS | CSF | Energy metabolism, amino acid metabolism | [60] |
| AD (N = 15)/healthy controls (N = 15) | RPLC-MS (ion pairing) | CSF | Neurotransmission, nucleotide metabolism, antioxidant defense | [61] |
| AD (N= 40)/MCI (N = 36)/healthy controls (N = 38) | RPLC-MS (ion pairing) | CSF | Neurotransmission, nucleotide metabolism, antioxidant defense | [62] |
| MCI (N = 20)/healthy controls (N = 20) | RPLC-MS (derivatization) | saliva | Taurine | [63] |
| CRND8 (N = 12)/WT (N = 12) | RPLC-MS (derivatization) | urine | Taurine, amino acid metabolism | [64] |
| AD_younger (N = 4)/AD_older (N = 4)/healthy controls (N = 3) | RPLC-MS (derivatization) | frontal lobe | L-phenylalanine, L-lactate | [65] |
| AD (N = 17)/healthy controls (N = 17) | RPLC-MS (improved retention for polar metabolites) | CSF | 53 unidentified discriminant signals | [66] |
| AD I-II (N = 7)/AD III-IV (N = 4)/AD V-VI (N = 5)/healthy controls (N = 4) | RPLC-MS (improved retention for polar metabolites) | entorhinal cortex | Nucleotide metabolism | [67] |

## 2. Alzheimer's Disease and DMS-Based Metabolomics

DMS analysis has been repeatedly applied in various AD metabolomics studies as a first-pass screening tool for simultaneously measuring a wide range of metabolite classes, including hydrophilic metabolites and lipids, in a high-throughput manner [68]. Two-step extraction of serum samples from AD patients and subsequent DMS fingerprinting revealed significant perturbations in the circulating levels of energy-related metabolites (e.g., glucose, fatty acids, and carnitine involved in β-oxidation) and neurotransmitters (e.g., dopamine) [18]. Additionally, it also found an abnormal phospholipid homeostasis reflected in reduced levels of species containing polyunsaturated fatty acids, increased levels of phospholipids composed of saturated fatty acids, and increased content of breakdown products (e.g., choline). Interestingly, this was then corroborated in other DMS-based works focused on the serum AD-related lipidome [19,20] and phospholipidome [21]. Although the electrospray (ESI) source is the most common ionization technique employed in DMS analysis, the atmospheric pressure photoionization (APPI) source has demonstrated complementary performance and metabolomics coverage [22]. In this work, the authors reported an accumulation of diacylglycerols, free fatty acids, and ceramides in AD serum, which is in line with the upregulated degradation of membrane lipids that was hypothesized in previous DMS studies, as well as other disturbances related to the monoaminergic neurotransmission and the urea cycle. These DMS-based high-throughput metabolomics platforms have also been employed to investigate the AD-like pathology in the APP × PS1 transgenic mouse model by considering multiple biological matrices, namely serum [23], urine [24], brain [25], and other peripheral organs [26]. The analysis of serum samples evidenced comparable metabolic disturbances to those reported in human studies, thus corroborating the utility of this transgenic line to model AD [23]. A similar strategy was applied to investigate the effect of interleukin-4 depletion (i.e., IL4-KO) on AD pathology by using APP × PS1×IL4-KO mice [27]. The results showed reduced serum content of various amino acids and metabolites implicated in the urea cycle, and the accumulation of eicosanoids in the IL4-KO model, which supported the close link between AD and inflammatory processes. Metabolomics fingerprinting of brain tissue enabled the in situ and region-specific investigation of the neuropathological processes underlying this neurodegenerative disorder [25]. Hippocampus and cortex were characterized by profound alterations in the levels of numerous lipids (e.g., phospholipids, fatty acids, acyl-carnitines, steroids) and hydrophilic metabolites (e.g., amino acids and derivatives), whereas other brain areas such as the cerebellum and olfactory bulbs were less affected. Complementarily, other peripheral organs, including the liver, kidneys, spleen, and thymus, were also studied to evaluate the systemic manifestations of the molecular mechanisms behind the AD pathology [26]. In this line, Lin et al. applied DMS metabolomics to characterize the metabolic perturbations in hippocampus [28] and cerebellum [29] of the CRND8 transgenic mouse. Interestingly, the most important findings were related to an altered metabolism of arachidonic acid and eicosanoids, amino acids, nucleotides, and other metabolite classes, which were in great agreement with the studies performed on the APP × PS1 model.

## 3. Alzheimer's Disease and GC-MS Based Metabolomics

Metabolomics based on GC-MS has been successfully applied to various biological samples for investigating the impact of AD on primary metabolic pathways. Widespread disturbances related to the glucose metabolism, the urea cycle, and amino acid homeostasis were detected in seven brain regions from AD patients (hippocampus, entorhinal cortex, middle-temporal gyrus, cingulate gyrus, sensory cortex, motor cortex, cerebellum), including some regions traditionally considered not to be affected [30]. Similar alterations were observed in the hippocampus of the SAMP8 mouse along a 10-month follow-up, comprising energy-related metabolites, amino acids, lipids, and some others [31]. In this regard, Han et al. have demonstrated that these hippocampal metabolic perturbations may be sharpened by chronic unpredictable mild stress in APP × PS1 mice, particularly in relation to the metabolism of amino acids, ketone bodies, and sphingolipids [32]. Furthermore, comparative analysis of brain and plasma from TASTPM mice revealed the occurrence of similar disturbances in both biological matrices, thus reinforcing the utility of peripheral blood to mirror the neuropathological changes underlying AD [33]. In another study, these systemic manifestations on the AD-related metabolome were reflected in altered levels of 23 metabolites in serum from AD patients, indicating impaired neurotransmission, energy metabolism (e.g., TCA cycle), urea cycle, and some others [34]. Finally, other samples analyzed by GC-MS in AD metabolomics research included exhaled breath [35] and urine [36], with the aim of investigating the involvement of volatile compounds and odorants in its etiology.

The combination of GC-MS with RPLC-MS is nowadays one of the most common strategies to achieve comprehensive metabolomics analysis. This multiplatform was applied to serum samples from a prospective study among AD, mild cognitive impairment (MCI), and healthy subjects, uncovering profound lipidomics changes in AD patients at baseline and increased 2,4-dihydroxybutanoic acid along disease progression [37]. Wang et al. found that plasma metabolites measured through GC+RPLC-MS might serve to differentiate AD and amnesic MCI patients from control subjects [38]. The metabolic signatures associated with AD and MCI shared many metabolites participating in the metabolism of fatty acids, amino acids, nucleic acids, and one-carbon metabolism, thus suggesting the occurrence of common pathogenic mechanisms in both dementia disorders. In a more recent study, plasma metabolomics revealed that AD among the Down syndrome population is characterized by a shift in energy metabolism toward the upregulation of the anaerobic respiration [39]. In this line, it has been reported that mitochondrial stress and altered energy metabolism are major hippocampal disturbances occurring in three transgenic models of AD [40]. Metabolomics analysis of CSF has also been proposed to identify potential biomarkers for an improved diagnostic performance of AD. Czech et al. described that the combination of cortisol, cysteine, and uridine levels together with other amino acids yields predictive models with sensitivity and specificity above 80% [41]. Another study detected two CSF metabolic features with higher discrimination performance than that provided by traditional amyloid and tau biomarkers, but further confirmatory studies are needed [42]. To complement the DMS screening analyses that have been described in the previous section of this review article [18–27], González-Domínguez et al. conducted a comprehensive metabolomics characterization of the APP × PS1 model by applying combined GC-MS and RPLC-MS analysis to serum samples [43], various brain regions [44], metabolically active organs (i.e., liver, kidney) [45], and organs involved in the immune function (i.e., spleen, thymus) [46]. These studies validated most of the findings unveiled by DMS-based metabolomics fingerprinting with regard to the altered homeostasis of lipids (e.g., phospholipids, sphingolipids, cholesterol, fatty acids and acyl-carnitines), amino acids, nucleic acids, energy-related metabolism, and many others, both at the central and the systemic levels.

## 4. Alzheimer's Disease and HILIC-MS-Based Metabolomics

Although its use is not as widespread as other metabolomics platforms such as RPLC-MS and GC-MS, various published works have explored the potential of HILIC-MS to investigate the AD-related polar metabolome. Two preliminary studies demonstrated that the statistical modeling of HILIC-MS metabolomics data may provide satisfactory subject classification by using both brain [47] and plasma [48] samples, but the metabolites responsible for this discrimination were not identified. In another prospective study, the analysis of plasma samples from MCI patients, MCI patients who developed AD upon the follow-up and healthy controls revealed disturbances in 22 metabolic pathways, some of them traditionally associated with the pathogenesis of AD (e.g., metabolism of cholesterol, glucose, and amino acids), but also in relation to the polyamine and the L-arginine metabolism [49]. Recently, urinary metabolomics also highlighted the pivotal involvement of aromatic amino acids in the CRND8 mouse model, encompassing alterations in the tryptophan metabolism (e.g., upregulation of the serotonin pathway, downregulation of the kynurenine pathway), deficient aromatic L-amino acid decarboxylase activity (e.g., accumulation of N-acetylvanilalanine and 3-methoxytyrosine), and changes in microbiota-related and glycine conjugation processes [50].

Orthogonal RPLC and HILIC separations have also been used in combination to maximize the metabolomics coverage, as previously described for the RPLC+GC multiplatform. Trushina et al. accomplished a comprehensive investigation of the metabolic mechanisms behind the onset of AD and MCI by analyzing plasma and CSF samples, which revealed alterations in multiple pathways associated with energy metabolism, mitochondrial function, neurotransmission, amino acid and lipid metabolism, and many others [51]. A similar analytical approach was employed to predict the progression of AD along four diagnostic groups, namely healthy control subjects, stable MCI patients, MCI subjects who developed AD after a 2-year follow-up, and AD patients, which indicated significant alterations in the CSF levels of some amino acids and taurine-related metabolites [52]. Comparable findings have been obtained from brain metabolomics profiling, thus suggesting that modulating the metabolism of amino acids could be a possible therapeutic approach against AD [53]. Additionally, in the brain, Paglia et al. found profound cortical perturbations in the metabolism of glycerophospholipids and six central metabolic pathways, of which a significant impairment of the mitochondrial aspartate metabolism was noteworthy [54]. Conversely, other authors were surprisingly not able to differentiate AD patients and healthy controls by using combined RPLC+HILIC-MS plasma metabolomics, but a clear discrimination was achieved between MCI and control subjects [55].

## 5. Alzheimer's Disease and CE-MS Based Metabolomics

The application of CE-MS based metabolomics in AD research has only been reported in five studies published up to date. Ibáñez et al. identified a panel of CSF polar metabolites that was able to differentiate among subjects with different cognitive status, including patients with subjective cognitive impairment (SCI), MCI patients that remained stable within 2 years, MCI patients that progressed to AD after this follow-up period, and AD patients [56]. In another cohort, the analysis of serum samples evidenced similar alterations in metabolites related to oxidative stress, deficiencies in energy metabolism, and vascular risk factors [57]. Furthermore, the authors also found increased serum levels of proline betaine in AD patients, which is a marker of citrus consumption that has been recently validated in a prospective study on cognitive decline [69]. In this line, the analysis of brain tissue demonstrated that AD pathogenesis could be associated with dysregulated transmethylation and polyamine metabolism, abnormalities in neurotransmission, and impaired urea cycle and glutathione synthesis [58]. The two other studies published on CE-based metabolomics focused on the comparison of various neurodegenerative disorders. Tsuruoka et al. identified six serum metabolites and two saliva metabolites that were significantly altered in dementia patients (AD, frontotemporal lobe dementia, and Lewy body disease), whereas 45 metabolites detected in serum could differentiate at least one pair of these dementia groups [59]. More recently, the same methodology was employed to discriminate between AD and idiopathic normal pressure hydrocephalus patients by analyzing CSF [60].

## 6. Alzheimer's Disease and Other RPLC-MS Based Platforms to Explore Central Metabolites

As previously described, there are different strategies to reduce the polarity of hydrophilic metabolites for enabling their analysis by means of RPLC-MS. For instance, Kaddurah-Daouk et al. published various metabolomics studies based on ion pairing and subsequent electrochemical array detection for studying the involvement of redox-active CSF metabolites on AD and MCI [61,62]. Alternatively, dansylation has also been employed as a derivatization procedure for enhancing the resolving power of RPLC for the analysis of AD-related central metabolites in saliva [63] and urine [64] samples. In this regard, Takayama et al. developed an alternative approach for chiral metabolomics by using optically active derivatization reagents, which enabled determining chiral amines and carboxyls in brain samples as biomarker candidates for AD diagnosis [65]. To conclude, it should also be noted that various manufacturers have developed novel RPLC stationary phases with an improved retention of hydrophilic compounds, which have been successfully employed for analyzing cationic metabolites in CSF [66] and purine metabolites in brain [67] of AD patients.

## 7. Overview on the Involvement of Central Metabolic Pathways in Alzheimer's Disease

As shown in Table 1, hydrophilic-oriented MS-based metabolomics has demonstrated significant alterations in the levels of numerous polar metabolites in various biological matrices (e.g., serum/plasma, CSF, brain) and, consequently, the involvement of central metabolic pathways in the pathogenesis of AD (Figure 1). One of the most consistent findings across the metabolomics studies that have been reviewed here is the impairment of the energy-related metabolism. Altered glucose levels have been repeatedly reported in both the central nervous system and the peripheral system, suggesting an abnormal metabolic rate of carbohydrates, which are the main energy source in the brain. In turn, this was normally accompanied by perturbations in other metabolites participating in the glycolysis, the pentose phosphate pathway, ketogenesis and gluconeogenesis, the tricarboxylic (TCA) cycle, β-oxidation of fatty acids, and others (Table 1), thus evidencing profound disturbances affecting the entire energy metabolic system. Amino acids are involved in multiple central metabolic pathways, many of which have also been associated to the onset and progression of AD. It is noteworthy that failures in the homeostasis of aromatic amino acids and the synthesis of neurotransmitters (e.g., dopamine from tyrosine, serotonin from tryptophan) have been consistently reported in the literature. In this respect, growing evidence supports a role of branched chain amino acids in AD pathogenesis because these can compete with aromatic amino acids for entry into the brain but also due to their crucial involvement in the modulation of insulin resistance and energy metabolism. Moreover, various amino acids (e.g., arginine, glutamate/glutamine system) are closely linked to the nitrogen metabolism through the urea cycle and the polyamine system, which may also play a major role in brain health (e.g., hyperammonemia-induced neurotoxicity). Oxidative stress is another pivotal hallmark of AD with great impact on the metabolome, inducing the reduction of cerebral and circulating levels of numerous antioxidant metabolites (e.g., glutathione) and the accumulation of by-products derived from the oxidative damage to nucleic acids, proteins, and lipids. In this vein, various authors have reported important deregulations in the metabolism of purines and pyrimidines, which could be allocated not only to oxidative/nitrosative damage to nucleic acids but also to energy metabolism failures and impaired cellular signaling. In the crosstalk of many of the metabolic processes described above, including the homeostasis of amino acids, the synthesis of purines and redox defense, the one-carbon metabolism is also considered an essential piece of the AD pathology puzzle, in which hyperhomocysteinemia is one of the most important risk factors for cognitive decline and dementia. Altogether, the application of complementary metabolomics platforms for characterizing the polar metabolome stands out as a powerful strategy to decipher the molecular events behind the multifactorial pathogenesis and progression of AD.

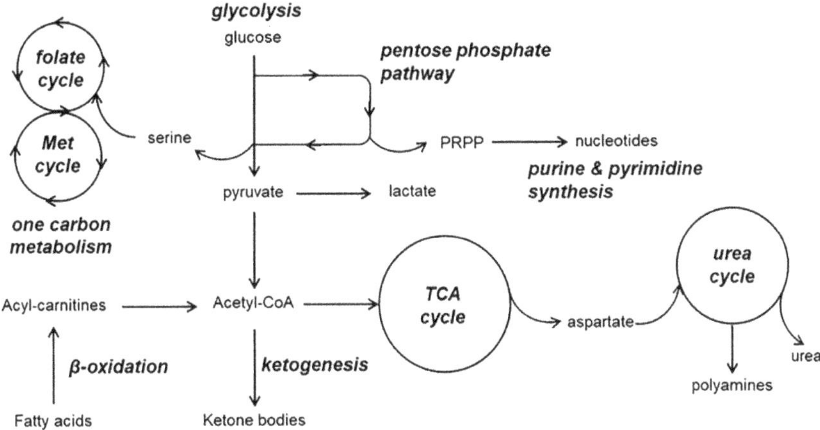


**Figure 1.** Overview of the central metabolic pathways altered in Alzheimer's disease.

## 8. Conclusions

Hydrophilic metabolites play an essential role in the central and primary pathways of the human metabolism (e.g., metabolism of carbohydrates, amino acids, and fatty acids). To approach this pivotal portion of the human metabolome, the coupling of mass spectrometry with gas chromatography (GC-MS), hydrophilic interaction liquid chromatography (HILIC-MS), and capillary electrophoresis (CE-MS) are currently the analytical techniques most commonly employed, together with direct mass spectrometry (DMS) analysis for comprehensive and high-throughput metabolomics. DMS can be regarded as a first-pass screening tool for rapid and simple metabolomics fingerprinting, but it usually requires being complemented with other hyphenated MS approaches to overcome its inherent analytical limitations (e.g., the impossibility of resolving isomeric metabolites, ion suppression) in order to get a deeper insight into the polar metabolome. In this respect, the coupling GC-MS is the most commonly used platform for profiling low molecular weight hydrophilic metabolites because of its sensitivity and reproducibility, despite the need for a derivatization step prior to analysis. As an alternative, HILIC and CE provide orthogonal separation performance for polar and ionic metabolites, but significant technical developments are still needed for increasing their robustness and high-throughput capacity. The application of these metabolomics platforms has demonstrated the great impact of the onset and progression of AD on central metabolites and associated metabolic pathways, encompassing disturbances in the energy-related metabolism (e.g., glycolysis, TCA cycle), nitrogen metabolism (e.g., urea cycle, polyamine metabolism), fatty acid metabolism (e.g., β-oxidation, eicosanoids), neurotransmission (e.g., serotonergic, dopaminergic), homeostasis of amino acids and nucleotides, and some others. These findings are of utmost importance for comprehensively understanding the pathogenesis of this neurodegenerative disorder with the aim of developing possible therapeutic and preventive approaches and for discovering potential diagnostic targets. However, it should be noted that unsatisfactory validation studies have been repeatedly reported in AD metabolomics [70–72]. These inconsistencies can in part arise from analytical issues related to the lack of proper standardization in metabolomics research but also to the enormous intra- and inter-individual variability of the human metabolome. Therefore, many authors have emphasized in recent years the great potential of metabolomics to comprehensively investigate biological pathways and the etiopathology of diseases but also the extreme difficulty of using metabolites as robust biomarkers for diagnosis/prognosis in the clinical practice [73].

**Author Contributions:** Conceptualization, R.G.-D.; writing—original draft preparation, R.G.-D., Á.G.-D.; writing—review and editing, R.G.-D., Á.G.-D., A.S., J.D.G.-S., A.M.L.-S., Á.F.-R. All authors have read and agreed to the published version of the manuscript.

**Funding:** This research received no external funding.

**Institutional Review Board Statement:** Not applicable.

**Informed Consent Statement:** Not applicable.

**Conflicts of Interest:** The authors declare no conflict of interest.

## References


1. Blennow, K.; de Leon, M.J.; Zetterberg, H. Alzheimer's disease. *Lancet* **2006**, *368*, 387–403. [CrossRef]
2. Maccioni, R.B.; Muñoz, J.P.; Barbeito, L. The molecular bases of Alzheimer's disease and other neurodegenerative disorders. *Arch. Med. Res.* **2001**, *32*, 367–381. [CrossRef]
3. González-Domínguez, R.; García-Barrera, T.; Gómez-Ariza, J.L. Characterization of metal profiles in serum during the progression of Alzheimer's disease. *Metallomics* **2014**, *6*, 292–300. [CrossRef] [PubMed]
4. González-Domínguez, R.; Sayago, A.; Fernández-Recamales, Á. Metabolomics in Alzheimer's disease: The need of complementary analytical platforms for the identification of biomarkers to unravel the underlying pathology. *J. Chromatogr. B* **2017**, *1071*, 75–92. [CrossRef]
5. Wilkins, J.M.; Trushina, E. Application of metabolomics in Alzheimer's disease. *Front. Neurol.* **2017**, *8*, 719. [CrossRef] [PubMed]
6. Emwas, A.H.M.; Salek, R.M.; Griffin, J.L.; Merzaban, J. NMR-based metabolomics in human disease diagnosis: Applications, limitations, and recommendations. *Metabolomics* **2013**, *9*, 1048–1072. [CrossRef]
7. González-Domínguez, R.; Jáuregui, O.; Queipo-Ortuño, M.I.; Andrés-Lacueva, C. Characterization of the human exposome by a comprehensive and quantitative large-scale multianalyte metabolomics platform. *Anal. Chem.* **2020**, *92*, 13767–13775. [CrossRef]
8. Wei, F.; Lamichhane, S.; Orešič, M.; Hyötyläinen, T. Lipidomes in health and disease: Analytical strategies and considerations. *Trends Anal. Chem.* **2019**, *120*, 115664. [CrossRef]
9. Zeng, Y.; Luo, L.; Hou, W.; Lu, B.; Gong, J.; Chen, J.; Zhang, X.; Han, B.; Xie, Z.; Liao, Q. Targeted metabolomics analysis of aromatic amino acids and their gut microbiota-host cometabolites in rat serum and urine by liquid chromatography coupled with tandem mass spectrometry. *J. Sep. Sci.* **2017**, *40*, 3221–3230. [CrossRef]
10. González-Domínguez, R.; Urpi-Sarda, M.; Jáuregui, O.; Needs, P.W.; Kroon, P.A.; Andrés-Lacueva, C. Quantitative Dietary Fingerprinting (QDF)-A novel tool for comprehensive dietary assessment based on urinary nutrimetabolomics. *J. Agric. Food Chem.* **2020**, *68*, 1851–1861. [CrossRef]
11. González-Domínguez, R.; Jáuregui, O.; Mena, P.; Hanhineva, K.; Tinahones, F.J.; Angelino, D.; Andrés-Lacueva, C. Quantifying the human diet in the crosstalk between nutrition and health by multi-targeted metabolomics of food and microbiota-derived metabolites. *Int. J. Obes.* **2020**, *44*, 2372–2381. [CrossRef]
12. González-Domínguez, R.; Sayago, A.; Fernández-Recamales, Á. Direct infusion mass spectrometry for metabolomic phenotyping of diseases. *Bioanalysis* **2017**, *9*, 131–148. [CrossRef]
13. Beale, D.J.; Pinu, F.R.; Kouremenos, K.A.; Poojary, M.M.; Narayana, V.K.; Boughton, B.A.; Kanojia, K.; Dayalan, S.; Jones, O.A.H.; Dias, D.A. Review of recent developments in GC-MS approaches to metabolomics-based research. *Metabolomics* **2018**, *14*, 152. [CrossRef] [PubMed]
14. Tang, D.Q.; Zou, L.; Yin, X.X.; Ong, C.N. HILIC-MS for metabolomics: An attractive and complementary approach to RPLC-MS. *Mass Spectrom. Rev.* **2016**, *35*, 574–600. [CrossRef]
15. Barbas, C.; Moraes, E.P.; Villaseñor, A. Capillary electrophoresis as a metabolomics tool for non-targeted fingerprinting of biological samples. *J. Pharm. Biomed. Anal.* **2011**, *55*, 823–831. [CrossRef]

16. Chen, K.; Baluya, D.; Tosun, M.; Li, F.; Maletic-Savatic, M. Imaging Mass Spectrometry: A New Tool to Assess Molecular Underpinnings of Neurodegeneration. *Metabolites* **2019**, *9*, 135. [CrossRef] [PubMed]
17. Gonzalez-Dominguez, A.; Duran-Guerrero, E.; Fernandez-Recamales, A.; Lechuga-Sancho, A.M.; Sayago, A.; Schwarz, M.; Segundo, C.; Gonzalez-Dominguez, R. An overview on the importance of combining complementary analytical platforms in metabolomic research. *Curr. Top. Med. Chem.* **2017**, *17*, 3289–3295. [CrossRef]
18. González-Domínguez, R.; García-Barrera, T.; Gómez-Ariza, J.L. Using direct infusion mass spectrometry for serum metabolomics in Alzheimer's disease. *Anal. Bioanal. Chem.* **2014**, *406*, 7137–7148. [CrossRef] [PubMed]
19. González-Domínguez, R.; García-Barrera, T.; Gómez-Ariza, J.L. Metabolomic approach to Alzheimer's disease diagnosis based on mass spectrometry. *Chem. Pap.* **2012**, *66*, 829–835. [CrossRef]
20. González-Domínguez, R.; García-Barrera, T.; Gómez-Ariza, J.L. Metabolomic study of lipids in serum for biomarker discovery in Alzheimer's disease using direct infusion mass spectrometry. *J. Pharm. Biomed. Anal.* **2014**, *98*, 321–326. [CrossRef] [PubMed]
21. González-Domínguez, R.; García-Barrera, T.; Gómez-Ariza, J.L. Combination of metabolomic and phospholipid-profiling approaches for the study of Alzheimer's disease. *J. Proteom.* **2014**, *104*, 37–47. [CrossRef]
22. González-Domínguez, R.; García-Barrera, T.; Gómez-Ariza, J.L. Application of a novel metabolomic approach based on atmospheric pressure photoionization mass spectrometry using flow injection analysis for the study of Alzheimer's disease. *Talanta* **2015**, *131*, 480–489. [CrossRef]
23. González-Domínguez, R.; García-Barrera, T.; Vitorica, J.; Gómez-Ariza, J.L. Application of metabolomics based on direct mass spectrometry analysis for the elucidation of altered metabolic pathways in serum from the APP/PS1 transgenic model of Alzheimer's disease. *J. Pharm. Biomed. Anal.* **2015**, *107*, 378–385. [CrossRef] [PubMed]
24. González-Domínguez, R.; Castilla-Quintero, R.; García-Barrera, T.; Gómez-Ariza, J.L. Development of a metabolomic approach based on urine samples and direct infusion mass spectrometry. *Anal. Biochem.* **2014**, *465*, 20–27. [CrossRef] [PubMed]
25. González-Domínguez, R.; García-Barrera, T.; Vitorica, J.; Gómez-Ariza, J.L. Metabolomic screening of regional brain alterations in the APP/PS1 transgenic model of Alzheimer's disease by direct infusion mass spectrometry. *J. Pharm. Biomed. Anal.* **2015**, *102*, 425–435. [CrossRef]
26. González-Domínguez, R.; García-Barrera, T.; Vitorica, J.; Gómez-Ariza, J.L. High throughput multiorgan metabolomics in the APP/PS1 mouse model of Alzheimer's disease. *Electrophoresis* **2015**, *36*, 2237–2249. [CrossRef] [PubMed]
27. González-Domínguez, R.; García-Barrera, T.; Vitorica, J.; Gómez-Ariza, J.L. Metabolomic research on the role of interleukin-4 in Alzheimer's disease. *Metabolomics* **2015**, *11*, 1175–1183. [CrossRef]
28. Lin, S.; Liu, H.; Kanawati, B.; Liu, L.; Dong, J.; Li, M.; Huang, J.; Schmitt-Kopplin, P.; Cai, Z. Hippocampal metabolomics using ultrahigh-resolution mass spectrometry reveals neuroinflammation from Alzheimer's disease in CRND8 mice. *Anal. Bioanal. Chem.* **2013**, *405*, 5105–5117. [CrossRef] [PubMed]
29. Lin, S.; Kanawati, B.; Liu, L.; Witting, M.; Li, M.; Huang, J.; Schmitt-Kopplin, P.; Cai, Z. Ultrahigh resolution mass spectrometry-based metabolic characterization reveals cerebellum as a disturbed region in two animal models. *Talanta* **2014**, *118*, 45–53. [CrossRef]
30. Xu, J.; Begley, P.; Church, S.J.; Patassini, S.; Hollywood, K.A.; Jüllig, M.; Curtis, M.A.; Waldvogel, H.J.; Faull, R.L.; Unwin, R.D.; et al. Graded perturbations of metabolism in multiple regions of human brain in Alzheimer's disease: Snapshot of a pervasive metabolic disorder. *Biochim. Biophys. Acta* **2016**, *1862*, 1084–1092. [CrossRef] [PubMed]
31. Wang, H.; Lian, K.; Han, B.; Wang, Y.; Kuo, S.H.; Geng, Y.; Qiang, J.; Sun, M.; Wang, M. Age-related alterations in the metabolic profile in the hippocampus of the senescence-accelerated mouse prone 8: A spontaneous Alzheimer's disease mouse model. *J. Alzheimers Dis.* **2014**, *39*, 841–848. [CrossRef]
32. Han, B.; Wang, J.H.; Geng, Y.; Shen, L.; Wang, H.L.; Wang, Y.Y.; Wang, M.W. Chronic stress contributes to cognitive dysfunction and hippocampal metabolic abnormalities in APP/PS1 mice. *Cell Physiol. Biochem.* **2017**, *41*, 1766–1776. [CrossRef] [PubMed]
33. Hu, Z.P.; Browne, E.R.; Liu, T.; Angel, T.E.; Ho, P.C.; Chan, E.C.Y. Metabonomic profiling of TASTPM transgenic Alzheimer's disease mouse model. *J. Proteome Res.* **2012**, *11*, 5903–5913. [CrossRef]
34. González-Domínguez, R.; García-Barrera, T.; Gómez-Ariza, J.L. Metabolite profiling for the identification of altered metabolic pathways in Alzheimer's disease. *J. Pharm. Biomed. Anal.* **2015**, *107*, 75–81. [CrossRef]
35. Ko, P.W.; Kang, K.; Yu, J.B.; Huh, J.S.; Lee, H.W.; Lim, J.O. Breath gas analysis for a potential diagnostic method of neurodegenerative diseases. *Sens. Lett.* **2014**, *12*, 1198–1202. [CrossRef]
36. Kimball, B.A.; Wilson, D.A.; Wesson, D.W. Alterations of the volatile metabolome in mouse models of Alzheimer's disease. *Sci. Rep.* **2016**, *6*, 19495. [CrossRef] [PubMed]
37. Orešič, M.; Hyötyläinen, T.; Herukka, S.K.; Sysi-Aho, M.; Mattila, I.; Seppänan-Laakso, T.; Julkunen, V.; Gopalacharyulu, P.V.; Hallikainen, M.; Koikkalainen, J.; et al. Metabolome in progression to Alzheimer's disease. *Transl. Psychiatry* **2011**, *1*, e57. [CrossRef]
38. Wang, G.; Zhou, Y.; Huang, F.J.; Tang, H.D.; Xu, X.H.; Liu, J.J.; Wang, Y.; Deng, Y.L.; Ren, R.J.; Xu, W.; et al. Plasma metabolite profiles of Alzheimer's disease and mild cognitive impairment. *J. Proteome Res.* **2014**, *13*, 2649–2658. [CrossRef]
39. Gross, T.J.; Doran, E.; Cheema, A.K.; Head, E.; Lott, I.T.; Mapstone, M. Plasma metabolites related to cellular energy metabolism are altered in adults with Down syndrome and Alzheimer's disease. *Dev. Neurobiol.* **2019**, *79*, 622–638. [CrossRef] [PubMed]

40. Trushina, E.; Nemutlu, E.; Zhang, S.; Christensen, T.; Camp, J.; Mesa, J.; Siddiqui, A.; Tamura, Y.; Sesaki, H.; Wengenack, T.M.; et al. Defects in mitochondrial dynamics and metabolomic signatures of evolving energetic stress in mouse models of familial Alzheimer's disease. *PLoS ONE* **2012**, *7*, e32737. [CrossRef]
41. Czech, C.; Berndt, P.; Busch, K.; Schmitz, O.; Wiemer, J.; Most, V.; Hampel, H.; Kastler, J.; Senn, H. Metabolite profiling of Alzheimer's disease cerebrospinal fluid. *PLoS ONE* **2012**, *7*, e31501. [CrossRef]
42. Motsinger-Reif, A.A.; Zhu, H.; Kling, M.A.; Matson, W.; Sharma, S.; Fiehn, O.; Reif, D.M.; Appleby, D.H.; Doraiswamy, P.M.; Trojanowski, J.Q.; et al. Comparing metabolomic and pathologic biomarkers alone and in combination for discriminating Alzheimer's disease from normal cognitive aging. *Acta Neuropathol. Commun.* **2013**, *1*, 28. [CrossRef]
43. González-Domínguez, R.; García-Barrera, T.; Vitorica, J.; Gómez-Ariza, J.L. Deciphering metabolic abnormalities associated with Alzheimer's disease in the APP/PS1 mouse model using integrated metabolomic approaches. *Biochimie* **2015**, *110*, 119–128. [CrossRef] [PubMed]
44. González-Domínguez, R.; García-Barrera, T.; Vitorica, J.; Gómez-Ariza, J.L. Region-specific metabolic alterations in the brain of the APP/PS1 transgenic mice of Alzheimer's disease. *Biochim. Biophys. Acta* **2014**, *1842*, 2395–2402. [CrossRef]
45. González-Domínguez, R.; García-Barrera, T.; Vitorica, J.; Gómez-Ariza, J.L. Metabolomic investigation of systemic manifestations associated with Alzheimer's disease in the APP/PS1 transgenic mouse model. *Mol. BioSyst.* **2015**, *11*, 2429–2440. [CrossRef]
46. González-Domínguez, R.; García-Barrera, T.; Vitorica, J.; Gómez-Ariza, J.L. Metabolomics reveals significant impairments in the immune system of the APP/PS1 transgenic mice of Alzheimer's disease. *Electrophoresis* **2015**, *36*, 577–587. [CrossRef] [PubMed]
47. Graham, S.F.; Chevallier, O.P.; Roberts, D.; Holscher, C.; Elliot, C.T.; Green, B.D. Investigation of the human brain metabolome to identify potential markers for early diagnosis and therapeutic targets of Alzheimer's disease. *Anal. Chem.* **2013**, *85*, 1803–1811. [CrossRef]
48. Inoue, K.; Tsuchiya, H.; Takayama, T.; Akatsu, H.; Hashizume, Y.; Yamamoto, T.; Matsukawa, N.; Toyo'oka, T. Blood-based diagnosis of Alzheimer's disease using fingerprinting metabolomics based on hydrophilic interaction liquid chromatography with mass spectrometry and multivariate statistical analysis. *J. Chromatogr. B* **2015**, *974*, 24–34. [CrossRef] [PubMed]
49. Graham, S.F.; Chevallier, O.P.; Elliot, C.T.; Hölscher, C.; Johnston, J.; McGuinness, B.; Kehoe, P.G.; Passmore, A.P.; Green, B.D. Untargeted metabolomic analysis of human plasma indicates differentially affected polyamine and L-arginine metabolism in mild cognitive impairment subjects converting to Alzheimer's disease. *PLoS ONE* **2015**, *10*, e0119452. [CrossRef] [PubMed]
50. Tang, Z.; Liu, L.; Li, Y.; Dong, J.; Li, M.; Huang, J.; Lin, S.; Cai, Z. Urinary metabolomics reveals alterations of aromatic amino acid metabolism of Alzheimer's disease in the transgenic CRND8 mice. *Curr. Alzheimer Res.* **2016**, *13*, 764–776. [CrossRef]
51. Trushina, E.; Dutta, T.; Persson, X.M.; Mielke, M.M.; Petersen, R.C. Identification of altered metabolic pathways in plasma and CSF in mild cognitive impairment and Alzheimer's disease using metabolomics. *PLoS ONE* **2013**, *8*, e63644. [CrossRef] [PubMed]
52. Ibañez, C.; Simo, C.; Barupal, D.K.; Fiehn, O.; Kivipelto, M.; Cedazo-Mínguez, A.; Cifuentes, A. A new metabolomic workflow for early detection of Alzheimer's disease. *J. Chromatogr. A* **2013**, *1302*, 65–71. [CrossRef]
53. Kim, Y.H.; Shim, H.S.; Kim, K.H.; Lee, J.; Chung, B.C.; Kowall, N.W.; Ryu, H.; Lee, J. Metabolomic analysis identifies alterations of amino acid metabolome signatures in the postmortem brain of Alzheimer's disease. *Exp. Neurobiol.* **2019**, *28*, 376–389. [CrossRef] [PubMed]
54. Paglia, G.; Stocchero, M.; Cacciatore, S.; Lai, S.; Angel, P.; Alam, M.T.; Keller, M.; Ralser, M.; Astarita, G. Unbiased metabolomic investigation of Alzheimer's disease brain points to dysregulation of mitochondrial aspartate metabolism. *J. Proteome Res.* **2016**, *15*, 608–618. [CrossRef]
55. Armirotti, A.; Basit, A.; Realini, N.; Caltagirone, C.; Bossù, P.; Spalletta, G.; Piomelli, D. Sample preparation and orthogonal chromatography for broad polarity range plasma metabolomics: Application to human subjects with neurodegenerative dementia. *Anal. Biochem.* **2014**, *455*, 48–54. [CrossRef] [PubMed]
56. Ibáñez, C.; Simó, C.; Martín-Álvarez, P.J.; Kivipelto, M.; Winblad, B.; Cedazo-Mínguez, A.; Cifuentes, A. Toward a predictive model of Alzheimer's disease progression using capillary electrophoresis–mass spectrometry metabolomics. *Anal. Chem.* **2012**, *84*, 8532–8540. [CrossRef]
57. González-Domínguez, R.; García, A.; García-Barrera, T.; Barbas, C.; Gómez-Ariza, J.L. Metabolomic profiling of serum in the progression of Alzheimer's disease by capillary electrophoresis-mass spectrometry. *Electrophoresis* **2014**, *35*, 3321–3330. [CrossRef]
58. Mahajan, U.V.; Varma, V.R.; Griswold, M.E.; Blackshear, C.T.; An, Y.; Oommen, A.M.; Varma, S.; Troncoso, J.C.; Pletnikova, O.; O'Brien, R.; et al. Dysregulation of multiple metabolic networks related to brain transmethylation and polyamine pathways in Alzheimer disease: A targeted metabolomic and transcriptomic study. *PLoS Med.* **2020**, *17*, e1003012. [CrossRef]
59. Tsuruoka, M.; Hara, J.; Hirayama, A.; Sugimoto, M.; Soga, T.; Shankle, W.R.; Tomita, M. Capillary electrophoresis-mass spectrometry-based metabolome analysis of serum and saliva from neurodegenerative dementia patients. *Electrophoresis* **2013**, *34*, 2865–2872. [CrossRef]
60. Nagata, Y.; Hirayama, A.; Ikeda, S.; Shirahata, A.; Shoji, F.; Maruyama, M.; Kayano, M.; Bundo, M.; Hattori, K.; Yoshida, S.; et al. Comparative analysis of cerebrospinal fluid metabolites in Alzheimer's disease and idiopathic normal pressure hydrocephalus in a Japanese cohort. *Biomark. Res.* **2018**, *6*, 5. [CrossRef]
61. Kaddurah-Daouk, R.; Rozen, S.; Matson, W.; Han, X.; Hulette, C.M.; Burke, J.R.; Doraiswamy, P.M.; Welsh-Bohmer, K.A. Metabolomic changes in autopsy-confirmed Alzheimer's disease. *Alzheimers Dement.* **2011**, *7*, 309–317. [CrossRef]

62. Kaddurah-Daouk, R.; Zhu, H.; Sharma, S.; Bogdanov, M.; Rozen, S.G.; Matson, W.; Oki, N.O.; Motsinger-Reif, A.A.; Churchill, E.; Lei, Z.; et al. Alterations in metabolic pathways and networks in Alzheimer's disease. *Transl. Psychiatry* **2013**, *3*, e244. [CrossRef]
63. Zheng, J.; Dixon, R.A.; Li, L. Development of isotope labeling LC-MS for human salivary metabolomics and application to profiling metabolome changes associated with mild cognitive impairment. *Anal. Chem.* **2012**, *84*, 10802–10811. [CrossRef]
64. Peng, J.; Guo, K.; Xia, J.; Zhou, J.; Yang, J.; Westaway, D.; Wishart, D.S.; Li, L. Development of isotope labeling liquid chromatography mass spectrometry for mouse urine metabolomics: Quantitative metabolomic study of transgenic mice related to Alzheimer's disease. *J. Proteome Res.* **2014**, *13*, 4457–4469. [CrossRef] [PubMed]
65. Takayama, T.; Mochizuki, T.; Todoroki, K.; Min, J.Z.; Mizuno, H.; Inoue, K.; Akatsu, H.; Noge, I.; Toyo'oka, T. A novel approach for LC-MS/MS-based chiral metabolomics fingerprinting and chiral metabolomics extraction using a pair of enantiomers of chiral derivatization reagents. *Anal. Chim. Acta* **2015**, *898*, 73–84. [CrossRef]
66. Myint, K.T.; Aoshima, K.; Tanaka, S.; Nakamura, T.; Oda, Y. Quantitative profiling of polar cationic metabolites in human cerebrospinal fluid by reversed-phase nanoliquid chromatography/mass spectrometry. *Anal. Chem.* **2009**, *81*, 1121–1129. [CrossRef] [PubMed]
67. Ansoleaga, B.; Jové, M.; Schlüter, A.; Garcia-Esparcia, P.; Moreno, J.; Pujol, A.; Pamplona, R.; Portero-Otín, M.; Ferrer, I. Deregulation of purine metabolism in Alzheimer's disease. *Neurobiol. Aging* **2015**, *36*, 68–80. [CrossRef] [PubMed]
68. González-Domínguez, R.; Sayago, A.; Fernández-Recamales, Á. High-throughput direct mass spectrometry-based metabolomics to characterize metabolite fingerprints associated with Alzheimer's disease pathogenesis. *Metabolites* **2018**, *8*, 52. [CrossRef] [PubMed]
69. Low, D.Y.; Lefèvre-Arbogast, S.; González-Domínguez, R.; Urpi-Sarda, M.; Micheau, P.; Petera, M.; Centeno, D.; Durand, S.; Pujos-Guillot, E.; Korosi, A.; et al. Diet-related metabolites associated with cognitive decline revealed by untargeted metabolomics in a prospective cohort. *Mol. Nutr. Food Res.* **2019**, *63*, e1900177. [CrossRef] [PubMed]
70. Casanova, R.; Varma, S.; Simpson, B.; Min, K.; An, Y.; Saldana, S.; Riveros, C.; Moscato, P.; Griswold, M.; Sonntag, D.; et al. Blood metabolite markers of preclinical Alzheimer's disease in two longitudinally followed cohorts of older individuals. *Alzheimers Dement.* **2016**, *12*, 815–822. [CrossRef] [PubMed]
71. Li, D.; Misialek, J.R.; Boerwinkle, E.; Gottesman, R.F.; Sharrett, A.R.; Mosley, T.H.; Coresh, J.; Wruck, L.M.; Knopman, D.S.; Alonso, A. Prospective associations of plasma phospholipids and mild cognitive impairment/dementia among African Americans in the ARIC Neurocognitive Study. *Alzheimers Dement.* **2017**, *6*, 1–10. [CrossRef] [PubMed]
72. Costa, A.C.; Joaquim, H.P.G.; Forlenza, O.; Talib, L.L.; Gattaz, W.F. Plasma lipids metabolism in mild cognitive impairment and Alzheimer's disease. *World J. Biol. Psychiatry* **2019**, *20*, 190–196. [CrossRef] [PubMed]
73. Johnson, C.H.; Ivanisevic, J.; Siuzdak, G. Metabolomics: Beyond biomarkers and towards mechanisms. *Nat. Rev. Mol. Cell Biol.* **2016**, *17*, 451–459. [CrossRef] [PubMed]

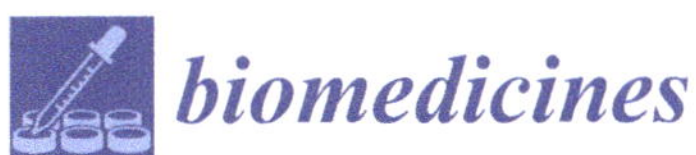

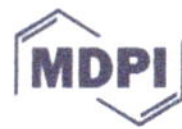

*Article*

# Determinants of Schizophrenia Endophenotypes Based on Neuroimaging and Biochemical Parameters

**Amira Bryll [1], Wirginia Krzyściak [2,*], Paulina Karcz [3], Maciej Pilecki [4], Natalia Śmierciak [4], Marta Szwajca [4], Anna Skalniak [5] and Tadeusz J. Popiela [1,*]**

1 Department of Radiology, Jagiellonian University Medical College, 31-501 Krakow, Poland; amira.bryll@uj.edu.pl
2 Department of Medical Diagnostics, Jagiellonian University Medical College, 30-688 Krakow, Poland
3 Department of Electroradiology, Jagiellonian University Medical College, 31-126 Krakow, Poland; paulina.karcz@uj.edu.pl
4 Department of Child and Adolescent Psychiatry, Faculty of Medicine, Jagiellonian University Medical College, 31-501 Krakow, Poland; maciej.pilecki@uj.edu.pl (M.P.); natalia.smierciak@uj.edu.pl (N.Ś.); marta.szwajca@uj.edu.pl (M.S.)
5 Department of Endocrinology, Faculty of Medicine, Jagiellonian University Medical College, 31-501 Krakow, Poland; anna.skalniak@uj.edu.pl
* Correspondence: wirginiakrzysciak@cm-uj.krakow.pl (W.K.); msjpopie@cyf-kr.edu.pl (T.J.P.)

**Citation:** Bryll, A.; Krzyściak, W.; Karcz, P.; Pilecki, M.; Śmierciak, N.; Szwajca, M.; Skalniak, A.; Popiela, T.J. Determinants of Schizophrenia Endophenotypes Based on Neuroimaging and Biochemical Parameters. *Biomedicines* **2021**, *9*, 372. https://doi.org/10.3390/biomedicines9040372

Academic Editor: Arnab Ghosh

Received: 26 February 2021
Accepted: 30 March 2021
Published: 1 April 2021



**Abstract:** Despite extensive research, there is no convincing evidence of a reliable diagnostic biomarker for schizophrenia beyond clinical observation. Disorders of glutamatergic neurotransmission associated with N-methyl-D-aspartate (NMDA) receptor insufficiency, neuroinflammation, and redox dysregulation are the principal common mechanism linking changes in the periphery with the brain, ultimately contributing to the emergence of negative symptoms of schizophrenia that underlie differential diagnosis. The aim of the study was to evaluate the influence of these systems via peripheral and cerebral biochemical indices in relation to the patient's clinical condition. Using neuroimaging diagnostics, we were able to define endophenotypes of schizophrenia based on objective laboratory data that form the basis of a personalized approach to diagnosis and treatment. The two distinguished endophenotypes differed in terms of the quality of life, specific schizophrenia symptoms, and glutamatergic neurotransmission metabolites in the anterior cingulate gyrus. Our results, as well as further studies of the excitatory or inhibitory balance of microcircuits, relating the redox systems on the periphery with the distant regions of the brain might allow for predicting potential biomarkers of neuropsychiatric diseases, including schizophrenia. To the best of our knowledge, our study is the first to identify an objective molecular biomarker of schizophrenia outcome.

**Keywords:** schizophrenia; endophenotypes; magnetic resonance spectroscopy; glutamatergic metabolites; anterior cingulate gyrus

## 1. Introduction

Schizophrenia is a severe mental disorder, the diagnosis of which is currently based solely on clinical criteria [1]. There is a lack of laboratory biomarkers related to the etiopathogenesis of this disease. A biomarker is 'an objectively measured trait that reflects a normal biological or pathological process, or response to a pharmacological intervention' [2]. Thus, it is a disease-specific indicator of the presence or intensity of a biological process directly related to the patient's clinical symptoms or the effects of a certain disorder [3].

Despite scientific progress in understanding the pathophysiological basis of schizophrenia, many potential emerging predictors do not meet the biomarker criteria. However, due to rapidly developing neuroimaging techniques, there is growing hope that those techniques might provide biomarkers in the future, which would correlate with the clinical outcome of the disease and predict the patients' endophenotypes [4].

Due to the complexity of the clinical picture of schizophrenia, the concept of endophenotypes is increasingly used in research on this disorder. An endophenotype is a quantitative measure based on neurobiological data that is created on the basis of laboratory measurements, which is not an estimate from clinical examination [5,6]. The clinical picture of schizophrenia might include classic subtypes [7] as well as a division, depending on the dominant component of negative and positive symptoms [8]. In addition, according to the latest International Classification of Diseases 11th classification, there is a division based on the stage of the illness (first episode/multiple episodes/solid course) and the severity of symptoms (currently symptomatic/partial remission/full remission) [8]. The boundaries between schizophrenia and schizoaffective and affective disorder with psychotic symptoms are also blurred. Schizophrenia might also manifest in a form with an expressed obsessive-compulsive component, obsessive-compulsive symptoms might be an initial stage in the development of schizophrenia, or both disorders could be comorbid [9]. The literature on the subject also includes descriptions of personality traits of schizotypes that predispose one to the development of schizophrenia or with a clinical picture similar to schizophrenia (schizotypal personality) [10]. As reported in the literature on the subject, this definition, as well as the progress made in research on the human genome and neuroimaging techniques in psychiatry, shows the polygenic nature of schizophrenia with its various causative factors, i.e., genetic, immunological, biochemical, and environmental [7–15].

Understanding the classic definition of endophenotypes and the Research Domains Criteria announced by the National Institute of Mental Health [16,17] allows us to assume that the matter concerning the boundaries of division is still open. As they emphasize, however, there are no data supporting this theory (only theoretical statements) [18,19], hence, the theory itself is purely an empirical question that should be solved by statistical methods designed to explain an existing scientific problem.

The starting point of the presented work was the hidden structure of endophenotypes underlying the classical understanding of this term. This gives an opportunity to build a model based on empirical laboratory data from neuroimaging and a number of other laboratory variables that connect the concept of pathology of schizophrenia with subtypes, thus outlining a new perspective on the classical understanding of its diagnosis.

Different studies suggest that several key brain regions involved in the pathophysiology of schizophrenia, such as the frontal cortex, dorsal anterior cingulate cortex (ACC), putamen, and temporal pole, share metabolic abnormalities or altered perfusion in patients with schizophrenia [20].

The progression of the disease also seems to be an important issue in this context. On the one hand, it is associated with the period of untreated psychosis, as we showed in our previous studies [21]. On the other hand, it might be related to the functioning of the ACC itself, which is seen especially in patients taking antipsychotic drugs who show greater ACC activation with associated better performance. It is, however, unclear whether this is directly caused by the influence of drugs, or by a reduction of symptoms [22]. Atrophy of the cerebral cortex, mainly related to the limited functional connectivity of the ACC, correlates with the most unpleasant predictors of disability in schizophrenia that do not respond to the classic form of treatment, i.e., negative symptoms. It also correlates with cognitive symptoms of schizophrenia but has no relation with the severity of positive symptoms [23,24]. Studies determining the concentration of metabolites proposed ACC as a potential source of biomarkers related to the risk of psychosis in early adolescence [25]. These data provide evidence of association between glutamatergic transmission metabolites and symptomatology, which might predict the development of psychosis in the future [26]. Thus, assessment of brain metabolites might thus play an important role as an early biomarker of schizophrenia risk, especially among young relatives of people with schizophrenia [27].

Therefore, the use of tools such as proton magnetic resonance spectroscopy (1H-MRS) might likely facilitate the identification of early predictors of schizophrenia, especially in the stage of juvenile psychosis, when the brain develops specific features related to changes in metabolite concentration, in particular reflecting changes in glutamatergic transmission [24].

Glutamate (also known as glutamic acid) is synthesized from glutamine by glutaminase in the central nervous system, and belongs to one of the main excitatory neurotransmitters changing neuronal activity and synaptic functions in the brain [28]. However, excessive glutamate release from presynaptic axon terminals can also cause neuronal death and permanent brain damage in a process known as excitotoxicity [29]. This phenomenon is associated with the pathogenesis of many debilitating human neurological diseases, such as stroke, amyotrophic lateral sclerosis, and epilepsy [30].

The concentration of glutamatergic metabolites determines higher or lower inhibitory connectivity in ACC and in the anterior part of the insula, shows a negative correlation with the inhibitory effect on excitatory neurons in ACC, and a negative correlation with the severity of social withdrawal in people with first-episode psychosis, as compared to healthy subjects [31]. Glutamate acts mainly postsynaptically by combining with ionotropic receptors (non-NMDA and NMDA), which leads, inter alia, to the depolarization of the cell membrane, and removal of $Mg^{2+}$ ions with simultaneous penetration of $Ca^{2+}$. This consequently contributes to the decarboxylation of glutamic acid and formation of a neurotransmitter with an inhibitory effect, i.e., $\gamma$-aminobutyric acid (GABA) (Figure 1). The imbalance between glutamate and brain GABA levels might be a marker of transition to psychosis in high-risk individuals [32]. The knowledge of GABA and glutamate levels at different stages of life of people at risk of developing psychosis might allow better assessment of the neurochemical phenomena underlying mental disorders [33].

The glutamatergic theory of psychosis (related to glutamatergic transmission metabolites), induced by ketamine or other NMDA receptor antagonists, allowed for the distinction between the classic psychosis of schizophrenia in a number of studies. It is mainly associated with positive symptoms, and the form of this disease is associated with additional negative and cognitive symptoms [34,35], which were not taken into account in the treatment of the commonly understood form of the disease [36], described in the early 1980s [37].

The mechanism of the observed changes might be concentrated on the increased ratio of glutamine to glutamate that is associated with an increased flow of excitatory neurotransmitters, and thus with glutamatergic hyperactivity or defective neural-glial coupling [38]. Abnormalities in glutamatergic neurotransmission are associated in this case with the function of glial cells in the prefrontal cortex (PFC) [39], abnormal volume of the brain ventricles [40], and abnormalities in the level of synaptic proteins [41]. These discoveries became the starting point of the latest pharmacological strategies based on NMDA antagonist models, to restore cognitive functions and reduce negative symptoms in schizophrenia [42]. However, cortical-limbic hyperactivity is induced by the administration of NMDA receptor antagonists, initiating the behavioral disturbances observed in schizophrenia, which is explained by the loss of glutamatergic function with excessive dopaminergic activity. Imbalance of the glutaminergic and dopaminergic systems in different regions of the brain might result in anti-kinetic effects or the development of psychosis [43]. The precise determination of the glutamatergic function related to Glu and Gln levels seems to be a limitation of the reported contradictory theories, due to signal-to-noise overlap and limitations of spectral resolution in magnetic resonance spectroscopy (MRS), therefore, in many works, the amounts of Glu–Gln are shown together as Glx [44]. For this reason, there might be misinterpretations of the observed changes, e.g., some studies report a decrease in the Glx levels during acute episodes of psychosis, while in others, the observed relationships are quite different. The physiological significance of the Glx results remains unclear, and MRS techniques distinguishing between the levels of Glu and Gln in different regions of the human brain could provide a solution to the existing problem and an important advance in the diagnosis of these debilitating diseases.

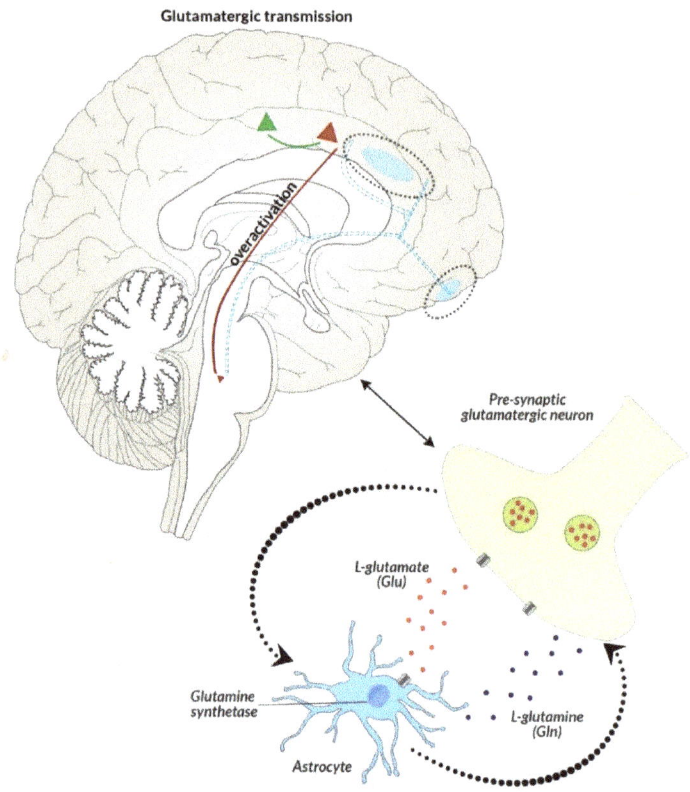


**Figure 1.** Potential mechanism explaining the occurrence of negative symptoms, and the developing resistance to classical neuroleptics due to the glutamatergic hypothesis and the NMDA receptor hypofunction. In addition to the glutamate projection pathway in the cortical brain stem, which is associated with the primary GLU neuron, the GABA interneuron, and the secondary GLU neuron, additional synapses in the midbrain with another GABA interneuron that targets neuronal DA projections that return to the frontal cortex, are involved in the projection of negative symptoms in schizophrenia. During normal psychiatric functioning, this circuit is balanced and sufficient DA reaches the frontal cortex without negative symptoms. However, when the pathway is modified with the formation of an additional GABA interneuron (originally: GLU-GABA-GLU-D; after modification: GLU-GABA-GLU-GABA-DA), this change might be associated with the appearance of negative symptoms. In the case of generating positive symptoms, glutamate from the primary GLU neuron reaches hypofunctional NMDA receptors located on the primary GABA interneuron, whose tone disappears in the absence of GLU stimulation and the secondary GLU neuron becomes hyperactive again. In contrast to the mechanism associated with the generation of positive symptoms, the main issue concerns the secondary GLU neuron, which hits another GABA interneuron, which, through a higher than normal GLU signal, releases much higher concentrations of GABA. This results in the inhibition of the final pathway of DA neurons derived from the midbrain and their lower release. This mesocortical DA pathway is now active and does not provide adequate amounts of DA in the frontal cortex, which causes hypofrontality and negative symptoms.

According to some of the research, glutamatergic-mediated excitotoxicity might be one of the mechanisms underlying resistance to classical neuroleptics seen in drug-resistant schizophrenia. The mentioned excitotoxicity associated with increased glutamatergic transmission metabolites levels would explain the weakened differentiation of oligodendrocytes with a higher sensitivity of the latter to inflammation and oxidative stress [45].

The most obvious evidence that oxidative stress might have an influence on the development of schizophrenia is prenatal exposure to hunger, which results in altered hippocampal morphology and impaired memory in the offspring, i.e., abnormalities consistent with the pathophysiology of schizophrenia [46].

Oxidative stress can be both a cause, an effect, and an attempt to combat pathological processes in the body [47]. The latter turned out to be particularly important in the context of parameters that form the so-called microcircuits, i.e., total cholesterol, triglycerides (TG), low-density lipoprotein cholesterol (LDL), high-density lipoprotein cholesterol (HDL), cortisol, and sodium ions, which play a significant role in the initiation of inflammation and assessment of cardiovascular risk in schizophrenics [48–50].

The role of oxidative stress related to oxidant–antioxidant imbalance in the pathophysiology of schizophrenia is emphasized by studies assessing the level of these indicators in the blood and peripheral tissues with clear differences between people with schizophrenia and healthy controls [51,52]. Nevertheless, it is unclear how biochemical changes in the periphery are related to neurochemical changes in the brain. There are few studies that point out a positive correlation between glutathione (which is the main intracellular non-enzymatic antioxidant) in plasma, with the levels of glutathione-dependent metabolites associated with glutamatergic transmission in the brains of schizophrenics, as compared to healthy controls [53]. The levels of these metabolites positively correlate with the neuropsychological assessment in patients with schizophrenia.

It could be assumed that oxidative stress and inflammation of the nervous system are the culmination of changes in the periphery [54,55], which, due to the increased permeability of the blood–brain barrier, might lead to increased infiltration of peripheral material into the brain, thus constituting a potential pathogenetic factor of the disease. Presumably, it is pro-inflammatory cytokines that modulate mood behavior and cognition by reducing the level of monoamines in the brain, or promoting glutamate excitotoxicity and, thus, affect the neuronal plasticity of the brain [56].

The potential mechanisms of the development of schizophrenia presented in the literature for us are now the starting points in the construction of a statistical model based on objective laboratory data, linking peripheral and cerebral biochemical indicators related to common inflammatory mechanisms in schizophrenia. Such a model might facilitate the prediction of the severity of schizophrenia symptoms and the assessment of the development of early psychosis.

In addition to assessing the usefulness of selected biomarkers in determining the importance of clinical endophenotypes, the aim of the research was to create a new perspective on the use of laboratory parameters in the diagnosis of different clinical types of schizophrenia. This could form the basis for a personalized approach to the diagnosis of the disease, based on a reliable etiopathogenetic factor.

## 2. Materials and Methods

### *2.1. Study Participants*

The research was approved by the Bioethics Committee of the Jagiellonian University (consent number: 1072.6120.152.2019 of 27 June 2019). The study included patients who gave informed written consent and additional consent was obtained in the case of legal guardians of participants under 18 years of age.

The study included patients with acute psychotic decompensation ($n$ = 40; 18 women and 22 men; mean age 22.68 $\pm$ 7.39 years), admitted to the In-Patient Unit for Adults and In-Patient Unit for Adolescents at the Psychiatry Department of the University Hospital in Krakow. Recruitment for the study lasted from January 2018 to December 2019. For 70% of patients, it was the first psychotic episode. In the remaining cases, it was the subsequent psychotic decompensation resulting in hospitalization. All patients met the diagnostic criteria for schizophrenia (F20) according to the International Statistical Classification of Diseases and Health Problems, 10th edition (ICD-10) [7]. For relapsing patients, the diagnosis was confirmed during the initial assessment by the consensus of two psychiatrists with extensive experience in psychiatric assessment. For the first time, psychotic patients experiencing acute multiform psychotic disorders (F23) due to the ICD-10 diagnosis of schizophrenia was confirmed in a 3-month follow up. The severity of various psychotic symptoms was assessed using the Positive and Negative Syndrome Scale (PANSS) [57].

Exclusion criteria from the study were—inability to express informed consent, intellectual disability, hospitalization without consent or due to presence of severe cardiovascular diseases, abuse of psychoactive substances or tobacco smoking within three months prior to admission, affective symptoms, history of other disorders of the central nervous system, past head injuries with loss of consciousness, alcohol addiction, hyperactivity, or psychomotor agitation, which make it difficult to perform Magnetic Resonance Imaging (MRI).

Demographic and clinical data were collected from each patient, including duration of untreated psychosis (DUP), the course of the first episode, the number and length of hospitalizations, treatment, and its intervals.

During the first week of hospitalization, after medical stability was achieved, routine blood tests and questionnaire assessment were performed. MRI and MRS imaging examinations were performed during the first two weeks of hospitalization in patients who showed no changes in the outpatient status and were not undergoing pharmacotherapy, 8 h before each brain imaging.

In the constructed model of a number of variables (clinical, neuronal, biochemical, psychosocial), the potential dependencies of the brain activity indicators, peripheral parameters, and the clinical condition of patients were assessed.

### 2.2. Routinely Performed Laboratory Tests

After the subjects were qualified for the study, blood samples were collected during admission (1st day of the examination) using the Sarstedt closed system [58]. The patients fasted overnight and the collection was performed in the early morning hours. Samples showing bilirubinemia, hemolysis, lipemia, and turbidity were rejected.

Routine laboratory blood tests were performed on the day of sample collection and included a complete blood count (5-diff) and a manual smear, biochemical markers (ionogram—sodium [mmol/L], potassium [mmol/L], chlorides [mmol/L]; metabolic markers—glucose [mmol/L], lipidogram—cholesterol [mmol/L], HDL [mmol/L], LDL [mmol/L], triglycerides [mmol/L]; renal markers—creatinine [µmol/L], estimated Glomerular Filtration Rate test eGFR according to MORD [mL/min/1.73 $m^2$]; inflammatory markers—C-Reactive Protein CRP [mg/L], cortisol [µg/dL], complement C3 [mg/dL], complement C4 [mg/dL]; thyroid markers—Thyroxine T4, Triiodothyronine T3, and Thyroid-Stimulating Hormone TSH), using the Sysmex XN-2000 automated analyzer (Kobe, Japan) for blood counts as well as the Cobas 6000 and Cobas 8000 biochemical analyzers (Roche Diagnostics, Mannheim, Germany) for the biochemical and hormonal parameters. Selection of the above-mentioned parameters is part of the obligatory routine management of patients admitted to the Psychiatry Department.

The excess of serum samples collected on the 1st day of the study was divided into aliquots and stored at −80 °C, and then used to evaluate the parameters of the oxidant–antioxidant balance (i.e., total antioxidant potential expressed as FRAP (ferric reducing ability of plasma))—paraoxonase 1 (PON-1, lipid peroxidation marker) and malondialdehyde (MDA).

### 2.3. Parameters of the Oxidant-Antioxidant Balance

#### 2.3.1. Rationale for the Assessment of the Efficiency of the Antioxidant System Expressed as FRAP in Schizophrenia

Activation of immune-inflammatory pathways is associated with oxidative stress and damage to lipids, nucleic acids, and proteins. Increased production of reactive oxygen species and weakening of the defense system associated with the action of antioxidants is the cause of oxidative stress (OxS) [59]. In turn, high antioxidant activity expressed as FRAP is associated with tardive dyskinesia, negative symptoms, neurological symptoms, dysfunction, and disturbances of total cholesterol metabolism in patients with schizophrenia [60,61].

#### 2.3.2. The Total Antioxidant Power Expressed as FRAP

The total antioxidant potential expressed as FRAP was determined by the spectrophotometric method of Benzie and Strain [62]. The spectrophotometric measurement provides information about the antioxidant capacity of plasma to counteract the effects of free oxygen radicals.

The reaction was performed in a 96-well microtiter plate on which 15 μL of the standard solution/test solution (serum) were placed, with water as the blank sample. Three hundred microliter of the working substrate solution (2,4,6-Tris(2-pyridyl)-s-triazine, TPTZ 0.01 mol/L, 0.02 mol/L $FeCl_3 \cdot 6H_2O$, 0.3 mol/L pH = 3.6) was added into each well, the contents were mixed, and the plate was incubated at 37 °C for 10 min. The absorbance for each tested sample was determined at the wavelength $\lambda_{max}$ = 593 nm. A standard curve was drawn ($FeSO_4 \cdot 7H_2O$, 0.1–1, mmol/L) and a simple regression equation was determined from which the concentrations of the test samples were calculated; the results are expressed in mmol/mL.

#### 2.3.3. Rationale for the Assessment the Activity of Paraoxonase-1 (PON-1)

Human serum paraoxonase (PON-1) is an enzyme synthesized by the liver, which shows both paraoxonase and arylesterase activity to prevent peroxidation of low-density lipoproteins, i.e., LDL. PON-1 is involved in the transport of high-density lipoproteins [63]. The activity of PON-1 is altered in diseases where oxidative or nitrosative stress develops. Reduced PON-1 activity seems to be a key component of the oxidative and nitrosative processes that accompany schizophrenia [64].

The activity of paroxonase-1 (PON-1) in the plasma was determined according to the method described by Eckerson et al. [65], with the authors' own modification. The absorbance of the resulting p-nitrophenol was recorded spectrophotometrically at $\lambda_{max}$ = 405 nm at 25 °C, using a FLUOstar Omega microplate reader (BMG Labtech, Ortenberg, Germany). Plasma samples were mixed with a buffer containing 1.2 mM paraoxone in 50 mM glycine buffer, containing 1 mM $CaCl_2$, pH = 10.5. Subsequently, samples were incubated for 15 min at 37 °C. In the next step, 20 μL of diluted plasma was measured, 200 μL of 1.2 mM paraoxone was added, and the absorbance value was monitored at 405 nm, every 15 s for 4 min, after prior gentle mixing.

The results were expressed in international units (U/L): PON-1 = OD/min × 11.4 = U/L.

#### 2.3.4. Rationale for the Assessment of the Lipid Peroxidation Product—MDA (Malondialdehyde)

Malondialdehyde (MDA) is one of the key indicators of oxidative stress and the end-product of lipid peroxidation. As a result of these processes, cell membranes are damaged and the amount of peroxygen polyunsaturated fatty acids in the brain is increased, which becomes a further easy target for an attack of reactive oxygen species (ROS), constituting one of the primary etiological mechanisms of schizophrenia [66,67].

The concentration of MDA was measured by the fluorimetric method described by Aust [68,69], in conjunction with the Gutteridge modification [70].

A working solution was prepared by dissolving the stock reagent, 2-Thiobarbituric acid, TBA/Trichloroacetic acid, TCA/Hydrochloric acid, HCl in water (on the assay day), thereby obtaining 3.5 mL TBA/TCA/HCl + 10.5 mL $H_2O$ + 0.21 mL BHT. The standard used was 1,1,3,3-tetramethoxypropane, which hydrolyzes in an acidic environment in a stoichiometric ratio to MDA. Hydrolysis was carried out in 0.05 mol/L hydrochloric acid at room temperature for 10 min, then standard solutions of 1,1,3,3-tetramethoxypropane were prepared in the range of 0.015–3.5 μmol/L. The working solution was prepared fresh daily from a solution containing TBA/TCA/HCl, by dissolution in water in a ratio of 1:3.

Test serum, blank, or reference samples were mixed with the working solution in the ratio—125 μL of the sample and 1000 μL of the working solution. The contents of the tubes were mixed for 10 s using a micro-shaker, and then heated in a boiling water bath for 15 min. The tubes were then immediately chilled on ice for 10 min, and 3 mL of butanol was added to each tube. The reaction mixtures were shaken for 30 s. After centrifugation for 10 min at 4000× $g$ at room temperature, 250 μL of the organic layer were carefully transferred to the wells of a black 96-well plate. Fluorimetric measurements were made at an excitation wavelength (Ex) of 536 nm and an emission wavelength (Em) of 549 nm. The readings of the results were performed using the FLUOstar Omega spectrophotometer (BMG Labtech, Germany), after 10 min.

The clinical significance of the determination of the oxidant–antioxidant indicators selected by us was related to the evaluation of the action of antioxidant systems with the inflammatory theory of schizophrenia [71,72]. This links the role of immunological factors with the oxidant–antioxidant balance and the action of glutamatergic systems in the brain, departing from a theory focused solely on dopamine and emphasizing the role of inflammation and related mechanisms of action of new drugs [73,74].

Among the inflammatory parameters we selected, those that were routinely assessed, i.e., CRP, HDL, LDL, fibrinogen, and others are described above. In the case of redox parameters, the following were selected—paroxonase-1, which is similarly responsible for some anti-inflammatory and antioxidant properties, especially in the context of e.g., HDL [75]. The total antioxidant capacity of the plasma expressed as FRAP was selected as a clinical indicator of oxidative stress [76]. The choice of malondialdehyde was dictated by the assessment of the intensity of the lipid peroxidation process, as an indicator of oxidative stress [77].

### 2.4. Clinical Evaluation

Clinical evaluation of patients was based on a detailed psychiatric assessment. Demographic data were also collected. The psychiatric assessment included a clinical interview, the review of systems by a psychiatrist, neuro-cognitive tests, and a thorough analysis of the patient's medical records and history. The severity of psychotic symptoms was assessed using the PANSS scale (Positive and Negative Syndrome Scale—PANSS positive, negative, general psychopathology, and PANSS total scores), which included the assessment of positive symptoms (e.g., delusions, hallucinations, excessive agitation, suspiciousness, hostility), negative symptoms (e.g., emotional withdrawal, poor communication, stereotypical thinking disorders, lack of spontaneity, and fluency in conversation), and general psychopathology [57]. The latter is an important addition to the assessment of basic positive and negative symptoms, providing information on the severity of schizophrenia, which constitutes a benchmark during the care of a psychotic patient.

### 2.5. Neuroimaging

MRI and MRS was performed using the 1,5T (General Electric Healthcare, Milwaukee, WI, USA) magnetic field induction MR system, with an 8-channel headcoil (receive only) in the supine position. The study was conducted with the use of a standard MR brain examination protocol, which included the following sequences: T2-weighted, FLAIR, Diffusion weighted imaging (DWI), and T1-weighted. Assessment of brain morphology was performed in order to exclude pathological or congenital lesions. Additional analysis of diffusion in the ACC region was performed using the Functool image analysis software (GE Healthcare; Chicago, IL, USA). For each subject, apparent diffusion coefficient maps were calculated. Region of interest (ROI) was placed in ACC, adjusted to the anatomical size of the ACC area, and it was approximately 2 $cm^2$. The value of the diffusion signal and ADC coefficient was automatically calculated from each ROI, given as mean value and standard deviation. DWI sequence was performed in axial plane (slice thickness 5.0 mm, spacing 1.5 mm, TR 8000 ms, TE 98 ms, FOV24 cm, and matrix 128 × 128). The diffusion weighted imaging for $b$ = 0, 1500, s/mm$^2$ was oriented in three directions.

Magnetic resonance spectroscopy (MRS) was performed using the single-voxel technique (SVS). The MRS spectra were acquired using the point-resolved spectroscopy sequence (PRESS Point- Resolved Spectroscopy Sequence). PRESS sequence utilizes one 900 and two 1800 radiofrequency pulses. For water suppression, the CHESS sequence (CHEmical shift Selective Imaging Sequence) was used with a frequency-selective 900 pulse to selectively excite the water signal, followed by a dephasing gradient. To obtain good quality spectra, automatic shimming was used. The magnetic resonance spectroscopy (MRS) acquisition parameters were—35 ms TE, 64 averages were acquired. In this study, the MRS signal was collected from the anterior cingulate cortex (ACC), parallel and superior to the dorsal anterior surface of the corpus callosum, and centered on the interhemispheric fissure. The volume of interest (VOI) was approximately 8 cm$^3$. The size of VOI was adjusted to the anatomical size of the area the spectrum was collected from. The duration of the sequence was 2 min and 12 s.

During the spectroscopic examination, frequency adjustment of the transmitter and receiver was performed, as well as general correction of the magnetic field (schimming). Automatic schimming was routinely used during the prepscan. Schimming corrects the non-uniformity of the magnetic field. In the case of spectroscopy, the heterogeneity of the magnetic field is the widening of the peaks in the spectrum, the decrease in their amplitude and the signal-to-noise ratio, that hinders the attenuation of the water signal. Lack of this homogeneity leads to different Larmor precession values for protons coming from the same molecule. This causes the broadening of successive peaks in the spectrum, which is of particular importance for distinguishing between two closely adjacent peaks. The shim coils are responsible for maintaining the best homogeneity of the magnetic field. Homogeneity was measured through the width of the water peak at half its height. This is called half width FWHM (= full width at half maximum—a measure of the magnetic field homogeneity). The value FWHM and SNR (signal-to-noise ratio) were used to exclude the MR spectra of poor quality. The PRESS sequence was performed only when the FWHM was about 3. If the FWHM value was above 3, correction of the VOI alignment for spectroscopy was performed, and re-schimming was carried out. In exceptional cases, manual schimming was performed.

The spectroscopic analysis was performed with the SAGE 7.0 software (Plano, TX, USA).

Analysis was performed in the following steps—(1) zero filling (always to a power of 2), (2) Fourier transformation, (3) baseline correction (4) automatic phase correction, and (5) curve fitting, performed on the basis of a Gaussian shape to calculate the peak area.

In the analysis of the spectrum, the highest peaks at the 2.1 and 2.45 ppm locations were chosen as glutamatergic transmission metabolites—GLU (2.1 ppm) and GLN (2.45 ppm)—glutamate and glutamine.

Taking into account the parameters of the PRESS sequence, the prepscan used, and the subsequent steps of the spectrum analysis in SAGE, these peaks were marked separately.

### 2.6. Statistical Analysis

The statistical analysis was performed with the use of the IBM SPSS Statistics 25 package. Statistical, unsupervised (without a priori available knowledge) data analysis was used to determine the endophenotypes. An algorithm was used that divided the data into groups (clusters) so that each group was as homogeneous as possible, and at the same time the clusters were as different as possible. The results of division into clusters are presented in the form of charts (Figure 2). The following indicators were used independently for unsupervised k-means cluster analysis:

1. Brain metabolites, i.e.,—lipids (lip 0.9–1.0 ppm), lactates (lac 1.33 ppm), alanine (ala 1.48 mm), N-acetyl-aspartate (NAA 2.02 ppm), glutamate (glu 2.1 and 3.7 ppm), $\gamma$-aminobutyric acid (GABA 2.3 ppm), glutamine (gln 2.45 and 3.7 ppm), creatine

(Cr 3.02 and 3.9 ppm), choline (Cho 3.22 ppm), glucose (glc 3.43 and 3.8 ppm), myo-inositol (mI 3.56 ppm), and glutathione (GSH 3.7 ppm), as well as the ratios of these metabolites in the frontal lobes—right, left, and ACC.

2. Biochemical parameters routinely determined as part of outpatient diagnostics, i.e.,: complete blood count (5-diff) and a manual smear, biochemical markers (ionogram—sodium [mmol/L], potassium [mmol/L], and chlorides [mmol/L]; metabolic markers—glucose [mmol/L], lipidogram—cholesterol [mmol/L], HDL [mmol/L], LDL [mmol/L], triglycerides [mmol/L]; renal markers—creatinine [μmol/L], eGFR according to MORD [mL/min/1.73 m$^2$]: inflammatory markers—CRP [mg/L], cortisol [μg/dL], complement C3 [mg/dL], complement C4 [mg/dL]; thyroid markers—T4, T3, TSH);
3. Biochemical parameters reflecting the formation and action of reactive oxygen species and the related excess of oxidative stress, which is a response to the breakdown of the elements of antioxidant defense, i.e., MDA, FRAP, and PON-1. Their selection was dictated by the redox balance and inflammation of the nervous system in altered glutamatergic transmission, associated with disease symptoms [54]. Changes in the peripheral redox microcircuits presented in the study, due to the increased permeability of BBB, might lead to increased infiltration of peripheral material into the brain, and consequently might be a potential pathogenetic factor of the disease [51]. The brain's susceptibility to stress, which leads to the overproduction of reactive forms of oxide, nitrogen, and sulfur, in conditions of impaired antioxidant defense, consequently causes damage to macromolecules, including extensive peroxidation of proteins, lipids, or nucleic acids, increased permeability of the blood–brain barrier and causes inflammation of the nervous system. Only when taken together, this can provide a reliable assessment of the centrally occurring changes in brain metabolism and morphology observed in mental disorders of a multifactorial nature [78].

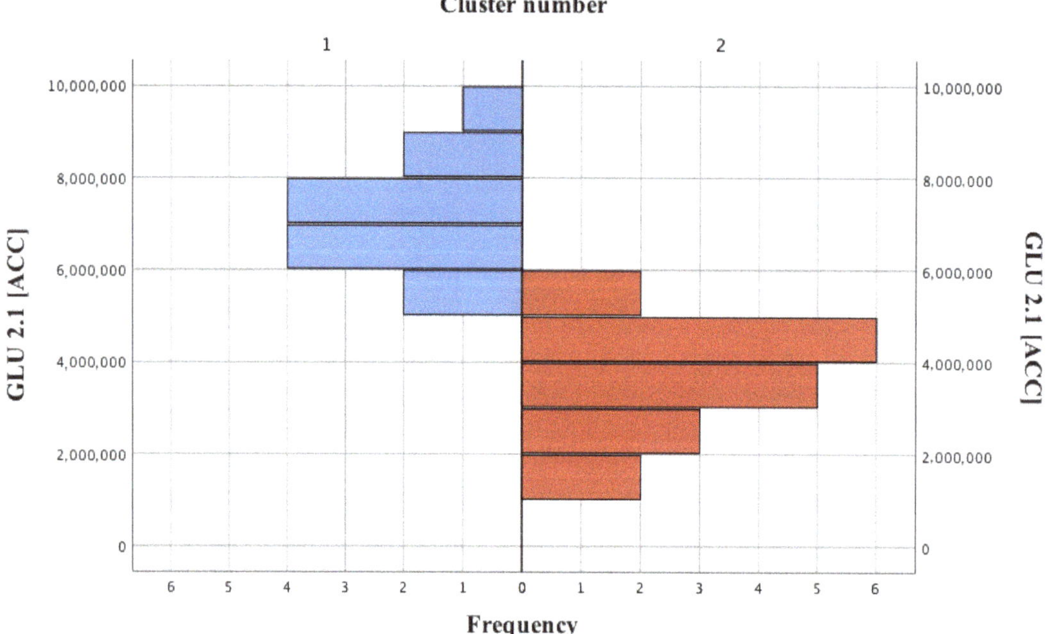


**Figure 2.** Separated clusters of subjects based on the GLU 2.1 (ACC) level, i.e., differing to the greatest possible extent in terms of the quality of life.

The k-means cluster analysis allowed to distinguish 2 clusters of patients, based on the parameter GLU 2.1 in ACC. Using the Mann–Whitney U test, it was verified whether there were statistically significant differences between the selected clusters. The analysis of the Spearman correlation allowed to assess whether there is a statistically significant relationship between the analyzed variables. A $p$-value below 0.05 was considered to be statistically significant.

## 3. Results

### 3.1. Endophenotypes

About 700 cluster analyzes were carried out. From our data it was observed that patients with schizophrenia could be differentiated on the basis of presence of GLU 2.1 in ACC. In this way, two clusters (endophenotypes) were obtained, using the k-means cluster analysis—the main branches of the tree in Figure 2 marked with red and blue colors. These were characterized by the highest differences in terms of clinical parameters. The groups contained 41.9% and 58.1% subjects, respectively. The clusters separated in this way were equal, $\chi^2$ (1) = 0.81; $p = 0.37$.

Glutamate was also the only biochemical parameter that showed a statistically significant relationship with the clinical assessment of schizophrenics, i.e., the PANSS total scores, PANSS positive, and PANSS negative scale.

Based on the separated equal clusters, a comparison was made in terms of clinical evaluation indicators related to symptomatic diagnosis currently used in the diagnosis of schizophrenia (according to the PANSS positive, negative, general psychopathology, and PANSS total scores from the PANSS classification).

Descriptive statistics for GLU 2.1 (ACC) in the clusters of patients are presented in Table 1. Patients from cluster 1 achieved a significantly higher mean GLU 2.1 (ACC), compared to the second group of participants in the study.

**Table 1.** Descriptive statistics for GLU 2.1 (ACC) in the selected clusters of patients with schizophrenia.

| Cluster Number | GLU 2.1 (ACC) (Mean ± SD) |
|---|---|
| I | 7,132,000 ± 1,167,008.62 |
| II | 3,574,438.89 ± 141,242.09 |
| Statistical result | U = 0; $p < 0.001$ |

### 3.2. Relationship of the Endophenotypes with the Clinical State of Patients with Schizophrenia

Patients from the second cluster, i.e., with a reduced level of GLU 2.1 (ACC), had significantly higher scores on the N, G, and T scales, as compared to the first cluster. In the case of the P scale, the score was also higher, but the difference was not significant (Table 2, Figure 3).

**Table 2.** Descriptive statistics on the quality of life of the two separate clusters of patients.

| Cluster Number | P Scale (Mean ± SD) | N Scale (Mean ± SD) | G Scale (Mean ± SD) | T Scale (Mean ± SD) |
|---|---|---|---|---|
| I | 25.85 ± 6.44 | 23.08 ± 6.03 | 50.35 ± 9.22 | 97.77 ± 19.46 |
| II | 28.94 ± 6.22 | 27.44 ± 4.71 | 57.22 ± 8.97 | 112.28 ± 19.15 |
| Statistical result | U = 85.5<br>$p = 0.21$ | U = 64<br>$p = 0.03$ | U = 69<br>$p = 0.049$ | U = 67.5<br>$p = 0.046$ |

Additionally, a receiver operating characteristic (ROC) curve was prepared. The T scale allows us to significantly predict the belonging to the second group of people suffering from schizophrenia, i.e., with a reduced level of GLU 2.1 (ACC); AUC = 0.71 (Figure 4).

### 3.3. Relationship of the Endophenotypes with Routinely Determined Parameters

There was a difference in the level of neutrophils in the separate clusters. In research conducted by Bryll et al., it turned out that the biochemical parameters that showed the most numerous and strong correlations with the quality of life of the respondents were neutrophils and lymphocytes [21]. Both clusters obtained in our study differed in a significant way in terms of both analyzed variables (Table 3).

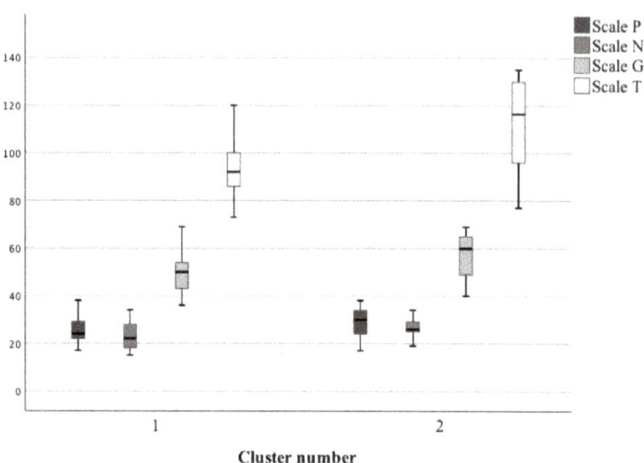


**Figure 3.** Scoring of the scales concerning the quality of life in selected clusters of patients.

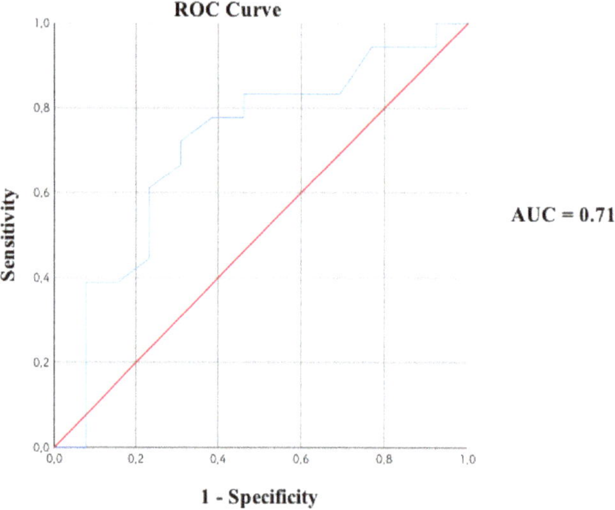


**Figure 4.** Predicting the membership of the second cluster on the basis of the T-scale scores. An ROC curve can be considered as the average value of the sensitivity for a test over all possible values of specificity or vice versa. A more general interpretation is that given the test results, the probability that for a randomly selected pair of patients with and without the disease/condition, the patient with the disease/condition has a result indicating greater suspicion. The area under the ROC (AUC) curve is bounded by the blue line and red baseline. The value of the AUC index is in the interval (0.1) delimited by two marked color lines. AUC, a high area under curve value limited by a blue line; ROC, a Receiver Operating Characteristic curve that includes all the possible decision thresholds from a diagnostic test result.

Patients from the second cluster, i.e., with a decreased GLU 2.1 (ACC) level, had a significantly higher percentage of neutrophils, as well as a lower percentage of lymphocytes, as compared to those from the first cluster. In our earlier studies, it turned out that the higher the percentage of neutrophils, the higher the scores of the individual scales [21]. A negative correlation was observed for the percentage of lymphocytes, which is presented in Table 4.

**Table 3.** The level of neutrophils and lymphocytes in the selected clusters of patients with schizophrenia.

| Cluster Number | Neutrophils [%] (Mean ± SD) | Lymphocytes [%] (Mean ± SD) |
|---|---|---|
| I | 48.34 ± 7.67 | 38.95 ± 6.66 |
| II | 59.14 ± 8.78 | 29.35 ± 7.39 |
| Statistical result | U = 44.5<br>$p = 0.003$ | U = 45<br>$p = 0.003$ |

**Table 4.** Relationship between the percentage of neutrophils and lymphocytes in the studied group of people and their scores for individual scales.

| Variable | P Scale | N Scale | G Scale | T Scale |
|---|---|---|---|---|
| Neutrophils [%] | 0.46<br>$p < 0.001$ | 0.47<br>$p < 0.001$ | 0.48<br>$p < 0.001$ | 0.55<br>$p < 0.001$ |
| Lymphocytes [%] | −0.4<br>$p < 0.001$ | −0.45<br>$p < 0.001$ | −0.46<br>$p < 0.001$ | 0.51<br>$p < 0.001$ |

The relationships of GLU 2.1 (ACC) with the percentage of neutrophils ($r = -0.49$) and lymphocytes ($r = 0.46$) were statistically significant ($p = 0.006$ and $p = 0.01$, respectively). The presence of two stronger relationships GLU 2.1 (ACC) with the percentage of neutrophils and lymphocytes was observed: (1) neutrophil level, $r = -0.49$; $p = 0.006$; The higher the neutrophil count, the lower the GLU 2.1 (ACC) score; (2) lymphocyte level, $r = 0.46$; $p = 0.01$; The higher the lymphocyte count, the higher the GLU 2.1 (ACC) score.

### *3.4. Relationship of the Endophenotypes with Biochemical Parameters and Diffusion in the Anterior Cingulate Area*

No other significant differences were observed between the biochemical parameters and diffusion in the anterior cingulate area in the clusters. The only significant difference was present in the level of GLU 2.1 (ACC) (Table 5).

In summary, two clusters of patients with schizophrenia were distinguished, based on the level of glutamatergic transmission metabolite in the anterior cingulate cortex (GLU 2.1 (ACC)), which differed in terms of symptoms, and also strongly differed in the percentage of neutrophils and lymphocytes (which, in turn, correlated with the quality of life).

No additional variables significantly differed between the two endophenotypes among those analyzed, i.e., parameters of oxidative stress (FRAP, MDA, and PON-1), diffusion (DWI), or biochemical indices.

**Table 5.** Descriptive statistics concerning the selected clusters of patients for biochemical parameters and diffusion in the anterior cingulate area.

| Cluster Number | GLU 2.1 (ACC) (Mean ± SD) | FRAP (Mean ± SD) | MDA (Mean ± SD) | DWI, Frontal Lobes (AVG) | | ADC, Right Frontal Lobe (DEV) (Mean ± SD) | PON-1 (Mean ± SD) |
|---|---|---|---|---|---|---|---|
| | | | | Left (Mean ± SD) | Right (Mean ± SD) | | |
| I | 7,132,000 ± 1,167,008.62 | 0.36 ± 0.22 | 0.7 ± 0.16 | 333.69 ± 27.53 | 325.13 ± 33.09 | 0.00073 ± 0.0001 | 102.69 ± 3.79 |
| II | 3,574,438.89 ± 141,242.09 | 0.4 ± 0.23 | 0.78 ± 0.14 | 342.07 ± 41.02 | 343.07 ± 37.1 | 0.00069 ± 0.00064 | 101.08 ± 5.35 |
| Statistical result | U = 0<br>$p < 0.001$ | U = 105<br>$p = 0.63$ | U = 114<br>$p = 0.92$ | U = 85<br>$p = 0.21$ | U = 99<br>$p = 0.49$ | U = 94<br>$p = 0.36$ | U = 101<br>$p = 0.52$ |

PON-1: Paraoxonase-1; MDA: malondialdehyde; FRAP: ferric reducing ability of plasma; DWI: diffusion-weighted imaging; AVG: average; ADC—apparent diffusion coefficient; and DEV: standard deviation.

## 4. Discussion

### 4.1. Endophenotypes

The medical world's attention to the importance of subtypes in schizophrenia is not a new topic. It was Bleuler who independently pointed out the importance of the so-called 'latent schizophrenia', which emphasized not only the classic manifestation of the disease but also the different clinical pictures, from personality disturbances to affective psychosis. Interestingly, researchers believed that the symptoms of 'latent schizophrenia' interact with the underlying disease or the classic phenotype of schizophrenia, in which the concept of a latent trait is the basis of both glaring psychosis and other disorders described in the introduction. Bleuler, in his clinical observations, drew attention to the understanding of the definition of schizophrenia as a set of various disorders, defining them with the common term 'group of schizophrenia' [79].

The efforts of the last decade represent a breakthrough in the discovery of biomarkers that enhance symptomatic diagnosis and facilitate the prognosis of disease progression. Advances in the field of neuroimaging (NMR, PET, SPECT, fMRI, and MRS) and genetic techniques, opened the door to the characterization of clinical endophenotypes, which enriches the diagnosis and might constitute the basis for personalized medicine, related to the construction of appropriate statistical models to facilitate the diagnosis and treatment of neuropsychiatric diseases, including schizophrenia [46].

As a result of our research, two clusters of patients with an initial diagnosis of schizophrenia were defined in an unsupervised manner, based on the glutamatergic transmission metabolites level—Type I was characterized by a higher level of GLU 2.1, and Type II by its reduced level.

From the clinical point of view, due to the similar severity of positive symptoms but greater negative symptoms in the second endophenotype as compared to the first endophenotype, the second endophenotype might include patients with a less favorable course of schizophrenia, with more severe functional deterioration and requiring more intensive treatment. The obtained results might also suggest different risk factors for the development of schizophrenia in patients from both groups.

The glutamatergic hypothesis is one of the mechanisms explaining the observed results. One theory is that the insufficiency of the N-methyl-D-aspartate (NMDA) receptor leads to excessive release of glutamate in the frontal cortex, which might affect the release of dopamine and other neurotransmitters [80,81], which, in turn, leads to the expression of positive symptoms characteristic of schizophrenia [82]. It could also be explained by a higher density of D2 receptors in the striatum or an increased release of dopamine [83,84]. The results from the literature regarding the increased Gln/Glu ratio, explained by the abnormalities in the neuro-glial coupling, confirmed our results concerning the increased level of Glu in the endophenotype I [41]. These changes were more clearly marked in bipolar disorder, while in patients with acute psychotic episode, they only showed a tendency to be abnormal. These abnormalities appeared in both areas of the brain, suggesting that the lesions spread throughout the entire cortex. According to the hypothesis presented by Ongür et al., neuro-glial coupling abnormalities result in changes in the Gln/Glu ratio during acute episodes in the prefrontal cortex (ACC) and the parieto-occipital cortex (POC). Therefore, according to our previous results and reports of other authors, glutamatergic disorders might be associated with the period of illness or, sometimes, untreated psychosis [85,86].

The theories of glutamatergic transmission in schizophrenia suggest that the loss of NMDA receptors, especially in GABAergic interneurons, leads to disturbances in the excitatory–inhibitory balance and abnormalities of neuro-glial coupling in the prefrontal cortex. Oxidative stress is one of the initiating factors of schizophrenia, however, antioxidant systems or glutathione precursors (needed for the synthesis of glutamate and glutamine) might prevent changes in the synaptic transmission in pyramidal cells that result from the developmental NMDAR blockade and mitochondrial dysfunction with further generation of mitochondrial superoxides [87]. N-acetylcysteine (NAC) alleviates changes caused by the administration of ketamine, which confirms the participation of antioxidant systems in the changes generated by free radicals, with altered synaptic function [88]. Ketamine causes changes in the NMDAR function in prefrontal cortex interneurons, due to the increased generation of mitochondrial superoxides, mitigated by competition for the binding sites on NMDAR with NAC, which is considered to be a strong antioxidant [89,90]. Moreover, NAC administered at the last stage of maturation was also able to restore normal mitochondrial function and inhibition in pyramidal cells. This confirmed the role of peripherally located oxidant–antioxidant microcircuits on central macrosystems, and thus the self-control ability in preventing or restoring central changes. Moreover, this proves the validity of future schizophrenia treatment strategies targeting NMDA receptors and glutamatergic transmission.

The causes of the pathological sequelae arise from increases and dysregulation of mitochondrial ROS production and bioenergetic failure, which moves them from the periphery to the central nervous system. The mechanism of observed changes is connected with Nicotinamide Adenine Dinucleotide (NAD+) depletion, which raises ROS production on adenosine 5′-triphosphate (ATP) and NADPH generation and consistently decreases antioxidants and the glutamate signaling cascade in the anterior cingulate cortex is influenced [61].

Mitochondria, as the main source of energy production in the form of ATP and free radicals, play a key role in this regulation. The close relationship between the appearance of negative symptoms in schizophrenia and mitochondrial dysfunction, suggests that mitochondrial defects are crucial for disease development [91]. Disturbed glutamatergic transmission causes a reduction in GABA release and subsequent disinhibition of pyramidal cells with excessive release of glutamate [92] is visible in the group of patients with endophenotype I.

Another mechanism explaining glutamate excitotoxicity in patients with endophenotype I might be a mechanism related to resistance to classic neuroleptics, which is in some way related to NMDA receptor failure, and results in a weakening of NMDA signaling, consequently leading to inhibition of stimulation due to insufficient activation of GABAergic neurons. As a result, weak negative feedback from GABAergic interneurons to pyramidal neurons increases glutamatergic neurotransmission, which then leads to glutamate excitotoxicity and develops resistance to drugs that act primarily on positive (not negative) symptoms (Figures 1 and 5).

Disorders of glutamatergic neurotransmission might relate to another aspect of the pathophysiology of schizophrenia associated with the NMDA-R and its insufficiency, especially in the prefrontal cortex. NMDA-R mediates many neurobiological processes, including glutamatergic stimulation, brain structure development, and the induction of synaptic neuroplasticity. It was found that the NMDA-R deficiency in GABAergic neurons in the early postpartum period results in the development of schizophrenia. This type of receptor dysfunction is influenced by environmental factors. These include perinatal hypoxia or oxidative stress as important elements of NMDA-R deficiency in interneurons, which could be observed in the pilot studies conducted by our team [21].

Increased glutamatergic transmission levels in the ACC, as compared to healthy controls and patients responding to treatment were associated with the clinical endophenotypes identified in this study—endophenotype I in patients with schizophrenia who showed higher levels of glutamate (7,132,000.00 ± 1,167,008.62), in comparison to endophenotype II (3,574,438.89 ± 141,242.09) with a significantly reduced level of glutamate compared to endophenotype I. Results presented by the above-mentioned group of researchers suggest a relationship between the increased levels of glutamatergic neurometabolites and treatment-resistant schizophrenia (our results—7,132,000 ± 1,167,008.62 for $n$ = 13 vs. the results of Demjaha et al. 8.87 ± 2.44, for $n$ = 8 patients with schizophrenia in remission; or 10.32 ± 1.41 for $n$ = 6 patients with treatment-resistant schizophrenia) [93]. In addition, the authors indicate the neurobiological foundations of resistance to treatment, suggesting their relationship with the action of glutamine in the ACC area [94].

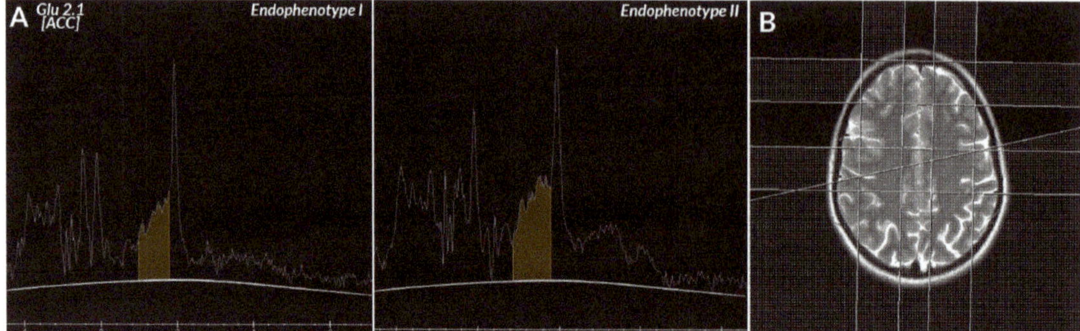


**Figure 5.** (**A**) On the MR spectrum, the yellow line is at the level of glutamatergic neurotransmission metabolites Glu, Gln (2.1–2.5 ppm) peak in endophenotype I, and the yellow line is at the level of Glu, Gln (2.1–2.5 ppm) peak in endophenotype II. (**B**) T2 weighted axial image, with the location of VOI in the ACC region.

In the work of Iwata et al., a similarly increased level of glutamate and glutamine in the ACC is explained by treatment-resistant schizophrenia. Consistent with the above-mentioned studies that showed higher levels of glutamine in ACC in patients with treatment-resistant schizophrenia, this study suggests that higher levels of ACC glutamatergic metabolites might be one of the common biological features of antipsychotic resistance in schizophrenic patients [95].

The phase of illness is not without significance, as the first episode of psychosis (FEP) and chronic schizophrenia constitute high-risk groups for which increased levels of glutamate and glutamine are found in the anterior and medial frontal cortex. Thus, higher levels of these metabolites occur in patients with more severe functional impairment, due to changes over time. The results of Dempster et al. showed no significant differences in the measurements of glutamatergic transmission metabolites in the ACC between patients who previously did not use drugs or used minimal treatment (FEP patients) and the control group [96]. This was consistent with our preliminary research, which was closer to explaining the importance of the glutamatergic theory in the pathophysiology of schizophrenia [21].

The levels of glutamate, glutamine, and other metabolites in the ACC showed an accelerated age-dependent decline [97]. Therefore, older people showed more pronounced decreases than the young. This additionally supported the clinical endophenotypes established in this study and their use in the group of younger people, who did not yet develop a visible difference from the healthy subjects [21] but showed likely changes before entering the psychotic phase, which could be considered to be a susceptibility to the disease [93,98].

The cluster II with a reduced glutamatergic transmission metabolites concentration selected in this study was explained in the works of Lutkenhoff et al. as a factor characterizing the obtained clinical endophenotype of patients with schizophrenia. This indicated the essential role of the reduced glutamate level in the quality of life in patients with schizophrenia [99]. This translated into clearly significant relationships between the decreased level of glutamate and negative, cognitive, and general symptoms obtained in this endophenotype, and a significantly smaller relationship with positive symptoms. This, in turn, confirmed the dopamine hypothesis of schizophrenia in eliminating the positive symptoms of the disease by classic neuroleptics, which left the negative symptoms unaffected.

The analysis of the relationships between the developed endophenotypes and the routinely measured parameters showed that neutrophils were most strongly associated with glutamate, while lymphocytes showed the opposite relationship. This confirmed the inflammatory hypothesis, which is often mentioned in the pathogenesis of schizophrenia. The positive relationship obtained in this study between cluster II (reduced glutamate level) and the level of neutrophils, as well as the negative relationship with lymphocytes, were confirmed in the study by Özdin and Böke [100]. The researchers observed that the ratio of neutrophils to lymphocytes (NLR) in patients during the exacerbation of the disease (the equivalent of our group with psychotic decompensation) was significantly higher, as compared to the control group. These studies confirmed the involvement of immunological and inflammatory mechanisms (outside the central one), emphasizing the role of the neutrophil–lymphocyte relationship with schizophrenia [101]. An additional explanation for the reduction of neutrophils in cluster I (increased glutamatergic transmission metabolites level) might be the response to the treatment of resistant schizophrenia, which could be interpreted as one of the side effects of polypharmacy. This would suggest additional phenotypic features of this endophenotype, such as greater exposure to neutropenia in the setting of polypharmacy and greater susceptibility to the effects of drug interactions [102].

In the group of patients with schizophrenia with a lower concentration of glutamatergic transmission metabolites (endophenotype II), we observed more severe clinical symptoms in all analyzed scales (P, N, G, T), and only the negative symptoms showed statistical significance. This might be associated with neurodegeneration or the consequences of chronic treatment usually linked with neutropenia [86,103]. However, this did not apply to our results characterizing patients with endophenotype II, for which a higher percentage of neutrophils than in the case of endophenotype I was observed. This rather indicated a substantial contribution of the inflammatory theory [71,72], which linked the role of immunological factors with the oxidant–antioxidant balance and the functioning of glutamatergic systems in the brain of schizophrenic patients [104].

Additional support for our results, emphasizing the role of the inflammatory theory related to altered glutamatergic transmission, was the lack of a relationship between local changes in the level of brain metabolites with the influence of previously used antipsychotic treatment, in a group of chronically schizophrenic patients [105].

An additional explanation for the reduced glutamatergic level observed in isolated subtype II and its statistically significant relationship with the symptoms (higher N, G, and T scores, compared to cluster I with elevated glutamatergic metabolites concentration) and the percentage of neutrophils, might be related to the release of inflammatory factors (such as chemokines, interleukins like MIP-2$\gamma$, or CXCL14). Their presence in the postsynaptic space reduced the expression of the glutamate-1 transporter on astrocytes and increased the sensitivity of neurons to glutamate excitotoxicity [106]. In addition, incorrect expression of glutamatergic transporters caused the accumulation of toxic concentrations of glutamatergic transmission metabolites and other free radical reaction products from the released neutrophils, which might also lead to inhibition of free diffusion (decrease in ADC, right frontal lobe, DEV) observed in the study in cluster II, as compared to cluster I. The degree of limitation of tissue diffusion was inversely proportional to cell density and cell membrane integrity. The higher the cell density, the number of intact cell membranes and, for example, the content of proteins/organelles (related to the infiltration of neutrophils), the more limited the free diffusion of water molecules, which could be seen in the study as an observed trend (without statistical significance). Consequently, changes in glutamatergic neurotransmission through reduced activity or expression of the glutamate transporter (GLT) might contribute to many observed neurological symptoms and the intensification of clinical symptoms. These results suggest that neutrophil-released inflammatory factors mediate the pathogenesis of CNS disorders associated with neutrophil infiltration into the brain and decreased GLT-1 activity. Overexpression of the toxic factors released by the infiltrating neutrophils, i.e., MIP-2$\gamma$, reduced the level of glutamate transporting proteins, i.e., GLT-1, resulting in glutamate excitotoxicity to neurons and astrocytes that removed excessive glutamate (observed increase in glutamate levels in cluster I).

### 4.2. Limitations

One of the limitations of the study was the use of a static model associated with a single measurement of the amount of metabolites (including glutamatergic transmission) in the 1H-MRS study, without the assessment of functional brain activation, allowing the assessment of changes in acquisition over time (1H-fMRS) [107]. This would give a more accurate assessment of the glutamatergic neurotransmission than the standard magnetic resonance spectroscopy [108].

The limitation of the methods used was conducting research related to MRS magnetic resonance spectroscopy on schizophrenia, at a relatively low-field strength of 1.5 T. A higher-field strength would provide a better signal-to-noise ratio (SNR) and thus a better spectral resolution, which in turn would allow for more precise quantification peaks of the studied metabolites of glutamatergic transmission. Field strengths, especially $\leq$3 T, have limited possibilities to quantify the overlapping glutamate and glutamine signals separately, which often makes their interpretation difficult. Multicenter cohort studies using high-field (7 T) MRS are planned, which would allow for improved detection of clear glutamate and glutamine signals in a group of patients at risk of developing schizophrenia and diseases from the differential diagnosis.

Additionally, the planned future research would determine the early response to the antipsychotic drugs, which seemed to determine the subsequent symptoms and functional outcomes of psychosis. Glutamate as an objective differential marker of patients with schizophrenia is a promising therapeutic target, especially for patients classified as endophenotype I, who are likely to show an insufficient response to classical treatment regimens.

We did not include the drugs used in the treatment of acute phase of schizophrenia in the analyses. These could affect both the glutamatergic activity of the brain and other investigated parameters, such as inflammatory markers, lipid profile, or blood morphology. There were several reasons for resigning from these analyses. The study was performed in the initial period of treatment of acute psychosis, accompanied by significant modifications of pharmacotherapy. Data on prior treatment were unreliable, due to the possibility of skipping prescription doses by patients, due to the increase in psychotic symptoms causing hospitalization. The study group was too small to analyze the effect of individual drugs or their groups. Difficulties with the use of drug equivalents in data mining were related to the use of both first- and second-generation drugs in the studied group that did not share pharmacokinetics, relations between dosage and effect, and affinity for various receptors, as well as the pro-inflammatory/anti-inflammatory effects [109].

The conducted study suggests that negative symptoms play an important role in young patients with an initial diagnosis of schizophrenia, especially in cluster II with low glutamatergic transmission metabolite levels in the MRS. The limitation of the obtained observations was the small sample size, however, due to the fact that our research provided strong evidence for linking the glutamatergic theory and a documented relationship with symptomatic diagnosis and inflammation (neutrophils/lymphocytes), we decided to present the results as the effect of research constituting a premise for further work on the endophenotypes identified in this research.

## 5. Conclusions

The multifactorial nature of schizophrenia and the lack of understanding of the role of biological factors in the etiopathogenesis of this disease, constitute the main limitation of the existence of an ideal biomarker. Thus, the introduction of new therapeutic approaches related to this disease is challenging.

Currently, there are no approved markers of risk stratification based on the multimodal bias of non-classical variants of schizophrenia and the proportion of rarer clinical endophenotypes with greater or lesser effect. We propose that the use of the glutamatergic marker(s) related to the functioning of the NMDA receptor in the anterior cingulate cortex could be used for diagnostic purposes in determining disease endophenotypes, which might lead to new diagnostic and therapeutic approaches and could provide more effective care for patients.

Personalized assessment based on the developed clinical endophenotypes of the disease seems to be highly justified in the stratification of young patients with schizophrenia. This should also be the main point of therapeutic activities related to the reduction of the severity of the axial symptoms of the disease. Negative symptoms of schizophrenia are often overlooked and difficult to treat, therefore, they are often accompanied by worse cognitive functioning or an increased risk of suicidal behavior. Glutamatergic transmission metabolites dysfunctions at the level of the anterior cingulate cortex appear first and spread to the prefrontal cortex [109], especially among adolescent patients with psychotic disorders, which is confirmed in the obtained endophenotypes (cluster II, which is most strongly associated with negative symptoms of the disease). Studies on a larger cohort might contribute to confirming the role of glutamatergic transmission in endophenotypes determination and might constitute an important premise for further research, especially among young people with an initial diagnosis of schizophrenia and negative symptoms.

Our study showed clear differences in the changes in the Glu level that objectively differentiate patients with schizophrenia (without a priori available knowledge), which is reflected in the different research hypotheses presented in the literature on the subject.

Further presentation of the results based on the influence of disease duration and phases (stable phase, decompensation, exacerbation, and symptomatic remission) on the level of Gln/Glu transmission seems justified.

**Author Contributions:** Conceptualization, W.K., A.B., T.J.P., M.P., and N.Ś.; methodology, A.B., W.K., and T.J.P.; software, W.K. and P.K.; validation, W.K. and A.B.; concept of data analysis and their interpretation as well as formal analysis and interpretation of all results, W.K. and T.J.P.; investigation, W.K. and T.J.P.; resources, T.J.P., A.B., and W.K.; data curation, A.B., W.K., P.K., N.Ś., M.S., M.P., and T.J.P.; participation in recruiting patients, N.Ś., M.P., and M.S.; writing (original draft preparation), W.K., A.B., M.S., M.P., N.Ś., and A.S.; revised the manuscript after reviews, W.K. and A.S.; visualization, W.K.; supervision, T.J.P.; project administration, A.B.; funding acquisition, A.B. and T.J.P. All authors have read and agreed to the published version of the manuscript.

**Funding:** This research was supported by the grant no. N41/DBS/000292 from the Jagiellonian University Medical College, Poland.

**Institutional Review Board Statement:** The study was conducted according to the guidelines of the Declaration of Helsinki, and approved by the Bioethics Committee of the Jagiellonian University (consent number: 1072.6120.152.2019 of 27 June 2019).

**Informed Consent Statement:** Written informed consent has been obtained from the patient(s) to publish this paper.

**Data Availability Statement:** Not applicable.

**Conflicts of Interest:** The authors declare no conflict of interest.

## References

1. World Health Organization. *International Statistical Classification of Diseases and Related Health Problems*; World Health Organization: Geneva, Switzerland, 2010.
2. Group, B.D.W. Biomarkers and surrogate endpoints: Preferred definitions and conceptual framework. *Clin. Pharmacol. Ther.* **2001**, *69*, 89–95.
3. Ritsner, M. *Neuropsychiatric Biomarkers, Endophenotypes and Genes: Promises, Advances and Challenges*; Springer: Berlin, Germany, 2009.
4. Schmitt, A.; Rujescu, D.; Gawlik, M.; Hasan, A.; Hashimoto, K.; Iceta, S.; Jarema, M.; Kambeitz, J.; Kasper, S.; Keeser, D.; et al. Consensus paper of the WFSBP Task Force on Biological Markers: Criteria for biomarkers and endophenotypes of schizophrenia part II: Cognition, neuroimaging and genetics. *World J. Biol. Psychiatry* **2016**, *17*, 406–428. [CrossRef] [PubMed]
5. Meehl, P.E. Toward an Integrated Theory of Schizotaxia, Schizotypy, and Schizophrenia. *J. Pers. Disord.* **1990**, *4*, 1–99. [CrossRef]

6. Lenzenweger, M. *Schizotypy and Schizophrenia: The View from Experimental Psychopathology*; Guilford Press: New York, NY, USA, 2010.
7. World Health Organization. *The ICD-10 Classification of Mental and Behavioural Disorders: Diagnostic Criteria for Research*; World Health Organization: Geneva, Switzerland, 1993; Volume 2.
8. Clark, L.A.; Cuthbert, B.; Lewis-Fernández, R.; Narrow, W.E.; Reed, G.M. Three Approaches to Understanding and Classifying Mental Disorder: ICD-11, DSM-5, and the National Institute of Mental Health's Research Domain Criteria (RDoC). *Psychol. Sci. Public Interest* **2017**, *18*, 72–145. [CrossRef] [PubMed]
9. Grover, S.; Dua, D.; Chakrabarti, S.; Avasthi, A. Factor analysis of symptom dimensions (psychotic, affective and obsessive compulsive symptoms) in schizophrenia. *Asian J. Psychiatry* **2018**, *38*, 72–77. [CrossRef] [PubMed]
10. Lenzenweger, M.F. Schizotypy, Schizotypic Psychopathology, and Schizophrenia: Hearing Echoes, Leveraging Prior Advances, and Probing New Angles. *Schizophr. Bull.* **2018**, *44*, S564–S569. [CrossRef]
11. Paksarian, D.; Merikangas, K.R.; Calkins, M.E.; Gur, R.E. Racial-ethnic disparities in empirically-derived subtypes of subclinical psychosis among a U.S. sample of youths. *Schizophr. Res.* **2016**, *170*, 205–210. [CrossRef]
12. Gross, G. Therapy of subclinical (subdiagnostic) syndromes of schizophrenia spectrum. *Fortschr. Neurol. Psychiatr.* **2001**, *69* (Suppl. 2), S95–S100. [CrossRef]
13. Rasmussen, A.R.; Nordgaard, J.; Parnas, J. Schizophrenia-spectrum psychopathology in obsessive-compulsive disorder: An empirical study. *Eur. Arch. Psychiatry Clin. Neurosci.* **2020**, *270*, 993–1002. [CrossRef]
14. Blokland, G.A.M.; Del Re, E.C.; Mesholam-Gately, R.I.; Jovicich, J.; Trampush, J.W.; Keshavan, M.S.; DeLisi, L.E.; Walters, J.T.R.; Turner, J.A.; Malhotra, A.K.; et al. The Genetics of Endophenotypes of Neurofunction to Understand Schizophrenia (GENUS) consortium: A collaborative cognitive and neuroimaging genetics project. *Schizophr. Res.* **2018**, *195*, 306–317. [CrossRef]
15. Gottesman, I.I.; Gould, T.D. The endophenotype concept in psychiatry: Etymology and strategic intentions. *Am. J. Psychiatry* **2003**, *160*, 636–645. [CrossRef]
16. National Institute of Mental Health. Available online: https://www-1nimh-1nih-1gov-1nb5yei5r0029.hanproxy.cm-uj.krakow.pl/research/research-funded-by-nimh/rdoc/index.shtml (accessed on 2 February 2021).
17. Smucny, J.; Iosif, A.-M.; Eaton, N.R.; Lesh, T.A.; Ragland, J.D.; Barch, D.M.; Gold, J.M.; Strauss, M.E.; MacDonald, A.W.; Silverstein, S.M.; et al. Latent Profiles of Cognitive Control, Episodic Memory, and Visual Perception Across Psychiatric Disorders Reveal a Dimensional Structure. *Schizophr. Bull.* **2020**, *46*, 154–162. [CrossRef] [PubMed]
18. Lenzenweger, M.F. Thinking clearly about schizotypy: Hewing to the schizophrenia liability core, considering interesting tangents, and avoiding conceptual quicksand. *Schizophr. Bull.* **2015**, *41* (Suppl. 2), S483–S491. [CrossRef] [PubMed]
19. Lenzenweger, M.F. Schizotaxia, schizotypy, and schizophrenia: Paul, E. Meehl's blueprint for the experimental psychopathology and genetics of schizophrenia. *J. Abnorm. Psychol.* **2006**, *115*, 195–200. [CrossRef] [PubMed]
20. Sukumar, N.; Sabesan, P.; Anazodo, U.; Palaniyappan, L. Neurovascular Uncoupling in Schizophrenia: A Bimodal Meta-Analysis of Brain Perfusion and Glucose Metabolism. *Front. Psychiatry* **2020**, *11*, 754. [CrossRef] [PubMed]
21. Bryll, A.; Krzyściak, W.; Karcz, P.; Śmierciak, N.; Kozicz, T.; Skrzypek, J.; Szwajca, M.; Pilecki, M.; Popiela, T.J. The Relationship between the Level of Anterior Cingulate Cortex Metabolites, Brain-Periphery Redox Imbalance, and the Clinical State of Patients with Schizophrenia and Personality Disorders. *Biomolecules* **2020**, *10*, 1272. [CrossRef]
22. Adams, R.; David, A.S. Patterns of anterior cingulate activation in schizophrenia: A selective review. *Neuropsychiatr. Dis. Treat.* **2007**, *3*, 87–101. [CrossRef]
23. Varea, O.; Martin-de-Saavedra, M.D.; Kopeikina, K.J.; Schürmann, B.; Fleming, H.J.; Fawcett-Patel, J.M.; Bach, A.; Jang, S.; Peles, E.; Kim, E.; et al. Synaptic abnormalities and cytoplasmic glutamate receptor aggregates in contactin associated protein-like 2/Caspr2 knockout neurons. *Proc. Natl. Acad. Sci. USA* **2015**, *112*, 6176–6181. [CrossRef]
24. Shukla, D.K.; Wijtenburg, S.A.; Chen, H.; Chiappelli, J.J.; Kochunov, P.; Hong, L.E.; Rowland, L.M. Anterior Cingulate Glutamate and GABA Associations on Functional Connectivity in Schizophrenia. *Schizophr. Bull.* **2019**, *45*, 647–658. [CrossRef]
25. Demro, C.; Rowland, L.; Wijtenburg, S.A.; Waltz, J.; Gold, J.; Kline, E.; Thompson, E.; Reeves, G.; Hong, L.E.; Schiffman, J. Glutamatergic metabolites among adolescents at risk for psychosis. *Psychiatry Res.* **2017**, *257*, 179–185. [CrossRef]
26. Vargas, T.; Damme, K.S.F.; Ered, A.; Capizzi, R.; Frosch, I.; Ellman, L.M.; Mittal, V.A. Neuroimaging Markers of Resiliency in Youth at Clinical High Risk for Psychosis: A Qualitative Review. *Biol. Psychiatry. Cogn. Neurosci. Neuroimaging* **2021**, *6*, 166–177. [CrossRef]
27. Tandon, N.; Bolo, N.R.; Sanghavi, K.; Mathew, I.T.; Francis, A.N.; Stanley, J.A.; Keshavan, M.S. Brain metabolite alterations in young adults at familial high risk for schizophrenia using proton magnetic resonance spectroscopy. *Schizophr. Res.* **2013**, *148*, 59–66. [CrossRef] [PubMed]
28. Chen, X.; Tamang, S.M.; Du, F.; Ongur, D. Glutamate diffusion in the rat brain in vivo under light and deep anesthesia conditions. *Magn. Reson. Med.* **2019**, *82*, 84–94. [CrossRef] [PubMed]
29. Bruno, V.; Scapagnini, U.; Canonico, P.L. Excitatory amino acids and neurotoxicity. *Funct. Neurol.* **1993**, *8*, 279–292. [PubMed]
30. Smith, Q.R. Transport of glutamate and other amino acids at the blood-brain barrier. *J. Nutr.* **2000**, *130*, 1016S–1022S. [CrossRef]
31. Limongi, R.; Jeon, P.; Mackinley, M.; Das, T.; Dempster, K.; Théberge, J.; Bartha, R.; Wong, D.; Palaniyappan, L. Glutamate and Dysconnection in the Salience Network: Neurochemical, Effective Connectivity, and Computational Evidence in Schizophrenia. *Biol. Psychiatry* **2020**, *88*, 273–281. [CrossRef] [PubMed]

32. Wenneberg, C.; Glenthøj, B.Y.; Hjorthøj, C.; Buchardt Zingenberg, F.J.; Glenthøj, L.B.; Rostrup, E.; Broberg, B.V.; Nordentoft, M. Cerebral glutamate and GABA levels in high-risk of psychosis states: A focused review and meta-analysis of (1)H-MRS studies. *Schizophr. Res.* **2020**, *215*, 38–48. [CrossRef] [PubMed]
33. Borgan, F.R.; Jauhar, S.; McCutcheon, R.A.; Pepper, F.S.; Rogdaki, M.; Lythgoe, D.J.; Howes, O.D. Glutamate levels in the anterior cingulate cortex in un-medicated first episode psychosis: A proton magnetic resonance spectroscopy study. *Sci. Rep.* **2019**, *9*, 8685. [CrossRef]
34. Moghaddam, B.; Adams, B.; Verma, A.; Daly, D. Activation of glutamatergic neurotransmission by ketamine: A novel step in the pathway from NMDA receptor blockade to dopaminergic and cognitive disruptions associated with the prefrontal cortex. *J. Neurosci.* **1997**, *17*, 2921–2927. [CrossRef]
35. Thompson, S.L.; Welch, A.C.; Iourinets, J.; Dulawa, S.C. Ketamine induces immediate and delayed alterations of OCD-like behavior. *Psychopharmacology* **2020**, *237*, 627–638. [CrossRef]
36. Howes, O.D.; Kambeitz, J.; Kim, E.; Stahl, D.; Slifstein, M.; Abi-Dargham, A.; Kapur, S. The nature of dopamine dysfunction in schizophrenia and what this means for treatment. *Arch. Gen. Psychiatry* **2012**, *69*, 776–786. [CrossRef] [PubMed]
37. Moghaddam, B.; Krystal, J.H. Capturing the angel in "angel dust": Twenty years of translational neuroscience studies of NMDA receptor antagonists in animals and humans. *Schizophr. Bull.* **2012**, *38*, 942–949. [CrossRef] [PubMed]
38. Michael, N.; Erfurth, A.; Ohrmann, P.; Gössling, M.; Arolt, V.; Heindel, W.; Pfleiderer, B. Acute mania is accompanied by elevated glutamate/glutamine levels within the left dorsolateral prefrontal cortex. *Psychopharmacology* **2003**, *168*, 344–346. [CrossRef]
39. Shevelkin, A.V.; Terrillion, C.E.; Hasegawa, Y.; Mychko, O.A.; Jouroukhin, Y.; Sawa, A.; Kamiya, A.; Pletnikov, M.V. Astrocyte DISC1 contributes to cognitive function in a brain region-dependent manner. *Hum. Mol. Genet.* **2020**, *29*, 2936–2950. [CrossRef]
40. Blumberg, H.P.; Krystal, J.H.; Bansal, R.; Martin, A.; Dziura, J.; Durkin, K.; Martin, L.; Gerard, E.; Charney, D.S.; Peterson, B.S. Age, rapid-cycling, and pharmacotherapy effects on ventral prefrontal cortex in bipolar disorder: A cross-sectional study. *Biol. Psychiatry* **2006**, *59*, 611–618. [CrossRef] [PubMed]
41. Ongür, D.; Jensen, J.E.; Prescot, A.P.; Stork, C.; Lundy, M.; Cohen, B.M.; Renshaw, P.F. Abnormal glutamatergic neurotransmission and neuronal-glial interactions in acute mania. *Biol. Psychiatry* **2008**, *64*, 718–726. [CrossRef] [PubMed]
42. Cadinu, D.; Grayson, B.; Podda, G.; Harte, M.K.; Doostdar, N.; Neill, J.C. NMDA receptor antagonist rodent models for cognition in schizophrenia and identification of novel drug treatments, an update. *Neuropharmacology* **2018**, *142*, 41–62. [CrossRef] [PubMed]
43. Del Arco, A.; Ronzoni, G.; Mora, F. Hypofunction of prefrontal cortex NMDA receptors does not change stress-induced release of dopamine and noradrenaline in amygdala but disrupts aversive memory. *Psychopharmacology* **2015**, *232*, 2577–2586. [CrossRef]
44. Govindaraju, V.; Young, K.; Maudsley, A.A. Proton NMR chemical shifts and coupling constants for brain metabolites. *NMR Biomed.* **2000**, *13*, 129–153. [CrossRef]
45. Kolomeets, N.S. Disturbance of oligodendrocyte differentiation in schizophrenia in relation to main hypothesis of the disease. *Zhurnal Nevrol. i Psikhiatrii Im. S. S. Korsakova* **2017**, *117*, 108–117. [CrossRef] [PubMed]
46. Marshall, C.R.; Howrigan, D.P.; Merico, D.; Thiruvahindrapuram, B.; Wu, W.; Greer, D.S.; Antaki, D.; Shetty, A.; Holmans, P.A.; Pinto, D.; et al. Contribution of copy number variants to schizophrenia from a genome-wide study of 41,321 subjects. *Nat. Genet.* **2017**, *49*, 27–35. [CrossRef]
47. Szczeklik, K.; Krzyściak, W. Od uszkodzeń miejscowych do narządowych-konsekwencje zaburzeń równowagi pomiędzy produkcją reaktywnych form tlenu a sprawnością układów antyoksydacyjnych w chorobie Leśniowskiego-Crohna. *Przegl. Lek.* **2019**, *76*, 36–42.
48. Lee, E.E.; Sears, D.D.; Liu, J.; Jin, H.; Tu, X.M.; Eyler, L.T.; Jeste, D.V. A novel biomarker of cardiometabolic pathology in schizophrenia? *J. Psychiatr. Res.* **2019**, *117*, 31–37. [CrossRef]
49. Devanarayanan, S.; Nandeesha, H.; Kattimani, S.; Sarkar, S.; Jose, J. Elevated copper, hs C-reactive protein and dyslipidemia in drug free schizophrenia: Relation with psychopathology score. *Asian J. Psychiatry* **2016**, *24*, 99–102. [CrossRef] [PubMed]
50. Rose, C.R.; Ziemens, D.; Untiet, V.; Fahlke, C. Molecular and cellular physiology of sodium-dependent glutamate transporters. *Brain Res. Bull.* **2018**, *136*, 3–16. [CrossRef]
51. Morris, G.; Walker, A.J.; Walder, K.; Berk, M.; Marx, W.; Carvalho, A.F.; Maes, M.; Puri, B.K. Increasing Nrf2 Activity as a Treatment Approach in Neuropsychiatry. *Mol. Neurobiol.* **2021**. [CrossRef] [PubMed]
52. KÖŞger, F.; YİĞİtaslan, S.; EŞsİzoĞlu, A.; GÜleÇ, G.; KarataŞ, R.D.; DeĞİrmencİ, S.S. Inflammation and Oxidative Stress in Deficit Schizophrenia. *Noro Psikiyatr. Ars.* **2020**, *57*, 303–307.
53. Coughlin, J.M.; Yang, K.; Marsman, A.; Pradhan, S.; Wang, M.; Ward, R.E.; Bonekamp, S.; Ambinder, E.B.; Higgs, C.P.; Kim, P.K.; et al. A multimodal approach to studying the relationship between peripheral glutathione, brain glutamate, and cognition in health and in schizophrenia. *Mol. Psychiatry* **2020**, 1–10. [CrossRef]
54. Kealy, J.; Greene, C.; Campbell, M. Blood-brain barrier regulation in psychiatric disorders. *Neurosci. Lett.* **2020**, *726*, 133664. [CrossRef]
55. Son, S.; Arai, M.; Miyata, J.; Toriumi, K.; Mizuta, H.; Hayashi, T.; Aso, T.; Itokawa, M.; Murai, T. Enhanced carbonyl stress and disrupted white matter integrity in schizophrenia. *Schizophr. Res.* **2020**, *223*, 242–248. [CrossRef] [PubMed]
56. Bauer, M.E.; Teixeira, A.L. Inflammation in psychiatric disorders: What comes first? *Ann. N. Y. Acad. Sci.* **2019**, *1437*, 57–67. [CrossRef] [PubMed]

57. Kay, S.R.; Fiszbein, A.; Opler, L.A. The positive and negative syndrome scale (PANSS) for schizophrenia. *Schizophr. Bull.* **1987**, *13*, 261–276. [CrossRef] [PubMed]
58. Szczeklik, K.; Krzysciak, W.; Domagala-Rodacka, R.; Mach, P.; Darczuk, D.; Cibor, D.; Pytko-Polonczyk, J.; Rodacki, T.; Owczarek, D. Alterations in glutathione peroxidase and superoxide dismutase activities in plasma and saliva in relation to disease activity in patients with Crohn's disease. *J. Physiol. Pharmacol.* **2016**, *67*, 709–715.
59. Albayrak, Y.; Ünsal, C.; Beyazyüz, M.; Ünal, A.; Kuloğlu, M. Reduced total antioxidant level and increased oxidative stress in patients with deficit schizophrenia: A preliminary study. *Prog. Neuropsychopharmacol. Biol. Psychiatry* **2013**, *45*, 144–149. [CrossRef]
60. Sarandol, A.; Sarandol, E.; Acikgoz, H.E.; Eker, S.S.; Akkaya, C.; Dirican, M. First-episode psychosis is associated with oxidative stress: Effects of short-term antipsychotic treatment. *Psychiatry Clin. Neurosci.* **2015**, *69*, 699–707. [CrossRef]
61. Yao, J.K.; Keshavan, M.S. Antioxidants, redox signaling, and pathophysiology in schizophrenia: An integrative view. *Antioxid. Redox Signal.* **2011**, *15*, 2011–2035. [CrossRef] [PubMed]
62. Benzie, I.F.; Strain, J.J. The ferric reducing ability of plasma (FRAP) as a measure of "antioxidant power": The FRAP assay. *Anal. Biochem.* **1996**, *239*, 70–76. [CrossRef]
63. Güneş, M.; Camkurt, M.A.; Bulut, M.; Demir, S.; İbiloğlu, A.O.; Kaya, M.C.; Atlı, A.; Kaplan, İ.; Sir, A. Evaluation of Paraoxonase, Arylesterase and Malondialdehyde Levels in Schizophrenia Patients Taking Typical, Atypical and Combined Antipsychotic Treatment. *Clin. Psychopharmacol. Neurosci.* **2016**, *14*, 345–350. [CrossRef] [PubMed]
64. Moreira, E.G.; Boll, K.M.; Correia, D.G.; Soares, J.F.; Rigobello, C.; Maes, M. Why Should Psychiatrists and Neuroscientists Worry about Paraoxonase 1? *Curr. Neuropharmacol.* **2019**, *17*, 1004–1020. [CrossRef]
65. Eckerson, H.W.; Wyte, C.M.; La Du, B.N. The human serum paraoxonase/arylesterase polymorphism. *Am. J. Hum. Genet.* **1983**, *35*, 1126–1138. [PubMed]
66. Bai, Z.-L.; Li, X.-S.; Chen, G.-Y.; Du, Y.; Wei, Z.-X.; Chen, X.; Zheng, G.-E.; Deng, W.; Cheng, Y. Serum Oxidative Stress Marker Levels in Unmedicated and Medicated Patients with Schizophrenia. *J. Mol. Neurosci.* **2018**, *66*, 428–436. [CrossRef] [PubMed]
67. Guidara, W.; Messedi, M.; Naifar, M.; Maalej, M.; Grayaa, S.; Omri, S.; Ben Thabet, J.; Maalej, M.; Charfi, N.; Ayadi, F. Predictive value of oxidative stress biomarkers in drug-free patients with schizophrenia and schizo-affective disorder. *Psychiatry Res.* **2020**, *293*, 113467. [CrossRef] [PubMed]
68. Aust, S. Thiobarbituric acid assay reactants. In *Methods in Toxicology. In Vitro Toxicity Indicators*; Tyson, C., Frazier, J., Eds.; Academic Press: San Diego, CA, USA, 1994; pp. 367–376.
69. Reilly, C.; Aust, S. Measurement of malondialdehyde. In *Current Methods in Toxicology. Assessment of Cell Toxicity*; John Wiley & Sons: Hoboken, NJ, USA, 2005.
70. Gutteridge, J.M. Aspects to consider when detecting and measuring lipid peroxidation. *Free Radic. Res. Commun.* **1986**, *1*, 173–184. [CrossRef] [PubMed]
71. Pedraz-Petrozzi, B.; Elyamany, O.; Rummel, C.; Mulert, C. Effects of inflammation on the kynurenine pathway in schizophrenia—A systematic review. *J. Neuroinflamm.* **2020**, *17*, 56. [CrossRef] [PubMed]
72. Roomruangwong, C.; Noto, C.; Kanchanatawan, B.; Anderson, G.; Kubera, M.; Carvalho, A.F.; Maes, M. The Role of Aberrations in the Immune-Inflammatory Response System (IRS) and the Compensatory Immune-Regulatory Reflex System (CIRS) in Different Phenotypes of Schizophrenia: The IRS-CIRS Theory of Schizophrenia. *Mol. Neurobiol.* **2020**, *57*, 778–797. [CrossRef] [PubMed]
73. Severance, E.G.; Dickerson, F.B.; Yolken, R.H. Autoimmune phenotypes in schizophrenia reveal novel treatment targets. *Pharmacol. Ther.* **2018**, *189*, 184–198. [CrossRef]
74. García-Bueno, B.; Pérez-Nievas, B.G.; Leza, J.C. Is there a role for the nuclear receptor PPARγ in neuropsychiatric diseases? *Int. J. Neuropsychopharmacol.* **2010**, *13*, 1411–1429. [CrossRef]
75. Mackness, M.I.; Mackness, B.; Durrington, P.N. Paraoxonase and coronary heart disease. *Atheroscler. Suppl.* **2002**, *3*, 49–55. [CrossRef]
76. Bryll, A.; Krzyściak, W.; Jurczak, A.; Chrzan, R.; Lizoń, A.; Urbanik, A. Changes in the Selected Antioxidant Defense Parameters in the Blood of Patients after High Resolution Computed Tomography. *Int. J. Environ. Res. Public Health* **2019**, *16*, 1476. [CrossRef]
77. Frijhoff, J.; Winyard, P.G.; Zarkovic, N.; Davies, S.S.; Stocker, R.; Cheng, D.; Knight, A.R.; Taylor, E.L.; Oettrich, J.; Ruskovska, T.; et al. Clinical Relevance of Biomarkers of Oxidative Stress. *Antioxid. Redox Signal.* **2015**, *23*, 1144–1170. [CrossRef]
78. Rossetti, A.C.; Paladini, M.S.; Riva, M.A.; Molteni, R. Oxidation-reduction mechanisms in psychiatric disorders: A novel target for pharmacological intervention. *Pharmacol. Ther.* **2020**, *210*, 107520. [CrossRef] [PubMed]
79. Beckmann, H. *Classification of Endogenous Psychoses and Their Differentiated Etiology*, 2nd ed.; Leonhard, K., Ed.; Springer: New York, NY, USA, 1999.
80. Egerton, A.; Murphy, A.; Donocik, J.; Anton, A.; Barker, G.J.; Collier, T.; Deakin, B.; Drake, R.; Eliasson, E.; Emsley, R.; et al. Dopamine and Glutamate in Antipsychotic-Responsive Compared with Antipsychotic-Nonresponsive Psychosis: A Multicenter Positron Emission Tomography and Magnetic Resonance Spectroscopy Study (STRATA). *Schizophr. Bull.* **2021**, *47*, 505–516. [CrossRef] [PubMed]
81. Veldman, E.R.; Svedberg, M.M.; Svenningsson, P.; Lundberg, J. Distribution and levels of 5-HT(1B) receptors in anterior cingulate cortex of patients with bipolar disorder, major depressive disorder and schizophrenia—An autoradiography study. *Eur. Neuropsychopharmacol.* **2017**, *27*, 504–514. [CrossRef] [PubMed]

82. Umino, M.; Umino, A.; Nishikawa, T. Effects of selective calcium-permeable AMPA receptor blockade by IEM 1460 on psychotomimetic-induced hyperactivity in the mouse. *J. Neural Transm.* **2018**, *125*, 705–711. [CrossRef] [PubMed]
83. Cumming, P.; Abi-Dargham, A.; Gründer, G. Molecular imaging of schizophrenia: Neurochemical findings in a heterogeneous and evolving disorder. *Behav. Brain Res.* **2021**, *398*, 113004. [CrossRef]
84. Shin, E.-J.; Dang, D.-K.; Tran, T.-V.; Tran, H.-Q.; Jeong, J.H.; Nah, S.-Y.; Jang, C.-G.; Yamada, K.; Nabeshima, T.; Kim, H.-C. Current understanding of methamphetamine-associated dopaminergic neurodegeneration and psychotoxic behaviors. *Arch. Pharm. Res.* **2017**, *40*, 403–428. [CrossRef]
85. Théberge, J.; Bartha, R.; Drost, D.J.; Menon, R.S.; Malla, A.; Takhar, J.; Neufeld, R.W.; Rogers, J.; Pavlosky, W.; Schaefer, B.; et al. Glutamate and glutamine measured with 4.0 T proton MRS in never-treated patients with schizophrenia and healthy volunteers. *Am. J. Psychiatry* **2002**, *159*, 1944–1946. [CrossRef]
86. Théberge, J.; Al-Semaan, Y.; Williamson, P.C.; Menon, R.S.; Neufeld, R.W.J.; Rajakumar, N.; Schaefer, B.; Densmore, M.; Drost, D.J. Glutamate and glutamine in the anterior cingulate and thalamus of medicated patients with chronic schizophrenia and healthy comparison subjects measured with 4.0-T proton MRS. *Am. J. Psychiatry* **2003**, *160*, 2231–2233. [CrossRef]
87. Phensy, A.; Driskill, C.; Lindquist, K.; Guo, L.; Jeevakumar, V.; Fowler, B.; Du, H.; Kroener, S. Antioxidant Treatment in Male Mice Prevents Mitochondrial and Synaptic Changes in an NMDA Receptor Dysfunction Model of Schizophrenia. *eNeuro* **2017**, *4*. [CrossRef]
88. Blanco-Ayala, T.; Sathyasaikumar, K.V.; Uys, J.D.; Pérez-de-la-Cruz, V.; Pidugu, L.S.; Schwarcz, R. N-Acetylcysteine Inhibits Kynurenine Aminotransferase II. *Neuroscience* **2020**, *444*, 160–169. [CrossRef]
89. Phensy, A.; Duzdabanian, H.E.; Brewer, S.; Panjabi, A.; Driskill, C.; Berz, A.; Peng, G.; Kroener, S. Antioxidant Treatment with N-acetyl Cysteine Prevents the Development of Cognitive and Social Behavioral Deficits that Result from Perinatal Ketamine Treatment. *Front. Behav. Neurosci.* **2017**, *11*, 106. [CrossRef]
90. Nakao, K.; Jeevakumar, V.; Jiang, S.Z.; Fujita, Y.; Diaz, N.B.; Pretell Annan, C.A.; Eskow Jaunarajs, K.L.; Hashimoto, K.; Belforte, J.E.; Nakazawa, K. Schizophrenia-Like Dopamine Release Abnormalities in a Mouse Model of NMDA Receptor Hypofunction. *Schizophr. Bull.* **2019**, *45*, 138–147. [CrossRef]
91. Kim, Y.; Vadodaria, K.C.; Lenkei, Z.; Kato, T.; Gage, F.H.; Marchetto, M.C.; Santos, R. Mitochondria, Metabolism, and Redox Mechanisms in Psychiatric Disorders. *Antioxid. Redox Signal.* **2019**, *31*, 275–317. [CrossRef]
92. Morris, G.; Walder, K.R.; Berk, M.; Marx, W.; Walker, A.J.; Maes, M.; Puri, B.K. The interplay between oxidative stress and bioenergetic failure in neuropsychiatric illnesses: Can we explain it and can we treat it? *Mol. Biol. Rep.* **2020**, *47*, 5587–5620. [CrossRef]
93. Demjaha, A.; Egerton, A.; Murray, R.M.; Kapur, S.; Howes, O.D.; Stone, J.M.; McGuire, P.K. Antipsychotic treatment resistance in schizophrenia associated with elevated glutamate levels but normal dopamine function. *Biol. Psychiatry* **2014**, *75*, e11–e13. [CrossRef] [PubMed]
94. Mouchlianitis, E.; Bloomfield, M.A.P.; Law, V.; Beck, K.; Selvaraj, S.; Rasquinha, N.; Waldman, A.; Turkheimer, F.E.; Egerton, A.; Stone, J.; et al. Treatment-Resistant Schizophrenia Patients Show Elevated Anterior Cingulate Cortex Glutamate Compared to Treatment-Responsive. *Schizophr. Bull.* **2016**, *42*, 744–752. [CrossRef] [PubMed]
95. Iwata, Y.; Nakajima, S.; Plitman, E.; Caravaggio, F.; Kim, J.; Shah, P.; Mar, W.; Chavez, S.; De Luca, V.; Mimura, M.; et al. Glutamatergic Neurometabolite Levels in Patients With Ultra-Treatment-Resistant Schizophrenia: A Cross-Sectional 3T Proton Magnetic Resonance Spectroscopy Study. *Biol. Psychiatry* **2019**, *85*, 596–605. [CrossRef] [PubMed]
96. Dempster, K.; Jeon, P.; MacKinley, M.; Williamson, P.; Théberge, J.; Palaniyappan, L. Early treatment response in first episode psychosis: A 7-T magnetic resonance spectroscopic study of glutathione and glutamate. *Mol. Psychiatry* **2020**, *25*, 1640–1650. [CrossRef] [PubMed]
97. Chen, T.; Wang, Y.; Zhang, J.; Wang, Z.; Xu, J.; Li, Y.; Yang, Z.; Liu, D. Abnormal Concentration of GABA and Glutamate in The Prefrontal Cortex in Schizophrenia.-An in Vivo 1H-MRS Study. *Shanghai Arch. Psychiatry* **2017**, *29*, 277–286. [PubMed]
98. Romeo, B.; Petillion, A.; Martelli, C.; Benyamina, A. Magnetic resonance spectroscopy studies in subjects with high risk for psychosis: A meta-analysis and review. *J. Psychiatr. Res.* **2020**, *125*, 52–65. [CrossRef] [PubMed]
99. Lutkenhoff, E.S.; van Erp, T.G.; Thomas, M.A.; Therman, S.; Manninen, M.; Huttunen, M.O.; Kaprio, J.; Lönnqvist, J.; O'Neill, J.; Cannon, T.D. Proton MRS in twin pairs discordant for schizophrenia. *Mol. Psychiatry* **2010**, *15*, 308–318. [CrossRef] [PubMed]
100. Özdin, S.; Böke, Ö. Neutrophil/lymphocyte, platelet/lymphocyte and monocyte/lymphocyte ratios in different stages of schizophrenia. *Psychiatry Res.* **2019**, *271*, 131–135. [CrossRef]
101. Yüksel, R.N.; Ertek, I.E.; Dikmen, A.U.; Göka, E. High neutrophil-lymphocyte ratio in schizophrenia independent of infectious and metabolic parameters. *Nord. J. Psychiatry* **2018**, *72*, 336–340. [CrossRef]
102. Simon, L.; Cazard, F. Clozapine rechallenge after neutropenia in resistant schizophrenia: A review. *L'encephale* **2016**, *42*, 346–353. [CrossRef] [PubMed]
103. Pisciotta, A.V.; Konings, S.A.; Ciesemier, L.L.; Cronkite, C.E.; Lieberman, J.A. On the possible mechanisms and predictability of clozapine-induced agranulocytosis. *Drug Saf.* **1992**, *7* (Suppl. 1), 33–44. [CrossRef] [PubMed]
104. Yang, A.C.; Tsai, S.-J. New Targets for Schizophrenia Treatment beyond the Dopamine Hypothesis. *Int. J. Mol. Sci.* **2017**, *18*, 1689. [CrossRef] [PubMed]

105. Kraguljac, N.V.; Morgan, C.J.; Reid, M.A.; White, D.M.; Jindal, R.D.; Sivaraman, S.; Martinak, B.K.; Lahti, A.C. A longitudinal magnetic resonance spectroscopy study investigating effects of risperidone in the anterior cingulate cortex and hippocampus in schizophrenia. *Schizophr. Res.* **2019**, *210*, 239–244. [CrossRef] [PubMed]
106. Fang, J.; Han, D.; Hong, J.; Tan, Q.; Tian, Y. The chemokine, macrophage inflammatory protein-2γ, reduces the expression of glutamate transporter-1 on astrocytes and increases neuronal sensitivity to glutamate excitotoxicity. *J. Neuroinflamm.* **2012**, *9*, 267. [CrossRef]
107. Stanley, J.A.; Burgess, A.; Khatib, D.; Ramaseshan, K.; Arshad, M.; Wu, H.; Diwadkar, V.A. Functional dynamics of hippocampal glutamate during associative learning assessed with in vivo (1)H functional magnetic resonance spectroscopy. *Neuroimage* **2017**, *153*, 189–197. [CrossRef] [PubMed]
108. Goryawala, M.Z.; Sheriff, S.; Maudsley, A.A. Regional distributions of brain glutamate and glutamine in normal subjects. *NMR Biomed.* **2016**, *29*, 1108–1116. [CrossRef] [PubMed]
109. Dlabac-de Lange, J.J.; Liemburg, E.J.; Bais, L.; van de Poel-Mustafayeva, A.T.; de Lange-de Klerk, E.S.M.; Knegtering, H.; Aleman, A. Effect of Bilateral Prefrontal rTMS on Left Prefrontal NAA and Glx Levels in Schizophrenia Patients with Predominant Negative Symptoms: An Exploratory Study. *Brain Stimul.* **2017**, *10*, 59–64. [CrossRef]

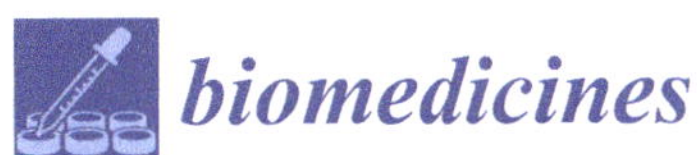

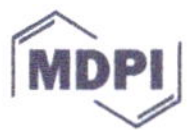

*Review*

# An Overview of ICA/BSS-Based Application to Alzheimer's Brain Signal Processing

**Wenlu Yang [1], Alexander Pilozzi [2] and Xudong Huang [2,*]**

[1] Department of Electrical Engineering, Information Engineering College, Shanghai Maritime University, Shanghai 200135, China; wlyang@shmtu.edu.cn
[2] Department of Psychiatry, Massachusetts General Hospital and Harvard Medical School, Charlestown, MA 02129, USA; apilozzi@mgh.harvard.edu
* Correspondence: Huang.Xudong@mgh.harvard.edu; Tel.: +1-617-724-49778; Fax: +1-617-726-4078

**Abstract:** Alzheimer's disease (AD) is by far the most common cause of dementia associated with aging. Early and accurate diagnosis of AD and ability to track progression of the disease is increasingly important as potential disease-modifying therapies move through clinical trials. With the advent of biomedical techniques, such as computerized tomography (CT), electroencephalography (EEG), magnetoencephalography (MEG), positron emission tomography (PET), magnetic resonance imaging (MRI), and functional magnetic resonance imaging (fMRI), large amounts of data from Alzheimer's patients have been acquired and processed from which AD-related information or "signals" can be assessed for AD diagnosis. It remains unknown how best to mine complex information from these brain signals to aid in early diagnosis of AD. An increasingly popular technique for processing brain signals is independent component analysis or blind source separation (ICA/BSS) that separates blindly observed signals into original signals that are as independent as possible. This overview focuses on ICA/BSS-based applications to AD brain signal processing.

**Keywords:** Alzheimer's disease; blind signal separation; brain signal processing; fMRI; independent component analysis; MRI

**Citation:** Yang, W.; Pilozzi, A.; Huang, X. An Overview of ICA/BSS-Based Application to Alzheimer's Brain Signal Processing. *Biomedicines* **2021**, *9*, 386. https://doi.org/10.3390/biomedicines9040386

Academic Editor: Arnab Ghosh

Received: 27 February 2021
Accepted: 30 March 2021
Published: 6 April 2021



## 1. Introduction

Alzheimer's disease (AD), which was first recognized by Alois Alzheimer in 1906, is the most common cause of dementia in older adults [1,2]. According to the 2008 Alzheimer's Disease Facts and Figures [3], recently released by the Alzheimer's Association, an estimated 5.8 million people in the United States presently have AD, with projections indicating growth to as many as 13.8 million by mid-century. Understanding all behavioral, anatomical, and physiological aspects of this disease is vitally important to populations worldwide. Improving the accuracy of diagnosis of AD at its early stage is critical to finding a successful treatment.

AD has a presymptomatic phase, likely lasting years, during which neuronal degeneration is occurring but clinical symptoms have not yet appeared. Critical to the early treatment of AD is the ability to discriminate between older individuals who will and will not ultimately develop the disease during this preclinical stage. Early treatment is beneficial to prevent or at least slow down the onset of the clinical manifestations of disease [4]. Moreover, to aid in the development of these treatments, specifically drugs for the treatment of AD at its early stage, early diagnostic tools and techniques to monitor disease progression in the presymptomatic phases of the disease are needed.

With the advent of biomedical engineering techniques, more and more brain signals have been acquired and processed for AD diagnosis. These brain signals come from electroencephalography (EEG) [5], magnetoencephalography (MEG) [6], computerized tomography (CT) [7], single photon emission computed tomography (SPECT) [8], positron emission tomography (PET) [9], magnetic resonance imaging (MRI) [10], and functional magnetic resonance imaging (fMRI) [11].

Correspondingly, a number of signal processing approaches have been proposed to process these brain signals for diagnosing patients with AD. These include: wavelet transformation (WT) [12], principal component analysis (PCA) [13], independent component analysis (ICA) [14], also known as blind source separation (BSS), parallel factor analysis (PARAFAC) [15], and so on. In this review, we will focus on applications of ICA/BSS/in processing of brain signals for potential AD diagnosis.

## 2. Alzheimer's Disease

Since the end of the 19th and the beginning of the 20th century, it has been recognized that two classic silver-positive lesions occur in the Alzheimer's brain: the intraneuronal neurofibrillary tangles and extracellular deposits of amyloid called senile plaques [16]. Plaques are made primarily of the amyloid β peptide, Aβ-40, and Aβ-42, derived from the amyloid precursor protein [17]. Neurofibrillary tangles, by contrast, are stained by β-pleated sheet histological reagents but are made of a different proteinaceous substance. These intracellular lesions are composed primarily of the microtubular-associated protein, tau, which changes from its normal neuronal localization in axons to occupy and dominate the somatic and dendritic compartments of a subpopulation of the large projection neurons in neocortex and limbic systems [18]. Gomez-Isla et al. introduced the concept of a third type of lesion, focusing on the neuritic changes that occur in dendrites and axons that are not (necessarily) silver-positive, but which reflect changes in morphology, trajectories, and post-synaptic structures that may also contribute to the breakdown of neural system function.

Clinical features of AD include a decline in memory and other cognitive functions. AD is the most common form of dementia, with prominent symptoms of memory loss, language difficulties (aphasia, anomia), and deficits in visual spatial skills (agnosia) and motor spatial skills (apraxia) [1]. General complaints of visual problems (difficulty reading, blurry vision, vague complaints of poor visual acuity) may be the presenting symptoms in AD, but patients may lack objective signs on ophthalmological examination [19–21]. Most research suggests that visual dysfunction is caused by neuropathology of the visual association cortices [22], rather than by changes in the retina, optic nerve or retino-calcarine pathways [23,24].

## 3. Biomedical Techniques for Detecting Alzheimer's Brain Signals

With advances in biomedical techniques, it is possible to obtain Alzheimer's brain signals to diagnose AD at an early stage. In this section, we will briefly introduce these biomedical techniques.

EEG [5] is a test used to detect abnormalities related to the electrical activity of the brain. Small metal discs with thin wires (electrodes) are placed on the scalp that sends signals to a computer for their recording. Normal electrical activity in the brain makes a recognizable pattern. Through an EEG, doctors can look for abnormal patterns that indicate seizures and other problems. EEG has good temporal resolution but relatively poor spatial resolution [25]. Since Hans Berger in 1931 first observed pathological EEG sequences in a historically verified AD patient, a large number of studies about the EEG of AD have been presented [26–29]. The primary EEG markers of AD include decreased alpha and beta activities, slower dominant-posterior rhythms, increased diffuse-slow activity, as well as a decrease in coherence [5].

MEG [30] is a complex reference-free non-invasive function brain imaging technique with millisecond temporal resolution that detects neuromagnetic signals produced by neuronal activity in the cortex of the brain. Compared to EEG, MEG is less distorted by the resistive properties of the skull, skin, and cerebral fluid, which act as a low pass filter. Several studies have been performed on AD and mild cognitive impairment (MCI) using MEG [31–43].

PET [9] and SPECT are two molecular imaging techniques that provide pictures of the brain that reflect the distribution of radioactive-labeled drugs (radioligands or tracers) injected into the body. Then, sensors that surround the injected body part detect the positrons emitted from the tracer in opposite directions, localizing the tracer. The most common tracer used is a glucose analogue, fluorodeoxyglucose (FDG), which measures regional cerebral glucose metabolism, a sign of neuronal activity. PET has been explored to determine its ability to differentiate between a diagnosis of AD and fronto-temporal dementia (FTD) [9,44–48]. SPECT also has been used to investigate functional alteration of the brain in patients with AD [46,49]. PET measurements of cerebral glucose metabolism also have been found to have superior accuracy compared to SPECT measurements of cerebral perfusion in differentiating AD from vascular dementia, regardless of dementia severity [50]. Klunk et al. presented the first human study of a novel amyloid-PET tracer, termed Pittsburgh Compound-B (PIB), in patients with diagnosed mild AD and controls and suggested that PIB can provide quantitative information on amyloid deposits [51] and detect cerebrovascular β-amyloid for identifying the extent of cerebral amyloid angiopathy (CAA) [52] in living subjects. More recent PET tracers have been found to be more effective than PIB for AD diagnosis, however [48].

CT and MRI are two biomedical imaging techniques that search for atrophy in the brain structure in vivo. With the use of CT, atrophy of medial temporal regions where AD pathology is seen early in the disease has been observed [7]. MRI techniques sensitive to changes in cerebral blood flow and blood oxygenation were developed by high-speed echo planar imaging. They allow one to obtain completely non-invasive tomographic maps of human brain activity through the use of visual and motor stimulus paradigms [53,54]. MRI has more recently surpassed CT in AD studies due to its greater accuracy, manipulability, and precision [55]. Moreover, compared to PET, MRI has the advantage of not using radioactively-labeled compounds and being non-invasive and safe for repeat studies. For AD diagnosis, MRI can act as a sensitive tool, detecting structural brain abnormalities, consistently revealing atrophy of hippocampus [56], entorhinal [10], and temporal–parietal cortices [57].

As discussed by Pekar [54], fMRI provides the opportunity to study brain function non-invasively. Since the early 1990s, it has been a powerful tool used in both research and clinical arenas [53]. The most popular form of fMRI uses blood-oxygenation-level-dependent (BOLD) contrast, that is based on the differing magnetic properties of oxygenated (diamagnetic) and deoxygenated (paramagnetic) blood. When brain neurons are activated, a localized change in blood flow and oxygenation results that causes a shift in the magnetic resonance (MR) decay parameter T2*. These blood flow and oxygenation (vascular or hemodynamic) changes are temporally delayed relative to the neural firing, a confounding factor known as hemodynamic lag. Although fMRI does not share the temporal resolution of EEG or MEG, it does have a spatial resolution of millimeters, and the experiments suggest that it may detect activations at the level of the cortical layers [58].

The detection of changes in neural activity using BOLD-fMRI [53,59] generally involves the identification of voxel signals that correlate with an imposed experimental paradigm [60].

## 4. Theory and Model of ICA/BSS

The essential problem of blind source separation is the isolation of original signals from their resulting mixture that is gathered from an array of sensors, without any information about the original signals or how they are mixed. BSS can be applied to a variety of fields, including audio processing, and is not unique to neuroimaging [61,62].

A fairly general BSS problem can be formulated as:

$$y(k) = Wx(k) \tag{1}$$

where $x(k) = [x_1(k), x_2(k), \ldots, x_m(k)]^T$ is the observed sensor signals, W is the unmixing matrix, $y(k) = [y_1(k), y_2(k), \ldots, y_n(k)]^T$ is the ouput signal, and $k$ is a discrete time. BSS assumes that $x(k)$ is the output signal from an unknown and inverse multiple-input/multiple-output (MIMO) mixing and filtering system, $x(k) = As(k)$ (A is the mixing matrix), in which the inputs are the source signals $s(k) = [s_1(k), s_2(k), \ldots, s_n(k)]^T$. It should be noted that $n$ will be less than $m$ if the system is not inversed.

The objective of BSS is to estimate the original source signals $s(k)$. To separate the source signals $s(k)$, a number of approaches have been developed such as ICA and its extensions, sparse component analysis (SCA), sparse principal component analysis (SPCA), non-negative matrix factorization (NMF), parallel factor analysis (PARAFAC), and so on.

PCA [63], one of well-known unsupervised analysis methods, projects the data into a new space spanned by the principal components. Each successive principal component is selected to be orthonormal to the previous ones and to capture the maximum variance that is not already present in the previous components.

ICA [64,65], as a specific embodiment of BSS, has been further developed in the last few decades. ICA, [66–68] as a generalization of PCA, separates the observed signals into statistically independent components using higher-order statistics whereas PCA obtains uncorrelated components using only second-order statistics. ICA is different from BSS; The basic goal of ICA is to solve the BSS problem by expressing a set of random variables (observations) as linear combinations of statistically independent component variables (source signals), whereas the objective of BSS is to estimate the original source signals, even if they are not all statistically independent. A more thorough description of ICA has been written by Comon (Comon, 1994 #58).

The technique of ICA was first used in 1982 for analyzing a problem pertaining to neurophysiology [69]. In the middle of the 1990s, after the term ICA was first coined by Comon [70], ICA received wide attention and growing interest when many efficient approaches were put forward, such as the Informax principle by Bell and Sejnowski [64], natural gradient-based infomax by Amri [71], and the fixed-point (FastICA) algorithm by Hyvärinen [72,73].

ICA [64,65] is becoming increasingly popular as a tool for analyzing biomedical data [14,74–76]. In the next section, we will introduce the basic model of ICA/BSS of fMRI and its variants for different purposes of application.

## 5. ICA/BSS Model for fMRI

Due to the spatial and temporal natures of fMRI data, the use of ICA can generally be grouped into two groups, namely, spatial ICA (sICA) and temporal ICA (tICA). These techniques are discussed in general terms, and the studies do not pertain to AD (or another specific neurological disorder) unless otherwise stated.

### 5.1. Spatial and Temporal ICA Models of fMRI

Makeig et al. [14] have first applied spatial instantaneous mixing ICA to the analysis of EEG data and event-related potential (ERP) data using the original Infomax algorithm [64]. Independently, Vigario et al. [77,78] have developed a method for artifact identification and noise removal from EEG and MEG through a FastICA algorithm [72].

Since then, ICA has become increasingly popular for analyzing biomedical data [14,74,75,79], especially for analysis of biomedical imaging, such as fMRI data [80]. A typical model for applying ICA to fMRI data, was introduced in a study [81] and provided a framework for understanding ICA as it applies to fMRI data and for introducing the various processing stages in ICA of fMRI data.

As an example, in the ICA processing of fMRI time series data by Calhoun et al, data was generated from a set of statistically independent (magnetic) hemodynamic source locations in the brain. These sources have weights that specify the contribution of each source plied by each source's hemodynamic time course [80,81]. The first stage of the data generation takes place within the brain, in which the sources are mixed. The second stage of data generation involves the fMRI scanner. The sources are sampled, and each represents a function of scan-specific MR parameters such as flip angle, slice thickness, pulse sequence, and field-of-view.

Data preprocessing consists of a number of possible preprocessing stages, including slice phase correction, motion correction, spatial normalization, and smoothing. After preprocessing, it is common to perform data reduction such as dimensionality-reductions using PCA or some other approach. The resultant estimated source, along with the unmixing matrix, can then be thresholded and presented as fMRI activation images and fMRI time courses, respectively [80,81].

Conventional ICA embodies the assumption that data can be decomposed into underlying sources that are independent over space (spatial) [79] or time (temporal) [14,82] and that the probability density functions (pdf) of these sources are highly kurtotic (distribution has heavy-tails) and symmetric [79,82,83]. Different assumptions can be made between sICA and tICA [82]; sICA seeks a set of mutually independent component (IC) source images and a corresponding (dual) set of unconstrained time courses [79]. By contrast, tICA seeks a set of IC source time courses and a corresponding (dual) set of unconstrained images [14]. In concrete fMRI data, sICA finds independent images and a corresponding set of dual unconstrained time courses and embodies the assumption that each image in $\mathbf{X}$ is composed of a linear combination of spatially and statistically independent images. Unlike sICA, tICA finds independent time courses and a corresponding set of dual unconstrained images and embodies the assumption that each eigensequence in $\mathbf{X}$ is a linear combination of temporally and statistically independent sequence $\mathbf{S}$ [83].

In addition, spatiotemporal ICA (stICA) [83] embodies the assumption that each eigenimage in $\boldsymbol{A}$ is a linear combination of spatially independent images, and each eigensequence in $\boldsymbol{S}$ is a linear combination of temporally independent sequences.

### 5.2. Variants of ICA Models for fMRI Data

Moreover, researchers have proposed many variants of ICA/BSS based on differently statistical characteristics [83,84] in fMRI data or on different purposes of analyzing fMRI data [15,85,86]. The variants include probabilistic ICA, skew-ICA, group ICA, tensor ICA, and cortex-based ICA.

***Probabilistic ICA***. To address the issues of what is attributable to the "real effects" of interest and what simply is due to observational noise, Beckmann et al. examined the probabilistic ICA (PICA) model [84,87] for fMRI data. PICA allows for a nonsquare mixing process and assumes that the data are confounded by additive Gaussian noise.

***Skew-ICA***. Stone et al. [83] combined spatiotemporal ICA and skew-ICA, to form skew-stICA to analyze synthetic data and data from an event-related, left-right visual hemifield fMRI experiment. Results [83] obtained with skew-stICA are superior to those of PCA, sICA, tICA, stICA, and skew-sICA. Here, skew-ICA is based on the assumption that images have skewed pdfs [88], an assumption consistent with spatially localized regions of activity. By contrast, conventional ICA is based on the physiologically unrealistic assumption that images have symmetric pdfs.

The skew-pdf can be described as:

$$p(y;a,b) \propto \exp\left(\frac{a-b}{2}y - \frac{a+b}{2}\sqrt{y^2+1}\right) \tag{2}$$

where the constants $a$ and $b$ define the skewness of the distribution.

***Group ICA***. ICA has been successfully utilized to analyze single-subject fMRI data sets and extended to group ICA for multi-subject analysis [15,85,86,89]. Group analysis of fMRI is important to study specific clinical and experimental conditions within or between groups of subjects [90].

Calhoun et al. [85] proposed a group ICA model that was a novel approach for drawing group inferences using ICA of fMRI data. The group ICA analysis revealed task-related components in the left and right visual cortex, a transiently task-related component in bilateral occipital/parietal cortex, and a non-task-related component in bilateral visual association cortex. The group ICA approach had been implemented in the Group ICA for fMRI data (GIFT) [91], in which PCA is used to whiten the data by performing an orthogonal transformation and to reduce the number of principal component present in the mixture.

Svensen et al. [86] used the extended ICA of fMRI data from single subjects to simultaneous analysis of data from a group of subjects. The results demonstrated that group ICA can extract nontrivial task-related components without any *a priori* information about the fMRI experiment and identify components common to the whole group in analysis of group data.

***Tensor ICA***. Beckmann et al. extended the single-session probabilistic ICA [84] to a higher dimension, called tensor PICA, to analyze multisubject or multisession fMRI data. The tensor PICA [15] is derived from parallel factor analysis (PARAFAC) [92] and has three-way, including temporal, spatial, and subject-dependent, variations. Real fMRI activation data was decomposed by the approach to extract plausible activation maps, time courses, and session/subject modes that give simple and useful representations of multisubject or multisession fMRI data.

***Cortex-based ICA***. Cortex-based ICA (cbICA) assumes that cortical data are different from non-cortical data and processes a subset of the data determined by *a priori* information [93]. Formisano et al. used the mesh of the white matter/gray matter boundary, automatically reconstructed from high-spatial-resolution anatomical MR images, to limit the sICA decomposition of a coregistered functional time series to those voxels that are within a specified region with respect to the cortical sheet.

Comparisons between cbICA and other methods showed that cortical surface maps and component time courses blindly obtained with cbICA reliably reflect task-related spatiotemporal activation patterns and that the cbICA improves the fitting of the ICA model in the gray matter voxels, the separation of cortical components, and the estimation of their time courses, particularly in the case of fMRI data sets with a complex spatiotemporal statistical structure.

## 6. ICA/BSS Applications to Brain Signal Processing for AD Diagnosis

In this section, we will present some problems associated with ICA/BSS applications to brain signal processing for AD diagnosis, such as why ICA/BSS is successful when applied to the diagnosis of AD, what are useful components and noises, how many components should be extracted, and which algorithms of ICA/BSS are most suitable. Applications of ICA to the development of machine learning models will also be discussed.

### 6.1. Why Apply ICA to Diagnosis of AD

The simplest and most robust technique for analyzing MRI brain scans is region-of-interest (ROI) analysis [94]. ROI [95,96] analysis of the brain structure is considered the gold standard against which new techniques are compared, but it has some drawbacks such as operator-dependency, being labor-consuming and time-intensive, and requiring *a priori* choice of regions to be investigated.

To overcome these shortcomings, another automated method of measuring brain atrophy has been developed [97–100]. The method of voxel-based morphometry (VBM) objectively maps gray matter loss on a voxel-by-voxel basis after anatomical standardization analogous to that used in functional neuroimaging. The advantage of VBM over analyses based on ROI analysis is that VBM produces an unbiased result from exploration of the whole brain. Testa et al. reported higher accuracy of discriminating AD and controls than ROI-based analysis [101]. One of these popular statistical tools based on the voxel is statistical parametric mapping (SPM) that refers to the construction and assessment of spatially extended statistical processes used to test hypotheses about functional imaging data (http://www.fil.ion.ucl.ac.uk/spm/, accessed on 29 March 2021). Statistical parametric mapping (SPM) [102], a univariate hypothesis-driven method, provides simple and computationally efficient approaches to produce maps of task-related activations with estimates of their levels of significance based on a statistical parameter of each voxel. However, it results in a loss of sensitivity if the fMRI experiment induces co-activation of spatially disparate areas with slightly different temporal behaviors.

Unlike univariate methods, multivariate data-driven techniques enable an exploratory analysis of fMRI datasets and may potentially separate meaningful activation by computing suitable statistical models independent of nay reference paradigm [103]. Furthermore, multivariate nature exploits the relationship between voxels and may possibly provide useful information about co-activation in spatially different areas of the brain. In general, multivariate analysis might have increased sensitivity compared to univariate analysis even when the disease-related changes in cerebral blood flow (CBF) originate in clearly circumscribed foci and spread spatially during the disease course. Multivariate analysis can detect these subtle, but robust changes, although univariate analysis might experience overly stringent false-positive corrections that tend to 'correct away' the true effects (as evidenced by the results of our voxel-wise analysis).

Habeck et al. reported that multivariate analysis might be more sensitive than univariate analysis for the early diagnosis of AD [44]. The multivariate techniques do not necessarily rely on underlying "networks" of pathology. Asllani et al. used multivariate approaches to evaluate correlation/covariance of CBF measurement across brain regions rather than proceeding on a region-by-region (or voxel-by-voxel) basis [104].

Among the multivariate data-driven techniques, ICA/BSS has been shown to provide a powerful method for the exploratory analysis of fMRI data [79,105–107]. ICA does not require the specification of temporal signal profiles or anatomical ROIs to generate meaningful spatiotemporal patterns of brain activity [108].

The multivariate statistical nature of ICA allows one to transform three-dimensional fMRI data sets into brain activity patterns starting from the spatial or temporal covariance of the measured signals and reveals multiple spatiotemporal 'modes' of signal variability [11]. This transformation is achieved by imposing the general, yet neurophysiologically plausible, constraint of removing the statistical dependence of the output modes [105]. To meet this constraint, the value distribution of the fMRI signals in space or time is to be considered: two variants called sICA and tICA. The former refers to the statistical distribution of signals across the sampled hemodynamic locations, while the latter refers to the statistical distribution of source signals across the sampled time-points [82].

### 6.2. Comparison of ICA/BSS Algorithms

As there are a variety of ICA algorithms, it is also important to compare their performance to better understand their strengths and limitations [108].

Correa et al. [91] had compared performances of five algorithms included in the toolbox GIFT: Informax [64], FastICA [67], Joint Approximate Diagonalization of Eigen Matrices (JADE) [109], Simultaneous Blind Extraction using Cumulants SIMBEC [110], and Algorithm for Multiple Unknown Signal Extraction (AMUSE) [4]. Based on their results of fMRI data, Informax emerged as a reliable choice for the task, followed by JADE as a close second. FastICA performed reliably for most cases as well whereas the performance of SMIBEC and AMUSE did not prove to be robust. SIMBEC may prove to be useful to identify sub-Gaussian sources. The performance of AMUSE is highly dependent on the differentiability of the spectra of the sources.

### 6.3. Spatial, Temporal, and Spatiotemporal ICA

ICA is a technique that attempts to separate data into maximally independent groups, achieving maximal independence in space or time to yield three varieties of ICA meaningful for fMRI applications: spatial ICA (sICA), temporal ICA (tICA), and spatiotemporal ICA.

Since the first application of ICA for fMRI analysis [105], it has been controversial to choose spatial or temporal independency. McKeown et al. argued on the sparsely distributed nature of the spatial pattern with sICA. The applications of temporal ICA to fMRI data have appeared [74,82]; however, spatial ICA has by far dominated the functional imaging literature to date. The most important reasons for this are that the spatial dimension is much larger than that of the temporal dimension in fMRI data [82].

Stone et al. proposed a method that attempts to maximize both spatial and temporal independence [83]. Seifritz et al. presented an interesting combination of sICA and tICA [111] and used an initial sICA to reduce the spatial dimensionality of the data by locating a ROI in which they then performed tICA to study in more detail the structure of the nontrivial temporal response in the human auditory cortex.

### 6.4. How Many Components Are There?

Before applying ICA/BSS to fMRI, characteristics of the independent components must be determined.

In general, fMRI data may be composed of signals of interest and signals not of interest (noises). Signals of interest include task-related, function-related, and transiently task-related signals [80]. Signals not of interest include physiology-related (breathing and heart rate), motion-related (mouth movement in the naming task), and scanner-related (scanner drift and system noise, susceptibility, and radio frequency artifacts) signals. In addition, there are several types of noise in an fMRI experiment, such as object variability, thermal noise, patient movement, brain movement, and so on. In the ICA model, these noises are often not explicitly modeled, but rather manifested as separate components [105,112].

Another problem is determining the number of components. Beckmann et al. and Calhoun et al. used different methods to estimate the number of components in fMRI data [87,113]. McKeown et al. [105] applied ICA to fMRI data and calculated the contribution of each component to fMRI data for extracting consistently task-related, transiently task-related, slowly varying, quasiperiodic, movement-related, and residual noise components. McKeown et al. also applied a combined PCA/ICA approach to estimate the number of spatially independent components contained in fMRI data [79]. Calhoun et al. used standard information theoretic methods for estimating the number of components from the aggregate data set [113]. The number of sources can be estimated using Akaike's information criterion or the minimum description length criterion [114,115].

### 6.5. Application of ICA/BSS to AD Diagnosis

Many applications of ICA/BSS to brain signal processing exist, such as removal artifact from EEG [14] and MEG [77,78], analysis of evoked magnetic fields [14,116,117], fMRI data [90], and in clinical research, for example the diagnosis of AD [118]. In this section, we will focus on application of ICA/BSS to the diagnosis of AD.

Chapman et al. [119] used PCA to identify and measure the ERP components. Their scores to relevant and irrelevant stimuli were used in discriminant analyses to develop functions that successfully classified individuals as belonging to an early-stage AD group or a like-aged control group, with probabilities of an individual belonging to each group. Additionally, 92% of the subjects were correctly classified into either the AD group or the control group with a sensitivity of 1.0. Besthorn et al. [120] used PCA as a postprocessing tool for compressing linear and nonlinear EEG features over channels. They obtained 95.9% correct classification using age as a moderator variable in the study.

A number of EEG studies [4,121] on AD and MCI have reported several typical findings such as a slowing and diffusing of the posterior dominant alpha activity, an unclear alpha attenuation after eye-opening, as well as an increase of delta and theta, and a decrease of beta and gamma activities [5]. For more details, see a review of signal processing techniques applied for revealing pathological changes in EEG associated with AD [5]. Cichocki et al. investigated the application of ICA/BSS methods as preprocessing tools with possible application for AD diagnosis. They propose an approach of filtering EEG data based on ICA/BSS that can significantly improve the sensitivity and specificity of EEG-based diagnosis of AD at the early stage [4]. The team employed a non-ICA based method of BSS: the algorithm for multiple unknown signals extraction (AMUSE [122]), on data from MCI patients who progressed to AD and age matched controls, achieving a classification rate of 80% for MCI based on linear discriminant analysis (LDA) [4].

Vialatte et al. explored the group differences between Mild AD patients and control subjects, finding that precleaning data with ICA using the improved weight-adjusted second-order blind identification (IWASOBI) algorithm amplified the differences between the groups [123]. Melissant et al. used ICA to reduce artifacts of EEG data to improve classification results for patients in an initial stage [121]. They made a conclusion that a more robust detection of AD-related EEG patterns may be obtained by employing ICA as ICA-based preprocessing of EEG data can improve classification results for AD patients in an initial stage. Jervis et al. applied ICA and cluster analysis to EEG P300 data obtained from healthy and AD subjects [27] showed that the latencies of the back-projected independent components (BICs) of the P300 differed between healthy participants and AD patients. They proposed that the latencies of the BIC associated with the P3b component may be a suitable biomarker for AD.

Escudero et al. [124] analyzed MEG background activity recordings acquired with a 148-channel whole-head magnetometer from 21 AD patients and 21 control subjects using the algorithm for multiple unknown signals extraction (AMUSE [4]) to blindly decompose artifact-free epochs of 20s. Their preliminary results showed that the proposed procedure based on BSS and selection of significant components may improve the classification of AD patients using straightforward features from MEG recordings. Fernandez et al. [125] applied PCA to the mean frequency from the MEG signals of 22 patients with AD, 22 patients with MCI, and 21 healthy controls. Results demonstrated the mean frequency score seem to be adequate and sensitive to detect differences between normal aging, cognitive deterioration, and AD.

Higdon et al. [9] applied PCA to FDG-PET for the diagnosis of AD from frontotemporal dementia and reported slightly better results with images preprocessed with principal least squares analysis than with PCA when using a classifier based on linear discriminant analysis Habeck et al. [44] examined the efficacy of multivariate and univariate analytic methods for the diagnosis of early AD. Using the extended PCA-approach to the FDG-PET data from two clinical populations, they analyzed the spatially correlated metabolism as a function of AD status and reported that the multivariate marker's diagnostic performance in the replication samples was superior to that of the univariate marker's. Kerrouche et al. first applied a novel voxel-based multivariate technique, such as PCA, to a large FDG-PET data set to investigate whether it is possible to distinguish vascular dementia from AD. They used PCA to remove PCs significantly correlated to age. Their results show the potential of voxel-based multivariate methods to highlight independent functional networks in dementing disease. By maximizing the separation between groups, this method extracted a metabolic pattern that efficiently differentiated vascular dementia and AD [126].

Chen et al. proposed a simple and automated method for the measurement of changes in brain volume from an individual's sequential MRIs using an iterative PCA (IPCA) [127]. The IPCA considered the voxel intensity pairs from coregistered MRIs and identified those pairs a sufficiently large distance away from the iteratively determined PCA major axis. Their results demonstrated IPCA's ability to characterize whole-brain atrophy rates in patients with AD [127,128].

Su et al. [12] presented the Hybrid wavelet-ICA to investigate the use of ICA dynamic PET data both in the image domain and in the wavelet domain, where the data had been transformed using Battle-Lemarie wavelets, as in the article [129].

Greicius et al. adapted ICA to derive the default-mode network [130,131] in a more data-driven fashion (i.e., without requiring a priori specification of a seed region). Examination of the default-mode network in these groups revealed three critical findings: a significant coactivation of the hippocampus in the default-mode network, the network is abnormal in the mildest stages of AD compared to healthy aging, and network activity holds potential as a non-invasive biomarker of incipient AD [131].

By using resting-state fMRI and combining correlation and ICA, Tang [132] explored a new method for resting-state functional connectivity [133,134] that was finally applied to seek the abnormality of the brain functional network under the pathophysiology of AD.

Celone et al. [118] used ICA to investigate memory-related fMRI activity in 52 individuals across the continuum of normal aging, MCI, and mild AD. Memory function is likely subserved by multiple distributed neural networks that are disrupted by the pathophysiological processes of AD. ICA revealed specific memory-related networks that activated or deactivated during an associative memory paradigm. Across all subjects, hippocampal activation and parietal deactivation demonstrated a strong reciprocal relationship. Less impaired MCI subjects showed paradoxical hyperactivation in the hippocampus compared with controls, whereas more impaired MCI subjects demonstrated significant hypoactivation, similar to the levels observed in the mild AD subjects.

Sorg et al. combined ICA and ROI-based correlation methods to investigate resting-state networks (RSNs) in patients with MCI [90]. They analyzed fMRI and structural MRI data from healthy elderly and patients with amnestic MCI, a syndrome of high risk for developing AD and concluded that, in individuals at risk for AD, a specific subset of RSNs is altered.

Rombouts et al. applied tensor PICA [15] to study fMRI signal during face encoding in 18 AD, 28 MCI patients, and 41 healthy elderly controls [135]. The tensor PICA showed activation in regions associated with motor, visual, and cognitive processing, and deactivation in the default mode network. They concluded that the tensor PICA is a promising tool to identify and detect differences in (de)activated brain networks in elderly controls and dementia patients.

### 6.6. *ICA as a Component of Machine Learning Models*

Computer aided diagnosis (CAD) is poised to be a considerable tool for identifying cases of Alzheimer's disease and a host of other diseases. CAD typically involves the application of a machine learning (ML) model onto features derived from neuroimaging, biomarkers, and others. ML can be used in tandem with expert review; in cases of MRI and other image analysis, for example, a ML model can ascertain details and features that are difficult for a human to identify by eye. Support vector machines, as well as other model types such as decision trees and neural networks have been developed to diagnose Alzheimer's disease based on MRI, PET, and other imaging methods with high accuracy [136–141]. Models have also been effective when trained on EEG feature data as well [142–146].

ICA, which can be used for signal separation and feature extraction, can be implemented as a component of a machine learning-based diagnostic system. ICA can be employed to initially extract and transform features of a dataset, which can then be fed into a machine learning model. Such systems have been shown to be more effective that direct ML in problems such as facial recognition [147] and classification based on microarray data [148].

Such methods can be similarly applied to applications of brain health and imaging. Artificial neural networks and support vector machines (SVMs) working with data preprocessed with ICA have been found to detect artifacts in EEGs with an accuracy/alignments between 89.13% and 95.20% compared to expert rating [149]. The non-ICA based algorithm AMUSE was used y Vialatte et al., to process data for input for sparse-bump modeling, which was fed into a neural network geared towards the classification of MCI cases (that later progressed to AD), achieving a 93% classifier rate [150], an improvement from the aforementioned LDA with an 80% implemented by the team [4]. Data suggests that perhaps ICA based methods are superior to some standard BSS methods for artifact removal. Cassani et al. tested statistical artifact rejection (SAR), blind source separation based on second order blind identification and canonical correlation analysis (BSS–SOBI–CCA), and wavelet-enhanced independent component analysis; the removal of artifacts by experts was also assessed as a standard. The resulting features were used to train an SVM based classifier. The ICA-model performed comparably to the standard in discriminating normal and mild AD, and slightly better than the standard in discriminating mild and moderate AD. BSS was generally inferior to ICA and SAR, possibly due to the removal of discriminatory data [151]. Other specific analyses of brain development and health have been examined with similar combined-methods [152–156].

With regard to Alzheimer's disease, CAD systems incorporating ICA-processed into a machine learning model have been developed with some success. Khedher et al. developed a SVM based CAD system trained with MRI data from the Alzheimer's disease neuroimaging initiative (ADNI) that was able to distinguish between cognitively normal individuals and those with MCI or AD that notably featured graphical representations of the input features that makes the basis of the system's decision making more clear. The system had 79% accuracy distinguishing MCI from NC, 89% accuracy distinguishing AD from normal controls (NC), and 85% accuracy distinguishing MCI from AD cases [157].

Yang et al. applied similar methods to data from open access MRI datasets such as the ADNI; features processed and extracted with FastICA [158] were applied to a SVM classifier. Applying the system to grey-matter only images achieved an accuracy of approximately 89% when distinguishing between NC and AD subjects, and 81% between NC and MCI subjects at a 90–10 training/testing split; whole-brain image performance was notably lower [159]. A later 2017 model by Yang et al., using two stage component number estimation and ICA combined with clinical features used as inputs for a SVM, achieved an accuracy of 97.7% and 87.8% in distinguishing AD and MCI from NC, respectively [160].

Qiao et al., developed a three-level hierarchical partner matching ICA method; functional MRI data was first processed with spatial ICA and group-mapping of IC groups, followed by partner matching group-map clusters and cluster-map generation, then partner mapping of cluster-maps. Tracing the optimal clusters derived from the cluster-maps backwards indicates the most stable ICs. Inputs were fed into a directed acyclic graph neural network incorporating convolutional layers; an accuracy of 95.59% was achieved in leave-one-out cross validation [161].

Basheera et al. used MRI grey matter images segmented with hybrid enhanced independent component analysis applied to a convolutional neural network. Training was done with ADNI image data and, on a sample of 21 independent MRI slices, the output of the network was compared to the decision of a physician, and an accuracy of 90.47% was achieved [162].

Other imaging methods beyond MRI have been used as well. Illán et al. conducted a comparison of SVM based CAD systems based on voxels-as-features, principal component analysis, and ICA processing on SPECT images. Models based on samples with NC and AD patients either grouped (method 1) or split into 3 subgroups based on disease severity/characteristics (method 2) were tested. Accuracies of PCA and ICA were similar for both method 1 (88.61% and 89.87%, respectively) and method 2 (88.61% and 91.14%, respectively) and both were greater than the VAF baseline (72.15% and 74.68% for method 1 and method 2, respectively) [136]. Toussaint et al. utilized spatial ICA of fluoro-deoxygenase (FDG) PET images, combined with other clinical features such as cognitive test scores. Good accuracies were noted in leave-one-out cross validation distinguishing NC from preclinical AD, but lower when attempting to distinguish between stable and converting MCI [163].

## 7. Conclusions

AD is a progressive neurodegenerative disorder and the most common cause of dementia associated with aging. The diagnosis of AD remains largely based upon clinical assessment, and is often made at relatively late stages of the pathophysiological process. As disease-modifying therapies are likely to be most efficacious at much earlier stages of the disease, it is important to develop markers for early disease detection in individuals who are at risk for AD. Fortunately, some biomedical techniques such as EEG, CT, PET, MRI, and fMRI, can non-invasively acquire brain signals to aid in a more objective assessment of AD pathology, even when AD is at an early stage. As mentioned above, we have introduced the applications of these biomedical techniques as potential AD diagnostic tools.

The brain signals sampled from individuals using these biomedical techniques are the mixture of many signals of interest or non-interest; collectively, AD-related signals or noises serve different purposes for analysis. A key challenge is to acquire useful AD-related signals and to discover biomarkers from the sampled brain signals. To address this challenge, many novel signal processing techniques have been developed. In this paper, we focused on reviewing applications of ICA/BSS approaches to the diagnosis of AD.

ICA/BSS is one of the data-driven, multivariate, and unsupervised methods without any *a priori* information. The quite fruitful applications of ICA/BSS to brain signals have shown that such technique is very useful and powerful. Its ability to represent the high-dimensional data, especially MRI or fMRI data, enables it to be a powerful tool for clinical AD neuroimaging biomarker discovery.

**Author Contributions:** Conceptualization, W.Y. and X.H.; methodology, W.Y.; investigation, W.Y.; resources, X.H.; writing—original draft preparation, W.Y.; writing—review and editing, A.P. and X.H.; supervision, X.H.; project administration, X.H.; funding acquisition, X.H. All authors have read and agreed to the published version of the manuscript.

**Funding:** This research was partially funded by NIH/NIA, grant number R01AG056614 (to X.H.).

**Institutional Review Board Statement:** Not applicable.

**Informed Consent Statement:** Not applicable.

**Data Availability Statement:** Not applicable.

**Acknowledgments:** W.Y. would like to express his gratitude for the supports from the Shanghai Maritime University. We thank Kimberly Lawson and Reisa Sperling for their wonderful editing of our manuscript.

**Conflicts of Interest:** The authors declare no conflict of interest.

## References

1. Holroyd, S.; Shepherd, M.L. Alzheimer's disease: A review for the ophthalmologist. *Surv. Ophthalmol.* **2001**, *45*, 516–524. [CrossRef]
2. Hendrie, H.C. Epidemiology of dementia and Alzheimer's disease. *Am. J. Geriatr. Psychiatry* **1998**, *6*, S3–S18. [CrossRef]
3. Alzheimer's Association. Alzheimer's Disease Facts and Figures. *Alzheimer's Dement* **2020**, *16*, 391–460.
4. Cichocki, A.; Shishkin, S.L.; Musha, T.; Leonowicz, Z.; Asada, T.; Kurachi, T. EEG filtering based on blind source separation (BSS) for early detection of Alzheimer's disease. *Clin. Neurophysiol.* **2005**, *116*, 729–737. [CrossRef] [PubMed]
5. Jeong, J.S. EEG dynamics in patients with Alzheimer's disease. *Clin. Neurophysiol.* **2004**, *115*, 1490–1505. [CrossRef]
6. Babiloni, C.; Babiloni, F.; Carducci, F.; Cincotti, F.; Eusebi, F.; Ferri, R.; Miniussi, C.; Moretti, D.V.; Nobili, F.; Pasqualetti, P.; et al. Quantitative EEG/MEG analysis for objective assessment of Alzheimer disease: The project "Alzheimer database on-line". *Neuroimage* **2001**, *13*, S770. [CrossRef]
7. deLeon, M.J.; George, A.E.; Golomb, J.; Tarshish, C.; Convit, A.; Kluger, A.; DeSanti, S.; McRae, T.; Ferris, S.H.; Reisberg, B.; et al. Frequency of hippocampal formation atrophy in normal aging and Alzheimer's disease. *Neurobiol. Aging* **1997**, *18*, 1–11. [CrossRef]
8. Cohen, C.I.; Strashun, A.; Ortega, C.; Horn, L.; Magai, C. The effects of poverty and education on temporoparietal perfusion in Alzheimer's disease: A reconsideration of the cerebral reserve hypothesis. *Int. J. Geriatr. Psychiatry* **1996**, *11*, 1105–1110. [CrossRef]
9. Higdon, R.; Foster, N.L.; Koeppe, R.A.; DeCarli, C.S.; Jagust, W.J.; Clark, C.M.; Barbas, N.R.; Arnold, S.E.; Turner, R.S.; Heidebrink, J.L.; et al. A comparison of classification methods for differentiating fronto-temporal dementia from Alzheimer's disease using FDG-PET imaging. *Stat. Med.* **2004**, *23*, 315–326. [CrossRef]
10. De Santi, S.; de Leon, M.J.; Rusinek, H.; Convit, A.; Tarshish, C.Y.; Roche, A.; Tsui, W.H.; Kandil, E.; Boppana, M.; Daisley, K.; et al. Hippocampal formation glucose metabolism and volume losses in MCI and AD. *Neurobiol. Aging* **2001**, *22*, 529–539. [CrossRef]
11. Friston, K.J. Modes or models: A critique on independent component analysis for fMRI. *Trends Cogn. Sci.* **1998**, *2*, 373–375. [CrossRef]
12. Su, H.R.; Aston, J.A.D.; Lion, M.; Cheng, P.E. A hybrid wavelet-ICA model for dynamic PET analysis. *Neuroimage* **2006**, *31*, T67–T68. [CrossRef]

13. Marcie, P.; Roudier, M.; Goldblum, M.-C.; Boller, F. Principal component analysis of language performances in Alzheimer's disease. *J. Commun. Disord.* **1993**, *26*, 53–63. [CrossRef]
14. Makeig, S.; Jung, T.P.; Bell, A.J.; Ghahremani, D.; Sejnowski, T.J. Blind separation of auditory event-related brain responses into independent components. *Proc. Natl. Acad. Sci. USA* **1997**, *94*, 10979–10984. [CrossRef]
15. Beckmann, C.F.; Smith, S.M. Tensorial extensions of independent component analysis for multisubject FMRI analysis. *Neuroimage* **2005**, *25*, 294–311. [CrossRef] [PubMed]
16. Katz, B.; Rimmer, S. Ophthalmologic manifestations of alzheimers-disease. *Surv. Ophthalmol.* **1989**, *34*, 31–43. [CrossRef]
17. Masters, C.L.; Beyreuther, K. Molecular neuropathology of alzheimers-disease. *Arzneim. Forsch. Drug Res.* **1995**, *45*, 410–412.
18. Gomez-ISLA, T.; Spires, T.; De Calignon, A.; Hyman, B.T. Neuropathology of Alzheimer's Disease. *Hankbook Clin. Neurol. Dement.* **2008**, *89*, 234–243.
19. Cogan, D.G. Visual disturbances with focal progressive dementing disease. *Am. J. Ophthalmol.* **1985**, *100*, 68–72. [CrossRef]
20. Cogan, D.G. Alzheimer syndromes. *Am. J. Ophthalmol.* **1987**, *104*, 183–184.
21. Sadum, A.A.; Bassi, C.J. The visual system in Alzheimer's disease. *Res. Publ. Assoc Res. Nerv. Ment. Dis.* **1990**, *67*, 331–347.
22. Mendez, M.F.; Mendez, M.A.; Martin, R.; Smyth, K.A.; Whitehouse, P.J. Complex visual disturbances in alzheimers-disease. *Neurology* **1990**, *40*, 439–443. [CrossRef]
23. Croningolomb, A.; Rizzo, J.F.; Corkin, S.; Growdon, J.H. Visual function in alzheimers-disease and normal aging. *Aging Alzheimers Dis.* **1991**, *640*, 28–35.
24. Rizzo, J.F.; Croningolomb, A.; Growdon, J.H.; Corkin, S.; Rosen, T.J.; Sandberg, M.A.; Chiappa, K.H.; Lessell, S. Retinocalcarine function in alzheimers-disease—A clinical and electrophysiological study. *Arch. Neurol.* **1992**, *49*, 93–101. [CrossRef]
25. Fox, M.D.; Raichle, M.E. Spontaneous fluctuations in brain activity observed with functional magnetic resonance imaging. *Nat. Rev. Neurosci.* **2007**, *8*, 700–711. [CrossRef] [PubMed]
26. Adeli, H.; Ghosh-Dastidar, S.; Dadmehr, N. Alzheimer's disease: Models of computation and analysis of EEGs. *Clin. Eeg Neurosci.* **2005**, *36*, 131–140. [CrossRef]
27. Jervis, B.; Belal, S.; Camilleri, K.; Cassar, T.; Bigan, C.; Linden, D.E.; Michalopoulos, K.; Zervakis, M.; Besleaga, M.; Fabri, S.; et al. The independent components of auditory P300 and CNV evoked potentials derived from single-trial recordings. *Physiol. Meas.* **2007**, *28*, 745–771. [CrossRef] [PubMed]
28. Cassani, R.; Estarellas, M.; San-Martin, R.; Fraga, F.J.; Falk, T.H. Systematic review on resting-state EEG for Alzheimer's disease diagnosis and progression assessment. *Dis. Markers* **2018**, *2018*. [CrossRef] [PubMed]
29. Horvath, A.; Szucs, A.; Csukly, G.; Sakovics, A.; Stefanics, G.; Kamondi, A. EEG and ERP biomarkers of Alzheimer's disease: A critical review. *Front. Biosci. (Landmark Ed.)* **2018**, *23*, 183–220. [CrossRef] [PubMed]
30. Kurimoto, R.; Ishii, R.; Canuet, L.; Ikezawa, K.; Azechi, M.; Iwase, M.; Yoshida, T.; Kazui, H.; Yoshimine, T.; Takeda, M. Event-related synchronization of alpha activity in early Alzheimer's disease and mild cognitive impairment: An MEG study combining beamformer and group comparison. *Neurosci. Lett.* **2008**, *443*, 86–89. [CrossRef]
31. Osipova, D.; Rantanen, K.; Ahveninen, J.; Ylikoski, R.; Happola, O.; Strandberg, T.; Pekkonen, E. Source estimation of spontaneous MEG oscillations in mild cognitive impairment. *Neurosci. Lett.* **2006**, *405*, 57–61. [CrossRef]
32. Fernandez, A.; Hornero, R.; Mayo, A.; Poza, J.; Maestu, F.; Ortiz Alonso, T. Quantitative magnetoencephalography of spontaneous brain activity in Alzheimer disease: An exhaustive frequency analysis. *Alzheimer Dis. Assoc. Disord.* **2006**, *20*, 153–159. [CrossRef] [PubMed]
33. Maestu, F.; Garcia-Segura, J.; Ortiz, T.; Montoya, J.; Fernandez, A.; Gil-Gregorio, P.; Campo, P.; Fernandez, S.; Viano, J.; Portera, A. Evidence of biochemical and biomagnetic interactions in Alzheimer's disease: An MEG and MR spectroscopy study. *Dement Geriatr. Cogn. Disord.* **2005**, *20*, 145–152. [CrossRef] [PubMed]
34. Maestu, F.; Arrazola, J.; Fernandez, A.; Simos, P.G.; Amo, C.; Gil-Gregorio, P.; Fernandez, S.; Papanicolaou, A.; Ortiz, T. Do cognitive patterns of brain magnetic activity correlate with hippocampal atrophy in Alzheimer's disease? *J. Neurol. Neurosurg. Psychiatry* **2003**, *74*, 208–212. [CrossRef]
35. Fernandez, A.; Maestu, F.; Amo, C.; Gil, P.; Fehr, T.; Wienbruch, C.; Rockstroh, B.; Elbert, T.; Ortiz, T. Focal temporoparietal slow activity in Alzheimer's disease revealed by magnetoencephalography. *Biol. Psychiatry* **2002**, *52*, 764–770. [CrossRef]
36. Stam, C.J.; van Walsum, A.M.V.; Pijnenburg, Y.A.L.; Berendse, H.W.; de Munck, J.C.; Scheltens, P.; van Dijk, B.W. Generalized synchronization of MEG recordings in Alzheimer's disease: Evidence for involvement of the gamma band. *J. Clin. Neurophysiol.* **2002**, *19*, 562–574. [CrossRef]
37. van Cappellen van Walsum, A.M.; Pijnenburg, Y.A.L.; Berendse, H.W.; van Dijk, B.W.; Knol, D.L.; Scheltens, P.; Stam, C.J. A neural complexity measure applied to MEG data in Alzheimer's disease. *Clin. Neurophysiol.* **2003**, *114*, 1034–1040. [CrossRef]
38. Azami, H.; Escudero, J.; Fernández, A. Refined composite multivariate multiscale entropy based on variance for analysis of resting-state magnetoencephalograms in Alzheimer's disease. In Proceedings of the 2016 International Conference for Students on Applied Engineering (ICSAE), Newcastle upon Tyne, UK, 10–21 October 2016; pp. 413–418.
39. Escudero, J.; Acar, E.; Fernández, A.; Bro, R. Multiscale entropy analysis of resting-state magnetoencephalogram with tensor factorisations in Alzheimer's disease. *Brain Res. Bull.* **2015**, *119*, 136–144. [CrossRef]

40. Gómez, C.; Poza, J.; Monge, J.; Fernández, A.; Hornero, R. Analysis of magnetoencephalography recordings from Alzheimer's disease patients using embedding entropies. In Proceedings of the 2014 36th Annual International Conference of the IEEE Engineering in Medicine and Biology Society, Chicago, IL, USA, 26–30 August 2014; pp. 702–705.
41. Bruña, R.; Poza, J.; Gomez, C.; Garcia, M.; Fernandez, A.; Hornero, R. Analysis of spontaneous MEG activity in mild cognitive impairment and Alzheimer's disease using spectral entropies and statistical complexity measures. *J. Neural Eng.* **2012**, *9*, 036007. [CrossRef]
42. Gómez, C.; Hornero, R. Entropy and complexity analyses in Alzheimer's disease: An MEG study. *Open Biomed. Eng. J.* **2010**, *4*, 223. [CrossRef]
43. Poza, J.; Gómez, C.; Bachiller, A.; Hornero, R. Spectral and non-linear analyses of spontaneous magnetoencephalographic activity in Alzheimer's disease. *J. Healthc. Eng.* **2012**, *3*, 299–322. [CrossRef]
44. Habeck, C.; Foster, N.L.; Perneczky, R.; Kurz, A.; Alexopoulos, P.; Koeppe, R.A.; Drzezga, A.; Stern, Y. Multivariate and univariate neuroimaging biomarkers of Alzheimer's disease. *Neuroimage* **2008**, *40*, 1503–1515. [CrossRef] [PubMed]
45. Minoshima, S.; Giordani, B.; Berent, S.; Frey, K.A.; Foster, N.L.; Kuhl, D.E. Metabolic reduction in the posterior cingulate cortex in very early Alzheimer's disease. *Ann. Neurol.* **1997**, *42*, 85–94. [CrossRef] [PubMed]
46. Matsuda, H. Cerebral blood flow and metabolic abnormalities in Alzheimer's disease. *Ann. Nucl. Med.* **2001**, *15*, 85–92. [CrossRef] [PubMed]
47. Fukai, M.; Hirosawa, T.; Kikuchi, M.; Hino, S.; Kitamura, T.; Ouchi, Y.; Yokokura, M.; Yoshikawa, E.; Bunai, T.; Minabe, Y. Different Patterns of Glucose Hypometabolism Underlie Functional Decline in Frontotemporal Dementia and Alzheimer's Disease: FDG-PET Study. *Neuropsychiatry* **2018**, *8*, 441–447. [CrossRef]
48. Maclin, J.M.A.; Wang, T.; Xiao, S. Biomarkers for the diagnosis of Alzheimer's disease, dementia Lewy body, frontotemporal dementia and vascular dementia. *Gen. Psychiatry* **2019**, *32*, e100054. [CrossRef]
49. Craig-Schapiro, R.; Fagan, A.M.; Holtzman, D.M. Biomarkers of Alzheimer's disease. *Neurobiol. Dis.* **2008**, in press, Corrected. Available online: https://www.ncbi.nlm.nih.gov/pmc/articles/PMC2747727/ (accessed on 28 October 2008).
50. Messa, C.; Perani, D.; Lucignani, G.; Zenorini, A.; Zito, F.; Rizzo, G.; Grassi, F.; Delsole, A.; Franceschi, M.; Gilardi, M.C.; et al. High-resolution technetium-99m-hmpao spect in patients with probable alzheimers-disease—comparison with fluorine-18-FDG PET. *J. Nucl. Med.* **1994**, *35*, 210–216.
51. Klunk, W.E.; Engler, H.; Nordberg, A.; Wang, Y.M.; Blomqvist, G.; Holt, D.P.; Bergstrom, M.; Savitcheva, I.; Huang, G.F.; Estrada, S.; et al. Imaging brain amyloid in Alzheimer's disease with Pittsburgh Compound-B. *Ann. Neurol.* **2004**, *55*, 306–319. [CrossRef]
52. Johnson, K.A.; Gregas, M.; Becker, J.A.; Kinnecom, C.; Salat, D.H.; Moran, E.K.; Smith, E.E.; Rosand, J.; Rentz, D.M.; Klunk, W.E.; et al. Imaging of amyloid burden and distribution in cerebral amyloid angiopathy. *Ann. Neurol.* **2007**, *62*, 229–234. [CrossRef]
53. Kwong, K.K.; Belliveau, J.W.; Chesler, D.A.; Goldberg, I.E.; Weisskoff, R.M.; Poncelet, B.P.; Kennedy, D.N.; Hoppel, B.E.; Cohen, M.S.; Turner, R.; et al. Dynamic magnetic-resonance-imaging of human brain activity during primary sensory stimulation. *Proc. Natl. Acad. Sci. USA* **1992**, *89*, 5675–5679. [CrossRef]
54. Pekar, J.J. A brief introduction to functional MRI—History and today's developments. *IEEE Eng. Med. Biol. Mag.* **2006**, *25*, 24–26. [CrossRef] [PubMed]
55. Frisoni, G.B. Structural imaging in the clinical diagnosis of Alzheimer's disease: Problems and tools. *J. Neurol. Neurosurg. Psychiatry* **2001**, *70*, 711–718. [CrossRef] [PubMed]
56. Hampel, H.; Teipel, S.J.; Alexander, G.E.; Pogarell, O.; Rapoport, S.I.; Moller, H.J. In vivo imaging of region and cell type specific neocortical neurodegeneration in Alzheimer's disease—Perspectives of MRI derived corpus callosum measurement for mapping disease progression and effects of therapy. Evidence from studies with MRI, EEG and PET. *J. Neural Transm.* **2002**, *109*, 837–855. [PubMed]
57. Josephs, K.A.; Whitwell, J.L.; Dickson, D.W.; Boeve, B.F.; Knopman, D.S.; Petersen, R.C.; Parisi, J.E.; Jack, C.R. Voxel-based morphometry in autopsy proven PSP and CBD. *Neurobiol. Aging* **2008**, *29*, 280–289. [CrossRef] [PubMed]
58. Silva, A.C.; Koretsky, A.P. Laminar specificity of functional MRI onset times during somatosensory stimulation in rat. *Proc. Natl. Acad. Sci. USA* **2002**, *99*, 15182–15187. [CrossRef] [PubMed]
59. Ogawa, S.; Menon, R.S.; Tank, D.W.; Kim, S.G.; Merkle, H.; Ellermann, J.M.; Ugurbil, K. Functional brain mapping by blood oxygenation level-dependent contrast magnetic-resonance-imaging—A comparison of signal characteristics with a biophysical model. *Biophys. J.* **1993**, *64*, 803–812. [CrossRef]
60. Bandettini, P.A.; Jesmanowicz, A.; Wong, E.C.; Hyde, J.S. Processing strategies for time-course data sets in functional mri of the human brain. *Magn. Reson. Med.* **1993**, *30*, 161–173. [CrossRef]
61. Jain, S.N.; Rai, C. Blind source separation and ICA techniques: A review. *Int. J. Eng. Sci. Technol.* **2012**, *4*, 1490–1503.
62. Comon, P.; Jutten, C. *Handbook of Blind Source Separation: Independent Component Analysis and Applications*; Academic Press: Cambridge, MA, USA, 2010.
63. Jolliffe, I.T. *Principal Component Analysis*; Springer: New York, NY, USA, 1986.
64. Bell, A.J.; Sejnowski, T.J. An information maximization approach to blind separation and blind deconvolution. *Neural Comput.* **1995**, *7*, 1129–1159. [CrossRef]
65. Jutten, C.; Herault, J. Independent Component Analysis versus pca. *Proc. Eusipco* **1988**, 643–648.
66. Cardoso, J.F. Blind signal separation: Statistical principles. *Proc. IEEE* **1998**, *86*, 2009–2025. [CrossRef]

67. Hyvarinen, A. The fixed-point algorithm and maximum likelihood estimation for independent component analysis. *Neural Process. Lett.* **1999**, *10*, 1–5. [CrossRef]
68. Lee, T.W.; Girolami, M.; Bell, A.J.; Sejnowski, T.J. A unifying information-theoretic framework for independent component analysis. *Comput. Math. Appl.* **2000**, *39*, 1–21. [CrossRef]
69. Jutten, C.; Taleb, A. Source separation: From dusk till dawn. In Proceedings of the International Workshop on Independent Component Analysis and Blind Signal Separation—ICA2000, Helsinki, Finland, 19–22 June 2000; pp. 15–26.
70. Comon, P. Independent component analysis, a new concept. *Signal Process.* **1994**, *36*, 287–314. [CrossRef]
71. Amari, S. Natural gradient learning for over- and under-complete bases in ICA. *Neural Comput.* **1999**, *11*, 1875–1883. [CrossRef]
72. Hyvarinen, A.; Oja, E. A fast fixed-point algorithm for independent component analysis. *Neural Comput.* **1997**, *9*, 1483–1492. [CrossRef]
73. Hyvarinen, A. Survey on independent component analysis. *Neural Comput. Surv.* **1999**, *2*, 94–128.
74. Biswal, B.B.; Ulmer, J.L. Blind source separation of multiple signal sources of fMRI data sets using independent component analysis. *J. Comput. Assist. Tomogr.* **1999**, *23*, 265–271. [CrossRef]
75. McKeown, M.J. Detection of consistently task-related activations in fMRI data with hybrid independent component analysis. *Neuroimage* **2000**, *11*, 24–35. [CrossRef] [PubMed]
76. Porrill, J.; Stone, J.V.; Berwick, J.; Mayhew, J.; Coffey, P. Analysis of optical imaging data using weak models and ica. In *Perspectives in Neural Computing*; Springer: New York, NY, USA, 2000; pp. 233–317.
77. Vigario, R.; Sarela, J.; Jousmaki, V.; Hamalainen, M.; Oja, E. Independent component approach to the analysis of EEG and MEG recordings. *IEEE Trans. Biomed. Eng.* **2000**, *47*, 589–593. [CrossRef] [PubMed]
78. Vigario, R.N. Extraction of ocular artefacts from EEG using independent component analysis. *Electroencephalogr. Clin. Neurophysiol.* **1997**, *103*, 395–404. [CrossRef]
79. McKeown, M.J.; Sejnowski, T.J. Independent component analysis of fMRI data: Examining the assumptions. *Hum. Brain Mapp.* **1998**, *6*, 368–372. [CrossRef]
80. Calhoun, V.D.; Adali, T. Unmixing fMRI with independent component analysis—Using ICA to characterize high-dimensional fMRI data in a concise manner. *IEEE Eng. Med. Biol. Mag.* **2006**, *25*, 79–90. [CrossRef]
81. Calhoun, V.; Pearlson, G.; Adali, T. Independent component analysis applied to fMRI data: A generative model for validating results. *J. Vlsi Signal Process. Syst. Signal Image Video Technol.* **2004**, *37*, 281–291. [CrossRef]
82. Calhoun, V.D.; Adali, T.; Pearlson, G.D.; Pekar, J.J. Spatial and temporal independent component analysis of functional MRI data containing a pair of task-related waveforms. *Hum. Brain Mapp.* **2001**, *13*, 43–53. [CrossRef] [PubMed]
83. Stone, J.V.; Porrill, J.; Porter, N.R.; Wilkinson, I.D. Spatiotemporal independent component analysis of event-related fMRI data using skewed probability density functions. *Neuroimage* **2002**, *15*, 407–421. [CrossRef] [PubMed]
84. Beckmann, C.F.; Smith, S.A. Probabilistic independent component analysis for functional magnetic resonance imaging. *IEEE Trans. Med Imaging* **2004**, *23*, 137–152. [CrossRef] [PubMed]
85. Calhoun, V.D.; Adali, T.; Pearlson, G.D.; Pekar, J.J. A method for making group inferences from functional MRI data using independent component analysis. *Hum. Brain Mapp.* **2001**, *14*, 140–151. [CrossRef] [PubMed]
86. Svensen, M.; Kruggel, F.; Benali, H. ICA of fMRI group study data. *Neuroimage* **2002**, *16*, 551–563. [CrossRef] [PubMed]
87. Beckmann, C.F.; Noble, J.A.; Smith, S.M. Investigating the intrinsic dimensionality of FMRI data for ICA. *Neuroimage* **2001**, *13*, S76. [CrossRef]
88. Suzuki, K.; Kiryu, T.; Nakada, T. Fast and precise independent component analysis for high field fMRI time series tailored using prior information on spatiotemporal structure. *Hum. Brain Mapp.* **2002**, *15*, 54–66. [CrossRef]
89. Calhoun, V.D.; Adali, T.; McGinty, V.B.; Pekar, J.J.; Watson, T.D.; Pearlson, G.D. fMRI activation in a visual-perception task: Network of areas detected using the general linear model and independent components analysis. *Neuroimage* **2001**, *14*, 1080–1088. [CrossRef]
90. Sorg, C.; Riedl, V.; Muhlau, M.; Calhoun, V.D.; Eichele, T.; Laer, L.; Drzezga, A.; Forstl, H.; Kurz, A.; Zimmer, C.; et al. Selective changes of resting-state networks in individuals at risk for Alzheimer's disease. *Proc. Natl. Acad. Sci. USA* **2007**, *104*, 18760–18765. [CrossRef] [PubMed]
91. Correa, N.; Adali, T.; Li, Y.-O.; Calhoun, V. Comparison of blind source separation algorithms for FMRI using a new Matlab toolbox: GIFT. In Proceedings of the IEEE International Conference on Acoustics, Speech, and Signal, Processing, (ICASSP'05), Philadelphia, PA, USA, 18–23 March 2005; pp. 18–23.
92. Harshman, R.A.; Lundy, M.E. Parafac—parallel factor-analysis. *Comput. Stat. Data Anal.* **1994**, *18*, 39–72. [CrossRef]
93. Formisano, E.; Esposito, F.; Di Salle, F.; Goebel, R. Cortex-based independent component analysis of fMRI time series. *Magn. Reson. Imaging* **2004**, *22*, 1493–1504. [CrossRef] [PubMed]
94. Jack, C.R.; Petersen, R.C.; Obrien, P.C.; Tangalos, E.G. Mr-based hippocampal volumetry in the diagnosis of alzheimers-disease. *Neurology* **1992**, *42*, 183–188. [CrossRef] [PubMed]
95. Giesel, F.L.; Thomann, P.A.; Hahn, H.K.; Wilkinson, I.D. Comparison of manual direct and automated indirect measurement of hippocampus using magnetic resonance imaging. *Eur. J. Radiol.* **2008**, *66*, 268–273. [CrossRef] [PubMed]
96. Hirata, Y.; Matsuda, H.; Nemoto, K.; Ohnishi, T.; Hirao, K.; Yamashita, F.; Asada, T.; Iwabuchi, S.; Samejima, H. Voxel-based morphometry to discriminate early Alzheimer's disease from controls. *Neurosci. Lett.* **2005**, *382*, 269–274. [CrossRef] [PubMed]

97. Ashburner, J.; Friston, K.J. Voxel-based morphometry—The methods. *Neuroimage* **2000**, *11*, 805–821. [CrossRef]
98. Baron, J.C.; Chetelat, G.; Desgranges, B.; Perchey, G.; Landeau, B.; de la Sayette, V.; Eustache, F. In vivo mapping of gray matter loss with voxel-based morphometry in mild Alzheimer's disease. *Neuroimage* **2001**, *14*, 298–309. [CrossRef]
99. Ohnishi, T.; Matsuda, H.; Tabira, T.; Asada, T.; Uno, M. Changes in brain morphology in Alzheimer disease and normal aging: Is Alzheimer disease an exaggerated aging process? *Am. J. Neuroradiol.* **2001**, *22*, 1680–1685.
100. Busatto, G.E.; Garrido, G.E.J.; Almeida, O.P.; Castro, C.C.; Camargo, C.H.P.; Cid, C.G.; Buchpiguel, C.A.; Furuie, S.; Bottino, C.M. A voxel-based morphometry study of temporal lobe gray matter reductions in Alzheimer's disease. *Neurobiol. Aging* **2003**, *24*, 221–231. [CrossRef]
101. Testa, C.; Laakso, M.P.; Sabattoli, F.; Rossi, R.; Beltramello, A.; Soininen, H.; Frisoni, G.B. Comparison between the accuracy of voxel-based morphometry and hippocampal volumetry in Alzheimer's disease. *J. Magn. Reson. Imaging* **2004**, *19*, 274–282. [CrossRef] [PubMed]
102. Friston, K.J. Statistical parametric mapping and other analyses of functional imaging data. *Brain Mapp. Methods* **1996**, 363–386.
103. Esposito, F.; Formisano, E.; Seifritz, E.; Goebel, R.; Morrone, R.; Tedeschi, G.; Di Salle, F. Spatial independent component analysis of functional MRI time-series: To what extent do results depend on the algorithm used? *Hum. Brain Mapp.* **2002**, *16*, 146–157. [CrossRef] [PubMed]
104. Asllani, I.; Habeck, C.; Scarmeas, N.; Borogovac, A.; Brown, T.R.; Stern, Y. Multivariate and univariate analysis of continuous arterial spin labeling perfusion MRI in Alzheimer's disease. *J. Cereb. Blood Flow Metab.* **2008**, *28*, 725–736. [CrossRef] [PubMed]
105. McKeown, M.J.; Makeig, S.; Brown, G.G.; Jung, T.P.; Kindermann, S.S.; Bell, A.J.; Sejnowski, T.J. Analysis of fMRI data by blind separation into independent spatial components. *Hum. Brain Mapp.* **1998**, *6*, 160–188. [CrossRef]
106. Moritz, C.H.; Haughton, V.M.; Cordes, D.; Quigley, M.; Meyerand, M.E. Whole-brain functional MR imaging activation from a finger-tapping task examined with independent component analysis. *Am. J. Neuroradiol.* **2000**, *21*, 1629–1635.
107. McKeown, M.J.; Hansen, L.K.; Sejnowski, T.J. Independent component analysis of functional MRI: What is signal and what is noise? *Curr. Opin. Neurobiol.* **2003**, *13*, 620–629. [CrossRef] [PubMed]
108. Esposito, F.; Scarabino, T.; Hyvarinen, A.; Himberg, J.; Formisano, E.; Comani, S.; Tedeschi, G.; Goebel, R.; Seifritz, E.; Di Salle, F. Independent component analysis of fMRI group studies by self-organizing clustering. *Neuroimage* **2005**, *25*, 193–205. [CrossRef] [PubMed]
109. Cardoso, J.F.; Souloumiac, A. Blind beamforming for non-gaussian signals. *IEE Proc. F Radar Signal Process.* **1993**, *140*, 362–370. [CrossRef]
110. Cruces-alvarez, S.A.; Cichocki, A.; Amari, S.I. On a new blind signal extraction algorithm: Different criteria and stability analysis. *IEEE Signal Process. Lett.* **2002**, *9*, 233–236. [CrossRef]
111. Seifritz, E.; Esposito, F.; Hennel, F.; Mustovic, H.; Neuhoff, J.G.; Bilecen, D.; Tedeschi, G.; Scheffler, K.; Di Salle, F. Spatiotemporal pattern of neural processing in the human auditory cortex. *Science* **2002**, *297*, 1706–1708. [CrossRef]
112. Beckmann, C.F.; Neble, J.A.; Smith, S.M. Artefact detection in FMRI data using independent component analysis. *Neuroimage* **2000**, *11*, S614. [CrossRef]
113. Calhoun, V.; Adali, T.; Pearlson, G.; Pekar, J. A method for making group inferences using independent component analysis of functional MRI data: Exploring the visual system. *Neuroimage* **2001**, *13*, S88. [CrossRef]
114. Akaike, H. New look at statistical-model identification. *IEEE Trans. Autom. Control* **1974**, *AC19*, 716–723. [CrossRef]
115. Rissanen, J. A universal prior for integers and estimation by minimum description length. *Ann. Stat.* **1983**, *11*, 416–431. [CrossRef]
116. Vigario, R.; Sarela, J.; Oja, E. Independent component analysis inwave decomposition of auditory evoked fields. In Proceedings of the International Conference on Artificial Neural Networks (ICANN'98), Skovde, Sweden, 2–4 September 1998; pp. 287–292.
117. vigario, R.; Sarela, J.; Oja, E. Independent component analysis in decomposition of auditory and somatosensory evoked fields. In Proceedings of the International Workshop on Independent Component Analysis and Signal Separation (ICA'99), Aussois, France, 11–15 January 1999; pp. 167–172.
118. Celone, K.A.; Calhoun, V.D.; Dickerson, B.C.; Atri, A.; Chua, E.F.; Miller, S.L.; DePeau, K.; Rentz, D.M.; Selkoe, D.J.; Blacker, D.; et al. Alterations in memory networks in mild cognitive impairment and Alzheimer's disease: An independent component analysis. *J. Neurosci.* **2006**, *26*, 10222–10231. [CrossRef] [PubMed]
119. Chapman, R.M.; Nowlis, G.H.; McCrary, J.W.; Chapman, J.A.; Sandoval, T.C.; Guillily, M.D.; Gardner, M.N.; Reilly, L.A. Brain event-related potentials: Diagnosing early-stage Alzheimer's disease. *Neurobiol. Aging* **2007**, *28*, 194–201. [CrossRef] [PubMed]
120. Besthorn, C.; Zerfass, R.; GeigerKabisch, C.; Sattel, H.; Daniel, S.; SchreiterGasser, U.; Forstl, H. Discrimination of Alzheimer's disease and normal aging by EEG data. *Electroencephalogr. Clin. Neurophysiol.* **1997**, *103*, 241–248. [CrossRef]
121. Melissant, C.; Ypma, A.; Frietman, E.E.E.; Stam, C.J. A method for detection of Alzheimer's disease using ICA-enhanced EEG measurements. *Artif. Intell. Med.* **2005**, *33*, 209–222. [CrossRef]
122. Tong, L.; Soon, V.; Huang, Y.; Liu, R. AMUSE: A new blind identification algorithm. In Proceedings of the IEEE International Symposium on Circuits and Systems, New Orleans, LA, USA, 1–3 May 1990; pp. 1784–1787.
123. Vialatte, F.-B.; Solé-Casals, J.; Maurice, M.; Latchoumane, C.; Hudson, N.; Wimalaratna, S.; Jeong, J.; Cichocki, A. Improving the quality of EEG data in patients with Alzheimer's disease using ICA. In Proceedings of the International Conference on Neural Information Processing, Cambridge, MA, USA, 25–28 November 2008; pp. 979–986.

124. Escudero, J.; Hornero, R.; Poza, J.; Abasolo, D.; Fernandez, A. Assessment of classification improvement in patients with Alzheimer's disease based on magnetoencephalogram blind source separation. *Artif. Intell. Med.* **2008**, *43*, 75–85. [CrossRef] [PubMed]
125. Fernandez, A.; Hornero, R.; Mayo, A.; Poza, J.; Gil-Gregorio, P.; Ortiz, T. MEG spectral profile in Alzheimer's disease and mild cognitive impairment. *Clin. Neurophysiol.* **2006**, *117*, 306–314. [CrossRef]
126. Kerrouche, N.; Herholz, K.; Mielke, R.; Holthoff, V.; Baron, J.C. (18)FDG PET in vascular dementia: Differentiation from Alzheimer's disease using voxel-based multivariate analysis. *J. Cereb. Blood Flow Metab.* **2006**, *26*, 1213–1221. [CrossRef]
127. Chen, K.; Reiman, E.M.; Alexander, G.E.; Crum, W.R.; Fox, N.C.; Rossor, M.N. Automated method using iterative principal component analysis for detecting brain atrophy rates from sequential MRI in persons with Alzheimer's disease. *Soc. Neurosci. Abstr.* **2001**, *27*, 1216.
128. Chen, K.W.; Reiman, E.M.; Alexander, G.E.; Bandy, D.; Renaut, R.; Crum, W.R.; Fox, N.C.; Rossor, M.N. An automated algorithm for the computation of brain volume change from sequential MRIs using an iterative principal component analysis and its evaluation for the assessment of whole-brain atrophy rates in patients with probable Alzheimer's disease. *Neuroimage* **2004**, *22*, 134–143. [CrossRef]
129. Turkheimer, F.E.; Aston, J.A.D.; Banati, R.B.; Riddell, C.; Cunningham, V.J. A linear wavelet filter for parametric imaging with dynamic PET. *IEEE Trans. Med Imaging* **2003**, *22*, 289–301. [CrossRef]
130. Bai, F.; Zhang, Z.J.; Yu, H.; Shi, Y.M.; Yuan, Y.G.; Zhu, W.L.; Zhang, X.R.; Qian, Y. Default-mode network activity distinguishes amnestic type mild cognitive impairment from healthy aging: A combined structural and resting-state functional MRI study. *Neurosci. Lett.* **2008**, *438*, 111–115. [CrossRef] [PubMed]
131. Greicius, M.D.; Srivastava, G.; Reiss, A.L.; Menon, V. Default-mode network activity distinguishes Alzheimer's disease from healthy aging: Evidence from functional MRI. *Proc. Natl. Acad. Sci. USA* **2004**, *101*, 4637–4642. [CrossRef] [PubMed]
132. Tang, N.; Wang, Z.; Wu, X.; Li, K.; Yao, L. Functional connectivity methods based on ICA and correlation with fMRI data. *J. Beijing Norm. Univ. (Nat. Sci.)* **2008**, *44*, 54–58.
133. Calhoun, V.D.; Kiehl, K.A.; Pearlson, G.D. Modulation of temporally coherent brain networks estimated using ICA at rest and during cognitive tasks. *Hum. Brain Mapp.* **2008**, *29*, 828–838. [CrossRef] [PubMed]
134. Greicius, M. Resting-state functional connectivity in neuropsychiatric disorders. *Curr. Opin. Neurol.* **2008**, *21*, 424–430. [CrossRef] [PubMed]
135. Rombouts, S.A.; Damoiseaux, J.S.; Goekoop, R.; Barkhof, F.; Scheltens, P.; Smith, S.M.; Beckmann, C.F. Model-free group analysis shows altered BOLD FMRI networks in dementia. *Hum. Brain Mapp.* **2009**, *30*, 256–266. [CrossRef]
136. Illán, I.Á.; Górriz, J.; Ramírez, J.; Salas-Gonzalez, D.; López, M.; Segovia, F.; Padilla, P.; Puntonet, C.G. Projecting independent components of SPECT images for computer aided diagnosis of Alzheimer's disease. *Pattern Recognit. Lett.* **2010**, *31*, 1342–1347. [CrossRef]
137. Savio, A.; Graña, M. Deformation based feature selection for computer aided diagnosis of Alzheimer's disease. *Expert Syst. Appl.* **2013**, *40*, 1619–1628. [CrossRef]
138. Martínez-Murcia, F.J.; Górriz, J.M.; Ramirez, J.; Puntonet, C.G.; Salas-Gonzalez, D.; Initiative, A.s.D.N. Computer aided diagnosis tool for Alzheimer's disease based on Mann–Whitney–Wilcoxon U-test. *Expert Syst. Appl.* **2012**, *39*, 9676–9685. [CrossRef]
139. Chaves, R.; Ramírez, J.; Górriz, J.; López, M.; Salas-Gonzalez, D.; Alvarez, I.; Segovia, F. SVM-based computer-aided diagnosis of the Alzheimer's disease using t-test NMSE feature selection with feature correlation weighting. *Neurosci. Lett.* **2009**, *461*, 293–297. [CrossRef]
140. Salas-Gonzalez, D.; Górriz, J.M.; Ramírez, J.; López, M.; Alvarez, I.; Segovia, F.; Chaves, R.; Puntonet, C. Computer-aided diagnosis of Alzheimer's disease using support vector machines and classification trees. *Phys. Med. Biol.* **2010**, *55*, 2807. [CrossRef] [PubMed]
141. Bi, X.; Li, S.; Xiao, B.; Li, Y.; Wang, G.; Ma, X. Computer aided Alzheimer's disease diagnosis by an unsupervised deep learning technology. *Neurocomputing* **2020**, *392*, 296–304. [CrossRef]
142. Trambaiolli, L.R.; Lorena, A.C.; Fraga, F.J.; Kanda, P.A.; Anghinah, R.; Nitrini, R. Improving Alzheimer's disease diagnosis with machine learning techniques. *Clin. Eeg Neurosci.* **2011**, *42*, 160–165. [CrossRef]
143. Simpraga, S.; Alvarez-Jimenez, R.; Mansvelder, H.D.; Van Gerven, J.M.; Groeneveld, G.J.; Poil, S.-S.; Linkenkaer-Hansen, K. EEG machine learning for accurate detection of cholinergic intervention and Alzheimer's disease. *Sci. Rep.* **2017**, *7*, 1–11. [CrossRef] [PubMed]
144. Podgorelec, V. Analyzing EEG signals with machine learning for diagnosing Alzheimer's disease. *Elektron. Ir Elektrotechnika* **2012**, *18*, 61–64. [CrossRef]
145. Morabito, F.C.; Campolo, M.; Ieracitano, C.; Ebadi, J.M.; Bonanno, L.; Bramanti, A.; Desalvo, S.; Mammone, N.; Bramanti, P. Deep convolutional neural networks for classification of mild cognitive impaired and Alzheimer's disease patients from scalp EEG recordings. In Proceedings of the 2016 IEEE 2nd International Forum on Research and Technologies for Society and Industry Leveraging a better tomorrow (RTSI), Bologna, Italy, 7–9 September 2016; pp. 1–6.
146. Lehmann, C.; Koenig, T.; Jelic, V.; Prichep, L.; John, R.E.; Wahlund, L.-O.; Dodge, Y.; Dierks, T. Application and comparison of classification algorithms for recognition of Alzheimer's disease in electrical brain activity (EEG). *J. Neurosci. Methods* **2007**, *161*, 342–350. [CrossRef] [PubMed]

147. Qi, Y.; Doermann, D.; DeMenthon, D. Hybrid independent component analysis and support vector machine learning scheme for face detection. In Proceedings of the 2001 IEEE International Conference on Acoustics, Speech, and Signal Processing. Proceedings (Cat. No. 01CH37221), Salt Lake City, UT, USA, 7–11 May 2001; pp. 1481–1484.
148. Aziz, R.; Verma, C.; Srivastava, N. A fuzzy based feature selection from independent component subspace for machine learning classification of microarray data. *Genom. Data* **2016**, *8*, 4–15. [CrossRef] [PubMed]
149. Radüntz, T.; Scouten, J.; Hochmuth, O.; Meffert, B. Automated EEG artifact elimination by applying machine learning algorithms to ICA-based features. *J. Neural Eng.* **2017**, *14*, 046004. [CrossRef]
150. Vialatte, F.; Cichocki, A.; Dreyfus, G.; Musha, T.; Shishkin, S.L.; Gervais, R. Early detection of Alzheimer's disease by blind source separation, time frequency representation, and bump modeling of EEG signals. In Proceedings of the International Conference on Artificial Neural Networks, Warsaw, Poland, 11–15 September 2005; pp. 683–692.
151. Cassani, R.; Falk, T.H.; Fraga, F.J.; Kanda, P.A.; Anghinah, R. The effects of automated artifact removal algorithms on electroencephalography-based Alzheimer's disease diagnosis. *Front. Aging Neurosci.* **2014**, *6*, 55. [CrossRef] [PubMed]
152. Ball, G.; Aljabar, P.; Arichi, T.; Tusor, N.; Cox, D.; Merchant, N.; Nongena, P.; Hajnal, J.V.; Edwards, A.D.; Counsell, S.J. Machine-learning to characterise neonatal functional connectivity in the preterm brain. *Neuroimage* **2016**, *124*, 267–275. [CrossRef]
153. Welsh, R.C.; Jelsone-Swain, L.M.; Foerster, B.R. The utility of independent component analysis and machine learning in the identification of the amyotrophic lateral sclerosis diseased brain. *Front. Hum. Neurosci.* **2013**, *7*, 251. [CrossRef]
154. Xie, J.; Douglas, P.K.; Wu, Y.N.; Brody, A.L.; Anderson, A.E. Decoding the encoding of functional brain networks: An fMRI classification comparison of non-negative matrix factorization (NMF), independent component analysis (ICA), and sparse coding algorithms. *J. Neurosci. Methods* **2017**, *282*, 81–94. [CrossRef]
155. Sui, J.; Adali, T.; Pearlson, G.; Yang, H.; Sponheim, S.R.; White, T.; Calhoun, V.D. A CCA+ ICA based model for multi-task brain imaging data fusion and its application to schizophrenia. *Neuroimage* **2010**, *51*, 123–134. [CrossRef]
156. Vergara, V.M.; Ulloa, A.; Calhoun, V.D.; Boutte, D.; Chen, J.; Liu, J. A three-way parallel ICA approach to analyze links among genetics, brain structure and brain function. *Neuroimage* **2014**, *98*, 386–394. [CrossRef] [PubMed]
157. Khedher, L.; Illán, I.A.; Górriz, J.M.; Ramírez, J.; Brahim, A.; Meyer-Baese, A. Independent component analysis-support vector machine-based computer-aided diagnosis system for Alzheimer's with visual support. *Int. J. Neural Syst.* **2017**, *27*, 1650050. [CrossRef] [PubMed]
158. Hyvärinen, A. Fast and robust fixed-point algorithms for independent component analysis. *IEEE Trans Neural Netw* **1999**, *10*, 626–634. [CrossRef]
159. Yang, W.; Lui, R.L.; Gao, J.H.; Chan, T.F.; Yau, S.T.; Sperling, R.A.; Huang, X. Independent component analysis-based classification of Alzheimer's disease MRI data. *J Alzheimers Dis.* **2011**, *24*, 775–783. [CrossRef] [PubMed]
160. Yang, W.; Chen, X.; Cohen, D.S.; Rosin, E.R.; Toga, A.W.; Thompson, P.M.; Huang, X. Classification of MRI and psychological testing data based on support vector machine. *Int. J. Clin. Exp. Med.* **2017**, *10*, 16004–16026.
161. Qiao, J.; Lv, Y.; Cao, C.; Wang, Z.; Li, A. Multivariate deep learning classification of Alzheimer's disease based on hierarchical partner matching independent component analysis. *Front. Aging Neurosci.* **2018**, *10*, 417. [CrossRef]
162. Basheera, S.; Ram, M.S.S. Convolution neural network–based Alzheimer's disease classification using hybrid enhanced independent component analysis based segmented gray matter of T2 weighted magnetic resonance imaging with clinical valuation. *Alzheimer's Dement. Transl. Res. Clin. Interv.* **2019**, *5*, 974–986. [CrossRef] [PubMed]
163. Toussaint, P.-J.; Perlbarg, V.; Bellec, P.; Desarnaud, S.; Lacomblez, L.; Doyon, J.; Habert, M.-O.; Benali, H. Resting state FDG-PET functional connectivity as an early biomarker of Alzheimer's disease using conjoint univariate and independent component analyses. *Neuroimage* **2012**, *63*, 936–946. [CrossRef] [PubMed]

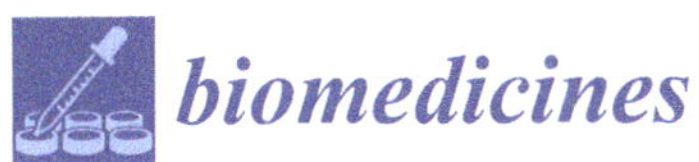

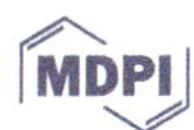

*Article*

# Alteration in the Cerebrospinal Fluid Lipidome in Parkinson's Disease: A Post-Mortem Pilot Study

**Joaquín Fernández-Irigoyen [1], Paz Cartas-Cejudo [1], Marta Iruarrizaga-Lejarreta [2] and Enrique Santamaría [1,*]**

[1] Clinical Neuroproteomics Unit, Navarrabiomed, Complejo Hospitalario de Navarra (CHN), Instituto de Investigación Sanitaria de Navarra (IdiSNA), Universidad Pública de Navarra (UPNA), 31008 Pamplona, Spain; jfernani@navarra.es (J.F.-I.); pazcarce@hotmail.com (P.C.-C.)

[2] Metabolomics Department, One Way Liver S.L. (OWL), 48160 Derio, Spain; miruarrizaga@owlmetabolomics.com

* Correspondence: esantamma@navarra.es; Tel.: +34-848-425-740; Fax: +34-848-422-200

**Abstract:** Lipid metabolism is clearly associated to Parkinson's disease (PD). Although lipid homeostasis has been widely studied in multiple animal and cellular models, as well as in blood derived from PD individuals, the cerebrospinal fluid (CSF) lipidomic profile in PD remains largely unexplored. In this study, we characterized the post-mortem CSF lipidomic imbalance between neurologically intact controls ($n = 10$) and PD subjects ($n = 20$). The combination of dual extraction with ultra-performance liquid chromatography-electrospray ionization quadrupole-time-of-flight mass spectrometry (UPLC-ESI-qToF-MS/MS) allowed for the monitoring of 257 lipid species across all samples. Complementary multivariate and univariate data analysis identified that glycerolipids (mono-, di-, and triacylglycerides), saturated and mono/polyunsaturated fatty acids, primary fatty amides, glycerophospholipids (phosphatidylcholines, phosphatidylethanolamines), sphingolipids (ceramides, sphingomyelins), N-acylethanolamines and sterol lipids (cholesteryl esters, steroids) were significantly increased in the CSF of PD compared to the control group. Interestingly, CSF lipid dyshomeostasis differed depending on neuropathological staging and disease duration. These results, despite the limitation of being obtained in a small population, suggest extensive CSF lipid remodeling in PD, shedding new light on the deployment of CSF lipidomics as a promising tool to identify potential lipid markers as well as discriminatory lipid species between PD and other atypical parkinsonisms.

**Keywords:** lipids; cerebrospinal fluid; Parkinson's disease; mass-spectrometry; lipidomics

**Citation:** Fernández-Irigoyen, J.; Cartas-Cejudo, P.; Iruarrizaga-Lejarreta, M.; Santamaría, E. Alteration in the Cerebrospinal Fluid Lipidome in Parkinson's Disease: A Post-Mortem Pilot Study. *Biomedicines* **2021**, *9*, 491. https://doi.org/10.3390/biomedicines9050491

Academic Editor: Arnab Ghosh

Received: 7 April 2021
Accepted: 27 April 2021
Published: 29 April 2021



## 1. Introduction

Due to the lipid heterogeneity, it has been estimated that the human lipidome may be composed by 100,000 different lipid species [1,2]. Lipids play multiple roles in brain function, affecting the elasticity and structural organization of synaptic membranes and modulating protein activity involved in cellular signaling dynamics [3–5]. In the context of PD, a genetic risk has been characterized between lipid/lipoproteins traits and the disease [6]. Mutations in lipid-producing enzymes, such as GBA, associated with familial PD and SNPs in multiple PD related-genes involved in lipid homeostasis [7–11] (*SREBF1*, *ASAH1*, *SMPD1*, *PLA2G6*, amongst others) have been linked to PD. Moreover, lipids not only influence in the aggregation potential of alpha-synuclein in vitro and in vivo [12], but they are also present in high concentration as components of crowded membranes, vesicle structures and dysmorphic organelles present in Lewy bodies (LB) [13]. All these data evidence that lipid metabolism should be tightly regulated to counteract the appearance and progression of PD. Systematic studies of cases with LB pathology have prompted a staging classification of PD based on the putative progression with time of LB pathology in the brain from the medulla oblongata and olfactory bulb to the neocortex.

Lipidomics is emerging as a powerful approach that complements protein and gene-centric workflows in the biomarker search to evaluate the neurodegenerative risk or the neurodegenerative progression [14]. Although the scientific community is on a continuous learning curve to obtain a comprehensive portrait of the human brain lipidome [15], the deployment of different variants of chromatographic separations coupled to mass-spectrometry is considered the gold standard approach to study lipid profiles in a high-throughput manner. However, multiple efforts are needed to solve and standardize the associated analytical challenges [16]. Several lipidomic platforms have recently been used to characterize the lipid composition of biofluids in neurological disorders such as amyotrophic lateral sclerosis, multiple sclerosis and Alzheimer's disease (AD) [17–21]. In this study, we applied a discovery workflow to determine the global lipidomic changes at the CSF level between PD and controls using ultra-performance liquid chromatography-electrospray ionization time-of-flight mass spectrometry (UPLC-ESI-ToF-MS), monitoring more than 250 lipid species and detecting a new metabolic signature associated with the disease that should be further validated in extensive sample cohorts in terms of biomarker sensitivity and specificity.

## 2. Materials and Methods

### 2.1. Materials

Internal standard (IS) compounds, nonadecanoid acid, dehydrocholic acid and tryptophan-(indole-d5), were purchased from Sigma-Aldrich-Merck KGaA (Darmstadt, Germany). 1-tridecanoyl-2-hydroxy-sn-glycero-3-phosphocholine (13:0 Lyso PC), N-hexanoyl-D-erythro-sphingosylphosphorylcholine SM (d18:1/6:0), 1,2-diheptadecanoyl-sn-glycero-3-phosphoethanolamine (17:0 PE), 1,2-dinonadecanoyl-sn-glycero-3-phosphocholine (19:0 PC) and N-heptadecanoyl-D-erythro-sphingosine Ceramide (d18:1/17:0) were purchased from Avanti Polar Lipids (Merck KGaA, Darmstadt, Germany). Tritridecanoylglycerol (13:0 TG), Triheptadecanoylglycerol (17:0 TG) and Cholesteryl Laurate ChoE (12:0) were purchased from Larodan Fine Chemicals (Solna, Sweden). All chemicals and solvents (acetonitrile, methanol, water, isopropanol, formic acid, ammonium formate) were of analytical, HPLC or HPLC-MS grade. See Appendix A for IS working solution preparations (Tables A1 and A2).

### 2.2. Metabolite Extraction from CSF

Control ($n$ = 10; mean age: 77.7 years; 4F/6M) and PD ($n$ = 20; mean age: 79.9 years; 7F/13M) post-mortem CSF samples were obtained from the Parkinson's UK Brain Bank funded by Parkinson's UK, a charity registered in England and Wales (258197) and in Scotland (SC037554) (Table 1). During the post-mortem brain removal (PMI < 24 h.), the CSF was obtained as follows. The tentorium cerebelli was cut close to its attachment to the skull base (on the petrous bone). CSF was obtained anteriorly to the brainstem. After a centrifugation step (3 min at 10,000 rpm), CSF aliquots were frozen at −80 °C. Metabolite extraction was performed as previously described [22]. Briefly, 150 µL of CSF was spiked with 600 µL and 570 µL of ice-cold IS working solution for lipidomics platforms 1 and 2, respectively. Once spiked with the extraction solvents, samples were mixed with 570 µL of ice-cold CHCl3, vortexed for 20 min at RT and incubated for 1 h at 4 °C. Then, a centrifugation step was carried out (18,000× $g$, 15 min, 4 °C) and 650 µL of supernatant were collected for each platform. Lipidomics platform 1:650 µL of supernatant were dried at 40 °C in a vacuum concentrator and reconstituted in 50 µL methanol with agitation for 20 min at RT. After centrifugation (18,000× $g$ for 5 min at 4 °C) to precipitate any particles, supernatants were transferred to a plate for UPLC®-MS analysis. Lipidomics platform 2:650 µL supernatant were mixed with 50 µL of $H_2O$ and vortexed for a few seconds. After centrifugation (18,000× $g$ for 5 min at 4 °C), 400 µL of the lower organic phase were dried at 40 °C in a vacuum concentrator. Dried samples were reconstituted in 50 µL of acetonitrile:isopropanol 1:1 and shaken vigorously at RT for 10 min. A centrifugation step (18,000× $g$ for 5 min at 4 °C) was performed to precipitate any particles, and supernatants were transferred to a plate for ultra-performance liquid chromatography UPLC®-MS analysis.

**Table 1.** Chromatographic and mass-spectrometric workflows used in this study.

| | Platform 1 | Platform 2 |
|---|---|---|
| Column type | UPLC BEH C18, 1.0 × 100 mm, 1.7 μm | UPLC BEH C18, 2.1 × 100 mm, 1.7 μm |
| Flow rate | 0.140 mL/min | 0.400 mL/min |
| Solvent A | 0.05% Formic Acid in water | Water:Acetronitrile (2:3) + 10 mM Ammonium Formate |
| Solvent B | 0.05% Formic Acid in acetonitrile | Acetonitrile:Isopropanol (1:9) + 10 mM Ammonium Formate |
| (%B), time | 0%, 0 min | 40%, 0 min |
| (%B), time | 50%, 2 min | 100%, 10 min |
| (%B), time | 100%, 13 min | 40%, 15 min |
| (%B), time | 0%, 18 min | 40%, 17 min |
| Column temperature | 40 °C | 60 °C |
| Injection volume | 2 μL | 3 μL |
| Autosampler temperature | 10 °C | 10 °C |
| Source temperature | 120 °C | 120 °C |
| Nebulisation $N_2$ flow | 600 L/hour | 1000 L/hour |
| Nebulisation $N_2$ temperature | 350 °C | 500 °C |
| Cone $N_2$ flow | 30 L/hour | 30 L/hour |
| Ionization | ESI −ve | ESI +ve |
| Capillary voltage | 2.8 kV | 3.2 kV |
| Cone voltage | 50 V | 30 V |
| Type of data | Centroid | Centroid |
| Scan time | 0.2 s | 0.2 s |
| Acquisition range | 50–1000 Da | 50–1200 Da |

Analysis of fatty acyls, bile acids, steroids and lysoglycerophospholipids was carried out with lipidomic platform 1, and analysis of glycerolipids, cholesterol esters, sphingolipids and glycerophospholipids was performed with lipidomic platform 2. Abbreviation: ESI, Electrospray ionization.

### 2.3. Chromatography and Mass-Spectrometry

Lipidomic profiling was carried out by OWL Metabolomics S.L. (Derio, Spain). Briefly, chromatographic separation and mass spectrometric detection conditions employed for each UHPLC-ToF-MS-based platform are indicated in Table 1. An Acquity-LCT Premier XE system and an Acquity-Xevo G2QTOF (Waters Corp., Milford, MA) were used as platform 1 and 2, respectively.

### 2.4. Data Processing and Normalization

TargetLynx application manager for MassLynx 4.1 software (Waters Corp. Milford, MA, USA) was used for data processing. A set of parameters associated to metabolites included in the analysis (Rt $m/z$, mass-to-charge ratio pairs, retention time) were incorporated into the program. Using a mass tolerance window of 0.05 Da and after peak detection and noise reduction (at LC and MS levels), only true metabolite related features were processed by the software. For each sample injection, a list of chromatographic peak areas was generated. Data normalization was performed following the procedure described by Barr et al. [23], where the ion intensity corresponding to each peak present in each

CSF sample was normalized in respect to the sum of peak intensities in each CSF sample. There were no significant differences ($t$-test = 0.1031) between the total intensities used for normalization of the sample groups compared in the study.

### 2.5. Data Analysis

Once normalized, the dimensionality of the complex data set was reduced to enable easy visualization of any metabolic clustering of the different groups of samples. This was achieved by multivariate data analysis, including the non-supervised principal components analysis (PCA) and/or supervised orthogonal partial least-squares to latent structures (OPLS) approaches. Univariate statistical analyses were also performed, calculating group percentage changes and unpaired Student's $t$-test $p$-value (or Welch's $t$-test where unequal variances were found) for the comparison between both experimental groups. To help in the interpretation of lipid changes in a biologically meaningful context, OWLStatApp was used (http://rstudio.owlmetabolomics.com:8031/OwlStatApp).

## 3. Results

During a neurodegenerative process, different types of molecules could be released and finally diffused into the CSF circuit, being considered as potential cerebrospinal fluid (CSF) biomarkers. Because cell membrane breakdown is a characteristic feature of a neurodegenerative process in brain syndromes, the deep characterization of CSF metabolomic profiles could reveal specific lipid molecules released by damaged neuronal or glial cell populations, establishing novel molecular panels to help us in the characterization of neurodegenerative diseases. In the current study, we have focused our attention on the metabolic profile of CSF lipids in PD.

### 3.1. Categorization of the Detected CSF Lipidome

Due to the wide concentration range of lipids and their extensive chemical diversity [1], it is not possible to analyze the full lipidomic profile in a single experiment. Therefore, lipid extraction was carried out by fractionating the post-mortem CSF samples into groups of species with similar physicochemical properties, using appropriate solutions of organic solvents (methanol, chloroform/methanol) and then analyzing the different extracts in specific analytical platforms [23]. In our case, two UHPLC-MS based platforms were used (Figure 1) to maximize the analysis of CSF lipidomic profiles derived from neurologically intact controls and PD subjects (Table 2), performing an optimal profiling of: (i) fatty acyls, bile acids, steroids and lysoglycerophospholipids; and (ii) glycerolipids, glycerophospholipids, sterol lipids and sphingolipids. Using this dual workflow, a total of 257 metabolic features were detected in all human CSF samples, including 6 bile acids, 10 fatty amides, 3 acylcarnitines, 65 glycerolipids, 111 glycerophospholipids, 22 non-esterified fatty acids, 33 sphingolipids and 7 sterols (Table S1).

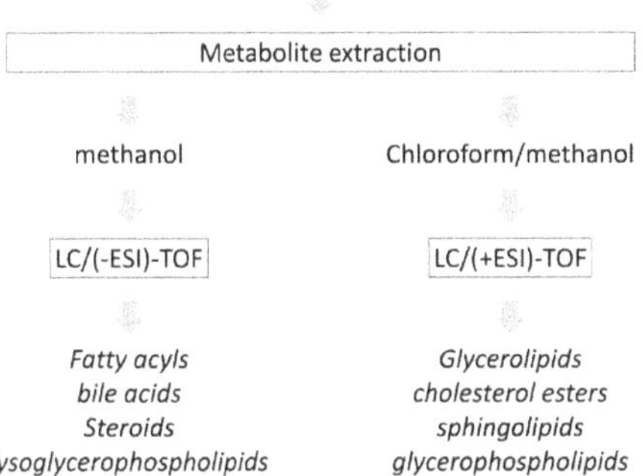


**Figure 1.** Lipidomic workflow applied in our pilot study.

**Table 2.** CSF samples included in the lipidomic study.

| SAMPLE.ID | Age | Sex | Onset | Duration | NPD |
|---|---|---|---|---|---|
| PD354 | 88 | F | 77 | 11 | LBDE |
| PD423 | 66 | F | 53 | 13 | LBDE |
| PD436 | 90 | M | 82 | 8 | LBDE |
| PD520 | 80 | M | 56 | 24 | LBDE |
| PD530 | 85 | M | 77 | 8 | LBDE |
| PD357 | 71 | M | 37 | 34 | LBDN |
| PD450 | 66 | M | 47 | 19 | LBDN |
| PD495 | 88 | F | 78 | 10 | LBDN |
| PD501 | 89 | F | 82 | 7 | LBDN |
| PD537 | 84 | M | 74 | 9 | LBDN |
| PD550 | 83 | F | 77 | 7 | LBDN |
| PD562 | 79 | M | 72 | 7 | LBDN |
| PD636 | 84 | M | 65 | 20 | LBDN |
| PD295 | 83 | M | 67 | 16 | LBDL |
| PD340 | 67 | M | 53 | 14 | LBDL |
| PD356 | 86 | F | 75 | 9 | LBDL |
| PD541 | 72 | M | 66 | 6 | LBDL |
| PD546 | 84 | F | 71 | 13 | LBDL |
| PD579 | 76 | M | 55 | 21 | LBDL |
| PD591 | 77 | M | 68 | 9 | LBDL |
| C022 | 65 | M | | | aging-related changes |
| C023 | 78 | F | | | aging-related changes |
| C030 | 77 | M | | | aging-related changes |
| C008 | 93 | F | | | aging-related changes |
| C015 | 82 | M | | | possible ischaemia |
| C026 | 78 | F | | | minimal leukostasis |
| C032 | 88 | M | | | aging-related changes |
| C054 | 66 | M | | | mild aging-related changes |
| C064 | 63 | F | | | microvascular pathology |
| C076 | 87 | M | | | aging-related changes |

PD: Parkinson's disease; C: controls. Duration (years). NPD: neuropathological diagnosis; LBDL: Lewy body disease limbic stage; LBDE: Lewy body disease early-neocortical stage; LBDN: Lewy body disease neocortical stage.

### 3.2. CSF Lipidomic Profiling in Parkinson's Disease

The 257 detected lipid features were analyzed across all CSF samples. Once normalized, the dimensionality of the complex dataset was reduced to enable easy visualisation of any metabolic clustering of the PD and control CSFs. The quality of the global experiment was assessed (see Appendix A).

3.2.1. Multivariate Analysis

A supervised OPLS model was also calculated in order to achieve the maximum separation between both experimental groups. Figure 2 (left panel) shows the score scatter plot of this model, in which a clear clustering of CSF samples according to the presence or absence of PD was observed. Similar to what was found for the loadings scatter plot displayed in Figure A4 (Appendix A), metabolites responsible for the differences observed were mainly glycerolipids (MAG, DAG, TAG), fatty acids (SFA, MUFA), FAA, glycerophospholipids (PC, PE) and sphingolipids (Cer, SM), which were increased in the PD group (Figure 2, right panel). However, this model had a low predictive ability (Q2X = 0.150), indicating it would be necessary to extend this pilot study to include additional sample cohorts.

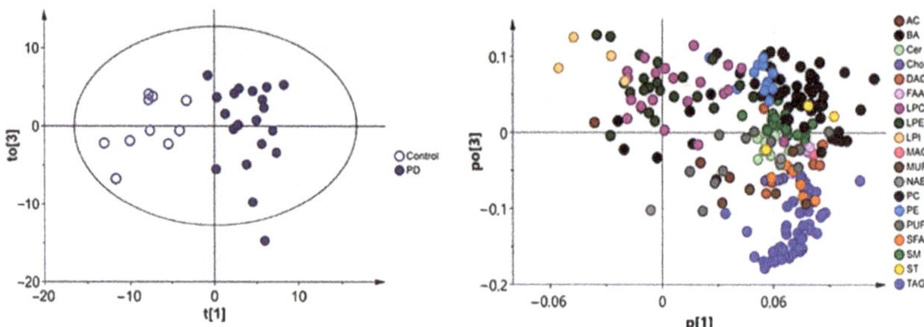


**Figure 2.** Score scatter plot (**left panel**) and loadings scatter plot (**right panel**) of the OPLS-DA model of CSF samples after square root transformation of the data. Model diagnostics (A = 9; R2X = 0.860; Q2X = 0.150).

3.2.2. Univariate Analysis

Univariate data analysis was also performed, calculating group percentage changes and unpaired Student's *t*-test *p*-value (or Welch's *t* test where unequal variances were found) for the PD vs. control comparison. As mentioned in Appendix A, a Shapiro–Wilk test revealed that the majority of the CSF metabolites measured from PD were not following a normal distribution. Then, in addition to the untransformed data analysis, a square root (sqrt) transformation of the data was also applied. Raw intensity data, average group intensities, fold changes and an unpaired Student's *t*-test of each individual metabolite and of each metabolic class for both untransformed and sqrt transformed data are included in Table S1. In order to correlate the alteration in specific lipid classes with Lewy body disease (LBD) staging, we classified the PD group according to the neuropathological staging: Lewy body disease (LBD) limbic stage (LBDL), LBD early-neocortical stage (LBDE) and LBD neocortical stage (LBDN) (Table 2). Moreover, to deepen our understanding of the lipid-dependent effects on PD duration, an additional analysis was performed, evaluating the correlation between the CSF lipidomic dysregulation and the disease duration in our sample cohort. To obtained balanced subgroups, we divided our PD cohort using a cutoff point of 10 years, generating two groups: (i) $<$10 years (9 subjects) and (ii) $\geq$10 years (11 subjects). The raw data per metabolic class was calculated as the sum of the normalized areas of all the metabolites with the same chemical characteristics. In order to help in the visualization of the results, a heatmap was generated. The heatmap in Figure 3 displays the log2 (fold-change) of the 257 metabolites included in all comparative analyses together with the unpaired Student's *t*-test obtained using the square root (Sqrt) transformation of the data.

According to disease duration, the deregulated lipid classes were highly similar between both groups, except for the phosphatidylcholines and sphingomyelins profiles that were most significantly deregulated in PD subjects with a disease duration of ≥10 years (Tables S2 and S3). According to the neuropathological classification and CSF lipidomic profiles (Tables S2 and S3), primary fatty amides (FAA), cholesteryl esters (ChoE) and sphingomyelins (SM) were most significantly increased in LBDL. A similar phosphatidylcholine profile was significantly elevated in CSF from LBDL and LBDE. However, the CSF lipid profile was reversed in LBDN, where a significant increment was mostly observed at the level of polyunsaturated fatty acids (PUFA) and triacylglycerols (TAG) (Figure 3).

A volcano plot was generated highlighting the most significant metabolites considered individually for the PD vs. control comparison (Figure 4).

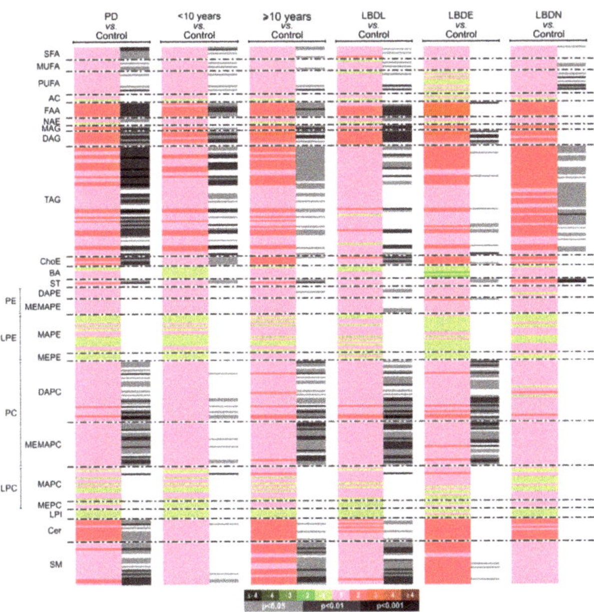


**Figure 3.** Heatmap representing differential individual metabolic features obtained from the global PD and control comparison and based on disease duration and neuropathological staging. Log transformed ion abundance ratios are depicted, as represented by the scale. Darker green and red colors indicate the change intensity of the metabolite levels, respectively. Grey lines correspond to significant fold-changes of individual metabolites; darker grey colors have been used to highlight higher significances ($p < 0.05$, $p < 0.01$ or $p < 0.001$). It is relevant to highlight that metabolites have been ordered in the heatmap according to their carbon number and unsaturation degree of their acyl chains. Heatmap color codes for log2 (fold change) and unpaired Student's $t$-test $p$-values are indicated at the bottom of the heatmap. Metabolite order is supplied in the "Heatmap datasheet" in Tables S1–S3.

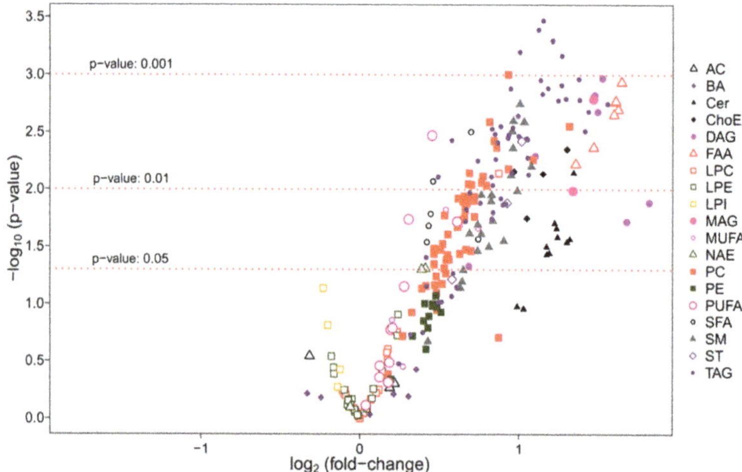


**Figure 4.** Volcano plot [−log10($p$-value) vs. log2(fold-change)] for the PD vs. control subjects comparison. This volcano plot highlights the significance $p$-value < 0.01 for glycerolipids and, more specifically, triacylglycerols (TAG).

Lipid classes were also calculated as the sum of the normalized areas of all the lipid metabolites with the same chemical characteristics (Table S1). Interestingly, all lipid classes significantly altered in PD subjects were increased. Changes in some of the most relevant metabolite classes are depicted in the boxplots shown in Figure 5.

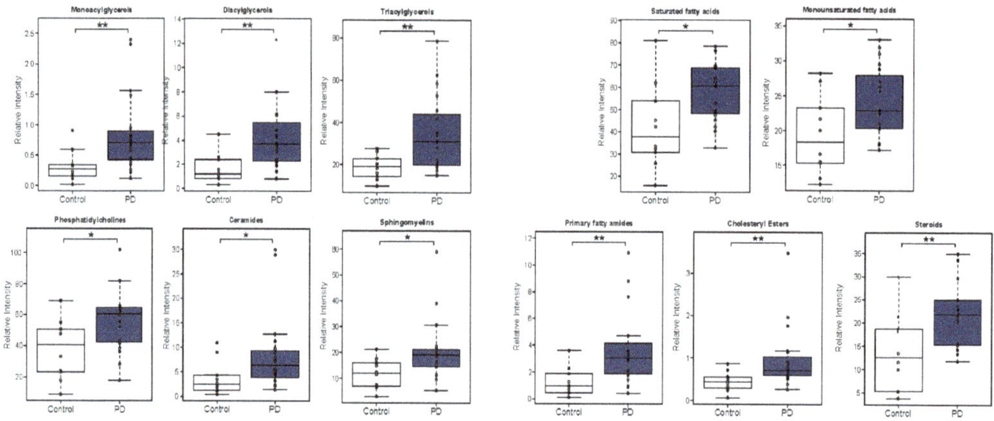


**Figure 5.** Boxplots of glycerolipids (monoacylglycerols (MAG), diacylglycerols (DAG), triacylglycerols (TAG)), phosphatidylcholines (PC) and sphingolipids (ceramides (Cer), sphingomyelins (SM)) (**left**). Boxplots of non-esterified fatty acids (NEFA) (saturated fatty acids (SFA), monounsaturated fatty acids (MUFA)), primary fatty amides (FAA) and sterol lipids (cholesteryl esters (ChoE), steroids (ST)) (**right**). significances (*; $p < 0.05$ and **; $p < 0.01$).

In order to help in the interpretation of the potential origin of the lipidomic changes in a biologically meaningful context, pathway analysis was performed, mapping the deregulated lipid species as well as the lipid metabolic enzymes involved in lipid biosynthetic routes (Figure 6).

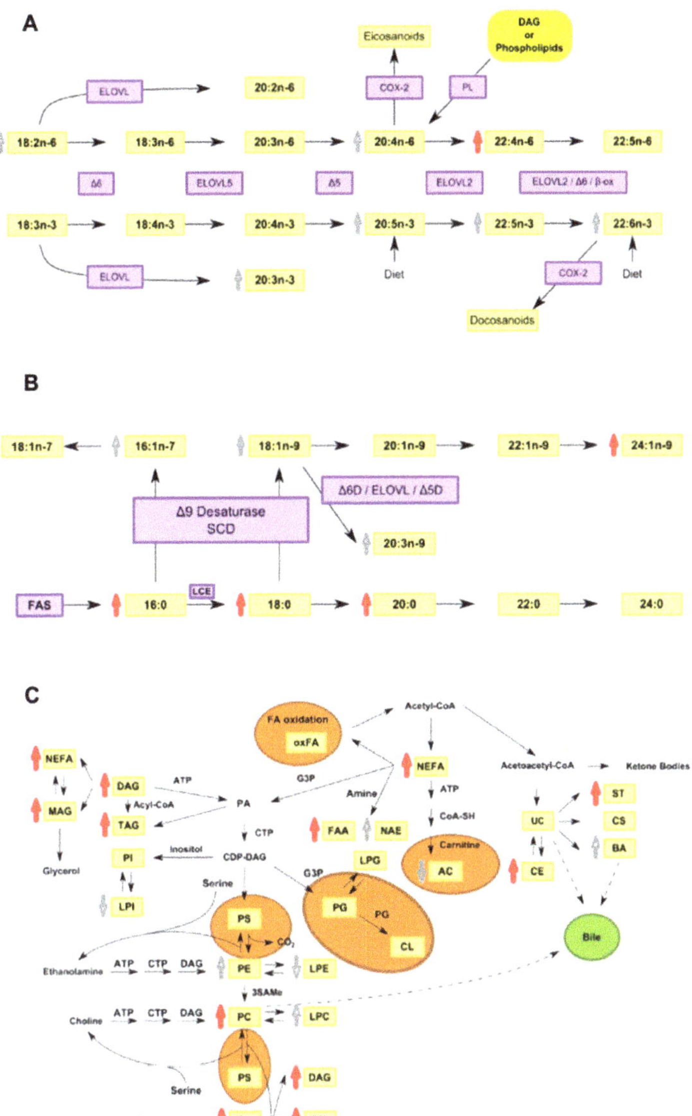


**Figure 6.** Pathway localization of deregulated lipid species detected in post-mortem CSF in PD. (**A**) Biosynthetic pathway of n-3 and n-6 fatty acids, (**B**) de novo lipogenesis and (**C**) lipid biosynthesis. Delta-6 desaturase (Δ6D), Delta-5 desaturase (Δ5D), elongase (ELOVL), beta-oxidation (β-ox), cyclooxygenase-2 (COX-2), phospholipases (PL). Fatty acid synthase (FAS), long-chain elongase (LCE), stearoyl-CoA desaturase (SCD), Glycerol 3-phosphate (G3P), phosphatidic acids (PA), phosphatidylinositols (PI), lysophosphatidylinositols (LPI), acyl carnitines (AC), unesterified cholesterol (UC), cholesterol sulfate (CS), cholesteryl esters (CE), steroids (ST), phodphatidylserines (PS), phosphatidylglycerols (PG), lysophosphatidylglycerols (LPG), cardiolipins (CL), S-adenosylmethionine (SAMe). Red arrows indicate significant increments in CSF lipid levels ($p < 0.05$). Grey arrows indicate non-significant increments in CSF lipid levels ($p > 0.05$). Orange areas represent routes carried out at the mitochondrial level.

## 4. Discussion

Brain lipids act as the major source of energy, provide insulation to cells and structural integrity to membranes and can be rapidly converted to signaling molecules or to inflammatory intermediates [24]. Thus, changes in lipid metabolism and its reflection on CSF lipid content might have a significant impact on brain function, contributing to PD pathogenesis [11,25]. Although the exact role of lipids in PD is not totally understood, the effects and/or levels of a subset of the lipidome have been partially characterized in plasma as well as in animal/cellular PD models [26]. However, brain levels of lipids may not correlate with plasma levels, so additional CSF measurements are needed to address the gap in knowledge about the potential pathological or compensatory composition of the brain lipidome in PD. In our case, all the lipid species which were found to be significantly increased in parkinsonian post-mortem CSF were: (i) several non-esterified fatty acids (NEFA), including the complete profile of saturated fatty acids (SFA), some monounsaturated fatty acids (MUFA) and a few polyunsaturated fatty acids (PUFA); (ii) various primary fatty amides (FAA) and N-acyl ethanolamines (NAE); (iii) almost the complete profile of glycerolipids, including monoacylglycerols (MAG), diacylglycerols (DAG) and triacylglycerols (TAG), (iv) several cholesteryl esters (ChoE) and steroids (ST), (v) almost the complete profile of phosphatidylcholines (PC) and (vi) the majority of ceramides (Cer) and sphingomyelins (SM). Moreover, our study demonstrated that CSF lipid homeostasis is differentially disrupted depending on neuropathological staging and disease duration. Several reasons may explain the over-representation of the characterized CSF lipidome in PD subjects. Lipid dyshomeostasis may be due to extensive synaptic dysfunction, severe lipid raft rearrangements and neuronal death, accompanied by membrane instability and tangled breakdown, contributing to an increment in lipid products in the CSF from PD subjects. Moreover, blood-brain-barrier (BBB) dysfunction is present in PD [27]. The opening of the BBB and the concomitant serum molecular infiltration inside the brain may trigger a multifactorial metabolic imbalance, leading to synaptic and neuronal dysfunction and adverse neuroinflammatory changes. One of these events may be the increment in lipid exchanges between CSF and the blood. However, bearing in mind that our workflow has allowed us to exclusively monitor around 250 lipid species, we cannot exclude the possibility that multiple lipid species not detected in this study may be underrepresented in parkinsonian CSFs. In fact, levels of some bile acids and multiple glycerophospholipids present a non-significant tendency to be lower in PD in respect to the control group (Table S1). Additional studies applying complementary lipidomic strategies in additional patient cohorts will facilitate the global interpretation about the lipid dyshomeostasis across biofluids in PD.

It has been speculated that SFA could exacerbate PD pathology [28]. Moreover, higher SFA levels are present in frontal cortical lipid rafts from PD subjects in respect to controls [29]. Using Drosophila mutant models, it has been shown that alpha-synuclein aggregation is facilitated by phospholipids with shorter acyl chains [30]. Interestingly, saturated phospholipids have been reported to improve alpha-synuclein aggregation and PD-like symptoms [31,32]. Although different CSF MUFA levels have been detected between several PD phenotypes, MUFA levels remain unchanged in the temporal cortex from PD subjects [33,34]. PUFA levels in the anterior cingulate cortex are increased in PD, although their CSF levels depend on the disease etiology [34,35]. At the molecular level, PUFA and alpha-synuclein are involved in the synaptic vesicle cycle [36]. Moreover, it has been evidenced that PUFA increase alpha synuclein oligomerization through the interaction with the N-terminal region [37,38]. With respect to glycerolipids, the exact function of MAG is unknown. While DAG is a secondary lipid messenger that plays a role in the synaptic vesicle cycle [39,40], TAG is directly involved in energy storage [41]. In the context of PD, plasma DAG and TAG tend to be diminished in PD, and higher serum TAG have been linked to a reduced risk of PD [42–44]. Alpha-synuclein overexpression has been directly related with intracellular TAG deposition [45,46].

In spite of CSF alterations in several cholesteryl esters (ChoE) and steroids (ST), little is known about the impact of sterols in PD pathogenesis. In general, sterols are known to play a role in immunity, membrane fluidity and serve as signaling mediators [47,48]. In PD, the cholesterol esterifying activity is reduced in fibroblasts and specific ChoE are reduced in the visual cortex [49,50]. Based on data obtained using several PD-related biological systems, it is not evident whether modulation of specific ChoE metabolic events may have a protective or pathological impact [51,52]. Phosphatidylcholine (PC), the most abundant glycerophospholipid in membranes, is involved in the control of inflammation, neuronal differentiation and cholesterol homeostasis [53–55]. Our data identified an increment in almost the complete profile of PCs at the level of CSF derived from PD subjects. However, decreased levels in multiple PCs have been observed in plasma, the frontal cortex and substantia nigra from PD patients [42,56,57]. This tendency has been also observed in substantia nigra and brain tissue derived from a mouse model of PD and from MPTP-treated goldfish, respectively [58,59]. Moreover, specific alpha-synuclein isoforms differentially interact with PC membranes [60–63].

Chronic neuroinflammation is a landmark of PD [64]. Sphingolipids, significantly increased in our study, have been recently proposed as potential diagnostic and therapeutic targets in PD, due to their direct involvement in neuroinflammation [65]. They are particularly relevant in immune-cell trafficking, cytokine signaling, production of pro-inflammatory eicosanoids and the regulation of cellular mechanisms involved in multiple inflammatory processes [66,67]. Specifically, an elevation in ceramide concentration can trigger neuronal apoptosis as well as astrocyte activation, playing a pro-inflammatory role [68,69]. However, the acyl chain length and the cell-type determine the functionality of ceramides as being long-chain ceramide mediators of pro-inflammatory phenotypes in microglial cells, whereas short-chain ones trigger anti-inflammatory mechanisms [65]. It has been proposed that different variations in ceramide (Cer) levels across brain areas may be linked to alpha-synuclein accumulation [26]. However, controversial data exist about the Cer plasma levels in PD patients [42,70,71]. In general, an increment in Cer levels is commonly observed in different studies performed in PD animal and cellular models [72–75]. However, the consequences associated with Cer increments are not fully understood, being potentially detrimental or beneficial for different PD-related mechanisms. It is important to note that CSF ceramides are also increased in other neurodegenerative diseases, such as AD and ALS, indicating that lipid imbalance may be partially common across neurological disorders [18,76]. Sphingomyelin (SM), a major myelin component, is considered a source of bioactive lipidic molecules which play a role in inflammation, autophagy and cell death [77–80]. According to our data obtained in CSF, SM accumulation has also been observed in: (i) LB aggregates [81], (ii) the primary visual cortex from PD subjects as well as in substantia nigra from males with PD [49,57] and (iii) PD patients with sphingomyelinase-1 mutations (risk factor) [82,83]. Although multiple factors suggest a potential role of SM accumulation in PD-associated neurodegeneration, more experimental evidence is needed to further elucidate the concise function of SM, not only in alpha-synuclein aggregation, but also in inflammatory balance.

In addition to the CSF Cer increment detected in PD, an increment in specific N-acylethanolamines and primary fatty amides (FAA) were also observed. N-acylethanolamines play an important role in various processes, from anti-inflammatory activities [84,85] to neuroprotective actions in PD models [86,87]. Specific FAA are sleep-inducing factors that may also affect memory processes, depress locomotor activity and are anti-inflammatory, anxiolytic and neuroprotective [88–91]. Interestingly, increased plasma FAA is associated with CSF beta-amyloids and clinical features [92]. The increment we observed in CSF FAA in PD was probably due to a dysfunctional synthesis-degradation efflux or transport. The major degradative step for FAA is the fatty acid amide hydrolase (FAAH) that degrades FAA to fatty acids and ammonia and also hydrolases the endocannabinoids. Pharmacological inhibition of FAAH leads to the inhibition of dopamine neuron death and reduces the immunoreactivity of microglial cells [93]. However, the precise role of FAA in alpha-synucleinopathies remains to be elucidated. Other lipid species with a pro-inflammatory role, such as platelet activating factors (PAFs) [94] or specific glycosphingolipids related to IL-1beta/IL-18 production, auto-antibody production and recruitment of peripheral immune cells within the CNS [95], were detected in our study, suggesting that additional workflows are needed to elucidate the full picture of inflammation-related CSF lipidome involved in PD.

It is important to note that our data obtained at the level of CSF partially corroborate previous associations between PD and the levels of fatty acyls, glycerolipids, glycerophospholipids, sphingolipids and sterols. Moreover, our pilot study established novel links between primary fatty amides (FAA) and N-acyl ethanolamines (NAE) with PD. However, although our untargeted lipidomic work has uncovered many intricacies in the CSF lipidomic homeostasis in the context of PD, there are potential limitations of our study that warrant discussion. First, due to the technological approach used, we failed to accurately monitor many lipid species present at low levels that might also participate in PD pathophysiology. Second, and based on the current knowledge, it is unclear whether the CSF lipid imbalance observed reflected pathological or compensatory mechanisms. Third, our study did not consider the effect of variables such as sex, age, PD etiology and/or mutational profiles.

Comparing our data with previously published works using early clinical PD biofluid samples, alteration of glycerophospholipid and sphingolipid metabolism was also observed at the plasma level [96]. However, the specific phosphatidylcholine, phosphatidylethanolamine and sphingomyelin profiles clearly differed with respect to our postmortem CSF data. Moreover, several studies have also indicated that sphingolipids (ceramides and sphingomyelins) are elevated in CSF derived from AD patients in respect to cognitively normal individuals [76,97]. Wood PL et al. [98] performed a lipidomic analysis in post-mortem CSF derived from AD subjects. In contrast, the differential lipidomic profile obtained was clearly different with respect to the lipid alterations we observed in post-mortem CSF from PD. Based on these data and taking into account the biomarker field, large cohorts of paired antemortem CSF and plasma samples should be used, not only from PD patients, but also from other synucleinopathies and tauopathies to obtain robust lipid-based conclusions in terms of biomarker specificity and sensitivity.

## 5. Conclusions

A CSF lipidomic approach performed in PD and control subjects ($n$ = 30) detected 257 metabolic features by ultra-high performance liquid chromatography-mass spectrometry (UHPLC-MS). A supervised OPLS model showed a clear separation between control and PD subjects, indicating that the lipids responsible for this separation were mainly glycerolipids (MAG, DAG, TAG), fatty acids (SFA, MUFA), primary fatty amides, glycerophospholipids (PC, PE) and sphingolipids (Cer, SM), which were increased in the PD group. Univariate data analysis also revealed a general increase in the CSF lipid metabolic profile in PD. Overall, these results suggest that: (i) multiple CSF lipid species tend to be increased in PD compared to control subjects and (ii) the dyshomeostasis observed in the parkinsonian CSF lipid profile varies depending on the disease duration and the neuropathological staging.

**Supplementary Materials:** The following are available online at https://www.mdpi.com/article/10.3390/biomedicines9050491/s1, Table S1: "Raw data per metabolite_1" and "Raw data per chemical class_1" contain raw intensity data per metabolites and per metabolite class of the untransformed data, respectively. "Raw data per metabolite_2" and "Raw data per chemical class_2" contain raw intensity data per metabolites and per metabolite class of the data after square root transformation of the data. These sheets also include: (i) "Individual notation", referring to the confirmed identification of the metabolites. Overlapping of two or more metabolites or non-confirmed identification is indicated in "Individual composition (or probable ID)", (ii) Average group intensities and standard errors, (iii) Shapiro test: used for testing the normality of data (Shapiro test ($p$) row is marked in red if the sample came from a normally distributed population), (iv) Fold-changes and unpaired Student's *t*-test *p*-values (or Welch´s *t* test where unequal variances were found) for the comparison PD vs. control and (v) "Heatmap" which contains the metabolites´ identification code, log2(fold-changes) and unpaired Student's *t*-test *p*-values illustrated in the heatmap. Table S2: "Raw data per metabolite" and "Raw data per chemical class" contain raw intensity data per metabolites and per metabolite class of the untransformed data, considering the neuropathological stage and the disease duration. Table S3: "Raw data per metabolite" and "Raw data per chemical class" contain raw intensity data per metabolites and per metabolite class after square root transformation of the data, considering the neuropathological stage and the disease duration.

**Author Contributions:** Conceptualization, E.S.; software, E.S., J.F.-I. and M.I.-L.; formal analysis, E.S., J.F.-I., P.C.-C. and M.I.-L.; investigation, E.S., J.F.-I. and P.C.-C.; resources, E.S. and J.F.-I.; funding acquisition, E.S. and J.F.-I.; writing—original draft preparation, E.S. All authors have read and agreed to the published version of the manuscript.

**Funding:** This work was funded by grants from the Spanish Ministry of Science Innovation and Universities (Ref. PID2019-110356RB-I00/AEI/10.13039/501100011033 to JF-I and ES) and the Department of Economic and Business Development from Government of Navarra (Ref. 0011-1411-2020-000028 to ES).

**Institutional Review Board Statement:** The study was conducted in accordance with the Declaration of Helsinki of 1975 (revised in 2013) and all assessments, post-mortem evaluations, and procedures were previously approved by the Local Clinical Ethics Committee (protocol code: 2016/36). Cerebrospinal fluid (CSF) samples and associated clinical and neuropathological data from patients with PD were supplied by the Parkinson's UK Brain Bank, funded by Parkinson's UK, a charity registered in England and Wales (258197) and in Scotland (SC037554).

**Informed Consent Statement:** According to the Spanish Law 14/2007 of Biomedical Research, informed written consent forms were obtained for research purposes from relatives of patients included in this study.

**Data Availability Statement:** Data available on request from the authors.

**Acknowledgments:** The authors are very grateful to the patients who generously donated the brain tissue and fluid samples for research purposes. The authors thank the collaboration of Parkinson's UK Brain Bank funded by Parkinson's UK, a charity registered in England and Wales (258197) and in Scotland (SC037554). The authors want to kindly thank Djordje Gveric (Centre for Brain Sciences, Imperial College London, London, UK) and technical personnel from OWL Metabolomics company (Derio, Spain) for their help in the management of associated clinical, neuropathological and molecular data. The Proteomics Unit of Navarrabiomed is a member of ProteoRed and PRB3-ISCIII and is supported by grant PT17/0019, of the PE I+D+I 2013–2016, funded by ISCIII and ERDF.

**Conflicts of Interest:** The authors declare no conflict of interest.

## Abbreviations

AC: acyl carnitines; BA: bile acids; Cer: ceramides; ChoE: cholesteryl esters; DAG: diacylglycerides; FAA: fatty acid amides (primary fatty amides); LPE: lysophosphatidylethanolamines; LPI: lysophosphatidylinositols; LPC: lysophosphatidylcholines; MAG: monoacylglycerides; MUFA: monounsaturated fatty acids; NAE: N-acyl ethanolamines; NEFA: non-esterified fatty acids; OPLS: orthogonal partial least-squares to latent structures; PC: phosphatidylcholines; PCA: Principal Component Analysis; PE: phosphatidylethanolamines; PUFA: polyunsaturated fatty acids; SFA: saturated fatty acids; SM: sphingomyelins; TAG: triacylglycerides; UFA: unsaturated fatty acids.

## Appendix A

**Table A1.** Internal Standard (IS) Solutions Platform 1.

| IS | IS Stock Solution (μg/mL) | IS Stock Solution | IS Intermediate Solution in $CHCl_3$:MeOH (2:1) (μg/mL) | IS Working Solution in MeOH (μg/mL) |
|---|---|---|---|---|
| **13:0 Lyso PC** | 10,000 | $CHCl_3$ | 10 | 0.1 |
| **Dehydrocholic acid** | 5000 | $CHCl_3$:MeOH (1:1) | 30 | 0.3 |
| **Nonadecanoic acid** | 10,000 | $CHCl_3$ | 500 | 5.0 |
| **Tryptophan-(indole-d5)** | 5000 | 0.05% Formic acid in water | 200 | 2.0 |

**Table A2.** Internal Standard Solutions Platform 2.

| IS | IS Stock Solution (μg/mL) | IS Stock Solution | Working IS Solution $CHCl_3$:MeOH (2:1) (μg/mL) |
|---|---|---|---|
| **SM (d18:1/6:0)** | 5000 | $CHCl_3$ | 5 |
| **PE (17:0/17:0)** | 10,000 | $CHCl_3$:MeOH:$H_2O$ | 50 |
| **PC (19:0/19:0)** | 10,000 | $CHCl_3$ | 10 |
| **TG (13:0/13:0/13:0)** | 10,000 | $CHCl_3$ | 5 |
| **TG (17:0/17:0/17:0)** | 10,000 | $CHCl_3$ | 5 |
| **Cer(d18:1/17:0)** | 10,000 | $CHCl_3$ | 10 |
| **ChoE(12:0)** | 10,000 | $CHCl_3$ | 250 |

Multivariate data analysis of all CSF samples, pool samples and quality control (QC) samples was initially performed. Score scatter plot corresponding to PCA analysis of these samples is shown in Figure 2. Proximity and overlap of the Pool and QC injections provides a good indication of the reproducibility and quality of the measurements.

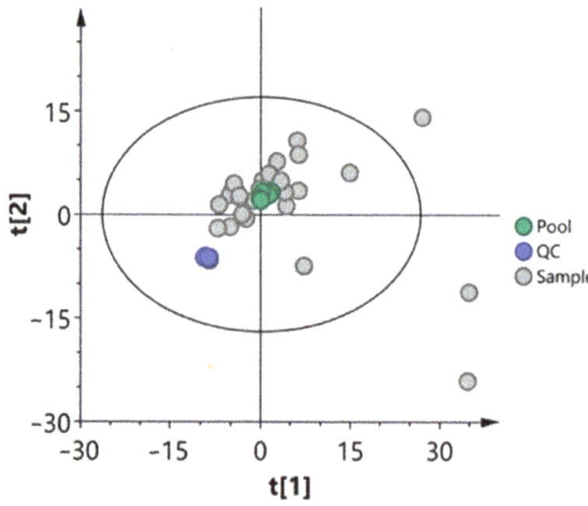


**Figure A1.** Score scatter plot of the PCA model of CSF, Pool and QC samples. Pool: 15 μl of each CSF sample was collected and pooled together. Model diagnostics (A = 6, R2X = 0.829, Q2X = 0.496).

After validating the quality of the experiment, the Pool and QC injections were removed from the analysis and a score scatter plot of the PCA model of all cerebrospinal fluid samples was generated.

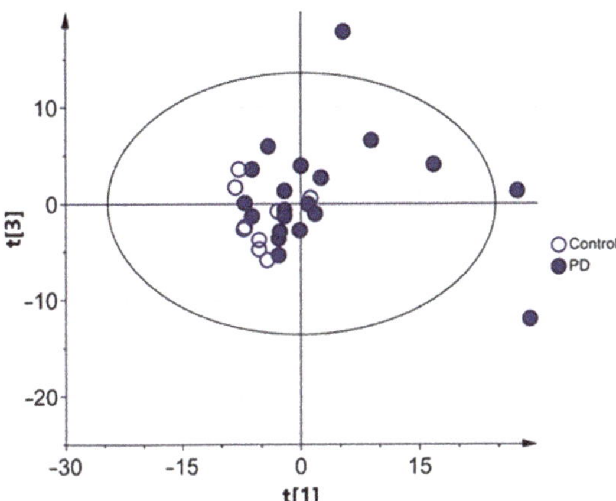


**Figure A2.** Score scatter plot of the PCA model of CSF samples. Model diagnostics (A = 6, R2X = 0.807, Q2X = 0.401).

The Shapiro–Wilk test was used for testing the normality of data (results included in Table S1), revealing that the majority of the metabolites measured in the CSF samples from PD patients were not following a normal distribution. Then, the Box–Cox method for correcting non-normally distributed data by variable transformations was applied, identifying the square root transformation as optimal for most of the metabolites. This kind of transformation is a common pre-treatment method in metabolomics for the conversion of the data, which corrects aspects that hinder the biological interpretation of data sets by emphasizing the biological information and thus, improving their physiological interpretability. Score scatter plot corresponding to PCA analysis of CSF samples after square root transformation of the data is shown in Figure A3.

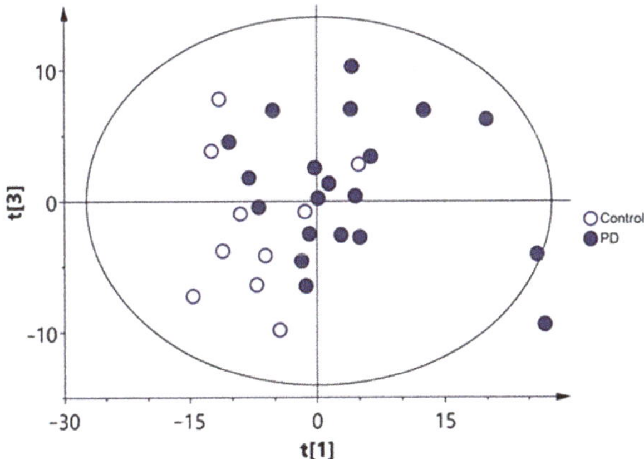


**Figure A3.** Score scatter plot of the PCA model of CSF samples after square root transformation of the data. Model diagnostics (A = 4, R2X = 0.752, Q2X = 0.505).

This score scatter plot showed certain clustering of samples according to the presence or absence of the disease and identified sample PD353 as a potential outlier, since it appeared outside the Hotelling´s T2 ellipse. Following Chauvenet's criterion, further inspection of the data relating to this sample revealed that it presented elevated levels of sphingolipids compared to the rest of the samples from the PD group. However, the levels of the majority of the metabolites in this sample were similar to those of the samples from the same group and thus, it was not excluded from the multivariate and univariate analyses. Metabolites responsible for this certain separation observed between CSF samples of PD and control subjects can be observed in the loadings scatter plot (Figure A4), which is a graph related to the score scatter plot shown in Figure A3.

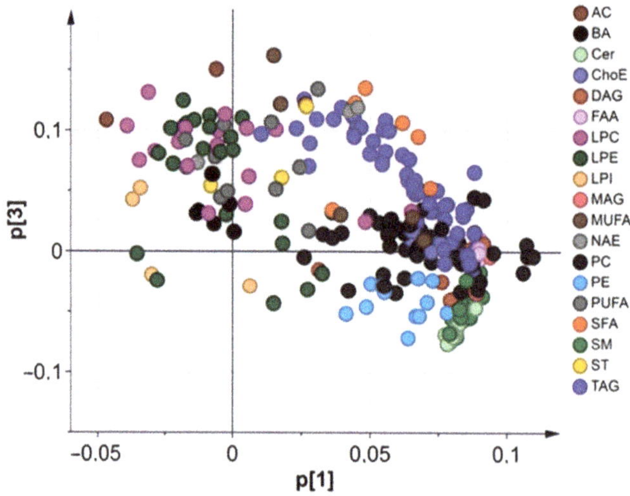


**Figure A4.** Loadings scatter plot of the PCA model of cerebrospinal fluid samples after square root transformation of the data. Model diagnostics (A = 4, R2X = 0.752, Q2X = 0.505).

Lipids lying away from the plot origin have a stronger impact on the model; besides, variables positively correlated are grouped together, while variables negatively correlated are positioned in the opposite sides of the plot origin. In this case, the metabolites responsible for the differences observed were mainly glycerolipids (monoacylglycerols (MAG), diacylglycerols (DAG), triacylglycerols (TAG)), fatty acids (saturated fatty acids (SFA), monounsaturated fatty acids (MUFA)), primary fatty amides (FAA), glycerophospholipids (phosphatidylcholines (PC), phosphatidylethanolamines (PE)) and sphingolipids (ceramides (Cer), sphingomyelins (SM)), which were increased in PD compared to the control group; and lysoglycerophospholipids (lysophosphatidylcholines (LP), lysophosphatidylethanolamines (LPE), lyshophosphatidylinositols (LPI)) and bile acids (BA), which seemed to be increased in controls compared to the PD group.

## References


1. Shevchenko, A.; Simons, K. Lipidomics: Coming to Grips with Lipid Diversity. *Nat. Rev. Mol. Cell Biol.* **2010**, *11*, 593–598. [CrossRef]
2. Brugger, B. Lipidomics: Analysis of the Lipid Composition of Cells and Subcellular Organelles by Electrospray Ionization Mass Spectrometry. *Annu. Rev. Biochem.* **2014**, *83*, 79–98. [CrossRef]
3. Piomelli, D.; Astarita, G.; Rapaka, R. A Neuroscientist's Guide to Lipidomics. *Nat. Rev. Neurosci.* **2007**, *8*, 743–754. [CrossRef]
4. Gross, R.W.; Han, X. Lipidomics at the Interface of Structure and Function in Systems Biology. *Chem. Biol.* **2011**, *18*, 284–291. [CrossRef]

5. Lauwers, E.; Goodchild, R.; Verstreken, P. Membrane Lipids in Presynaptic Function and Disease. *Neuron* **2016**, *90*, 11–25. [CrossRef]
6. Klemann, C.; Martens, G.J.M.; Sharma, M.; Martens, M.B.; Isacson, O.; Gasser, T.; Visser, J.E.; Poelmans, G. Integrated Molecular Landscape of Parkinson's Disease. *NPJ Parkinsons Dis.* **2017**, *3*, 14. [CrossRef]
7. Sidransky, E.; Lopez, G. The Link between the GBA Gene and Parkinsonism. *Lancet Neurol.* **2012**, *11*, 986–998. [CrossRef]
8. Do, C.B.; Tung, J.Y.; Dorfman, E.; Kiefer, A.K.; Drabant, E.M.; Francke, U.; Mountain, J.L.; Goldman, S.M.; Tanner, C.M.; Langston, J.W.; et al. Web-Based Genome-Wide Association Study Identifies Two Novel Loci and a Substantial Genetic Component for Parkinson's Disease. *PLoS Genet.* **2011**, *7*, e1002141. [CrossRef] [PubMed]
9. Pankratz, N.; Wilk, J.B.; Latourelle, J.C.; DeStefano, A.L.; Halter, C.; Pugh, E.W.; Doheny, K.F.; Gusella, J.F.; Nichols, W.C.; Foroud, T.; et al. Genomewide Association Study for Susceptibility Genes Contributing to Familial Parkinson Disease. *Hum. Genet* **2009**, *124*, 593–605. [CrossRef] [PubMed]
10. Robak, L.A.; Jansen, I.E.; van Rooij, J.; Uitterlinden, A.G.; Kraaij, R.; Jankovic, J.; Heutink, P.; Shulman, J.M. Excessive Burden of Lysosomal Storage Disorder Gene Variants in Parkinson's Disease. *Brain* **2017**, *140*, 3191–3203. [CrossRef]
11. Fanning, S.; Selkoe, D.; Dettmer, U. Vesicle Trafficking and Lipid Metabolism in Synucleinopathy. *Acta Neuropathol.* **2021**, *141*, 491–510. [CrossRef] [PubMed]
12. Galvagnion, C. The Role of Lipids Interacting with Alpha-Synuclein in the Pathogenesis of Parkinson's Disease. *J. Parkinsons Dis.* **2017**, *7*, 433–450. [CrossRef] [PubMed]
13. Shahmoradian, S.H.; Lewis, A.J.; Genoud, C.; Hench, J.; Moors, T.E.; Navarro, P.P.; Castano-Diez, D.; Schweighauser, G.; Graff-Meyer, A.; Goldie, K.N.; et al. Lewy Pathology in Parkinson's Disease Consists of Crowded Organelles and Lipid Membranes. *Nat. Neurosci.* **2019**, *22*, 1099–1109. [CrossRef]
14. Seyer, A.; Boudah, S.; Broudin, S.; Junot, C.; Colsch, B. Annotation of the Human Cerebrospinal Fluid Lipidome Using High Resolution Mass Spectrometry and a Dedicated Data Processing Workflow. *Metabolomics* **2016**, *12*, 91. [CrossRef]
15. Naudi, A.; Cabre, R.; Jove, M.; Ayala, V.; Gonzalo, H.; Portero-Otin, M.; Ferrer, I.; Pamplona, R. Lipidomics of Human Brain Aging and Alzheimer's Disease Pathology. *Int. Rev. Neurobiol.* **2015**, *122*, 133–189. [PubMed]
16. Liebisch, G.; Ahrends, R.; Makoto, A.; Masanori, A.; Bowden, J.A.; Ejsing, C.S.; Griffiths, W.J.; Holcapek, M.; Köfeler, H.; Mitchell, T.W. Lipidomics Needs More Standardization. *Nat. Metab.* **2019**, *1*, 745–747.
17. Proitsi, P.; Kim, M.; Whiley, L.; Simmons, A.; Sattlecker, M.; Velayudhan, L.; Lupton, M.K.; Soininen, H.; Kloszewska, I.; Mecocci, P.; et al. Association of Blood Lipids with Alzheimer's Disease: A Comprehensive Lipidomics Analysis. *Alzheimers Dement* **2017**, *13*, 140–151. [CrossRef]
18. Wong, M.W.; Braidy, N.; Poljak, A.; Pickford, R.; Thambisetty, M.; Sachdev, P.S. Dysregulation of Lipids in Alzheimer's Disease and Their Role as Potential Biomarkers. *Alzheimers Dement* **2017**, *13*, 810–827. [CrossRef] [PubMed]
19. Gonzalo, H.; Brieva, L.; Tatzber, F.; Jove, M.; Cacabelos, D.; Cassanye, A.; Lanau-Angulo, L.; Boada, J.; Serrano, J.C.; Gonzalez, C.; et al. Lipidome Analysis in Multiple Sclerosis Reveals Protein Lipoxidative Damage as a Potential Pathogenic Mechanism. *J. Neurochem.* **2012**, *123*, 622–634. [CrossRef]
20. Pieragostino, D.; Cicalini, I.; Lanuti, P.; Ercolino, E.; di Ioia, M.; Zucchelli, M.; Zappacosta, R.; Miscia, S.; Marchisio, M.; Sacchetta, P.; et al. Enhanced Release of Acid Sphingomyelinase-Enriched Exosomes Generates a Lipidomics Signature in CSF of Multiple Sclerosis Patients. *Sci. Rep.* **2018**, *8*, 3071. [CrossRef]
21. Blasco, H.; Veyrat-Durebex, C.; Bocca, C.; Patin, F.; Vourc'h, P.; Kouassi Nzoughet, J.; Lenaers, G.; Andres, C.R.; Simard, G.; Corcia, P.; et al. Lipidomics Reveals Cerebrospinal-Fluid Signatures of ALS. *Sci. Rep.* **2017**, *7*, 17652. [CrossRef]
22. Millan, L.; Fernandez-Irigoyen, J.; Santamaria, E.; Mayo, R. Mass Spectrometry Applied to Human Cerebrospinal Fluid Lipidome. *Methods Mol. Biol.* **2019**, *2044*, 353–361.
23. Barr, J.; Vazquez-Chantada, M.; Alonso, C.; Perez-Cormenzana, M.; Mayo, R.; Galan, A.; Caballeria, J.; Martin-Duce, A.; Tran, A.; Wagner, C.; et al. Liquid Chromatography-Mass Spectrometry-Based Parallel Metabolic Profiling of Human and Mouse Model Serum Reveals Putative Biomarkers Associated with the Progression of Nonalcoholic Fatty Liver Disease. *J. Proteome Res.* **2010**, *9*, 4501–4512. [CrossRef]
24. Fonteh, A.N.; Harrington, R.J.; Huhmer, A.F.; Biringer, R.G.; Riggins, J.N.; Harrington, M.G. Identification of Disease Markers in Human Cerebrospinal Fluid Using Lipidomic and Proteomic Methods. *Dis. Markers* **2006**, *22*, 39–64. [CrossRef] [PubMed]
25. Fanning, S.; Selkoe, D.; Dettmer, U. Parkinson's Disease: Proteinopathy or Lipidopathy? *NPJ Parkinsons Dis.* **2020**, *6*, 3. [CrossRef]
26. Xicoy, H.; Wieringa, B.; Martens, G.J.M. The Role of Lipids in Parkinson's Disease. *Cells* **2019**, *8*, 27. [CrossRef] [PubMed]
27. Sweeney, M.D.; Sagare, A.P.; Zlokovic, B.V. Blood-Brain Barrier Breakdown in Alzheimer Disease and Other Neurodegenerative Disorders. *Nat. Rev. Neurol.* **2018**, *14*, 133–150. [CrossRef] [PubMed]
28. Kamel, F.; Goldman, S.M.; Umbach, D.M.; Chen, H.; Richardson, G.; Barber, M.R.; Meng, C.; Marras, C.; Korell, M.; Kasten, M.; et al. Dietary Fat Intake, Pesticide Use, and Parkinson's Disease. *Parkinsonism Relat. Disord.* **2014**, *20*, 82–87. [CrossRef] [PubMed]
29. Fabelo, N.; Martin, V.; Santpere, G.; Marin, R.; Torrent, L.; Ferrer, I.; Diaz, M. Severe Alterations in Lipid Composition of Frontal Cortex Lipid Rafts from Parkinson's Disease and Incidental Parkinson's Disease. *Mol. Med.* **2011**, *17*, 1107–1118. [CrossRef] [PubMed]

30. Mori, A.; Hatano, T.; Inoshita, T.; Shiba-Fukushima, K.; Koinuma, T.; Meng, H.; Kubo, S.I.; Spratt, S.; Cui, C.; Yamashita, C.; et al. Parkinson's Disease-Associated iPLA2-VIA/PLA2G6 Regulates Neuronal Functions and Alpha-Synuclein Stability Through Membrane Remodeling. *Proc. Natl. Acad. Sci. USA* **2019**, *116*, 20689–20699. [CrossRef]
31. Imberdis, T.; Negri, J.; Ramalingam, N.; Terry-Kantor, E.; Ho, G.P.H.; Fanning, S.; Stirtz, G.; Kim, T.E.; Levy, O.A.; Young-Pearse, T.L.; et al. Cell Models of Lipid-Rich Alpha-Synuclein Aggregation Validate Known Modifiers of Alpha-Synuclein Biology and Identify Stearoyl-CoA Desaturase. *Proc. Natl. Acad. Sci. USA* **2019**, *116*, 20760–20769. [CrossRef] [PubMed]
32. Nuber, S.; Nam, A.Y.; Rajsombath, M.M.; Cirka, H.; Hronowski, X.; Wang, J.; Hodgetts, K.; Kalinichenko, L.S.; Muller, C.P.; Lambrecht, V.; et al. A Stearoyl-Coenzyme A Desaturase Inhibitor Prevents Multiple Parkinson Disease Phenotypes in alpha-Synuclein Mice. *Ann. Neurol.* **2021**, *89*, 74–90. [CrossRef] [PubMed]
33. Julien, C.; Berthiaume, L.; Hadj-Tahar, A.; Rajput, A.H.; Bedard, P.J.; Di Paolo, T.; Julien, P.; Calon, F. Postmortem Brain Fatty Acid Profile of Levodopa-Treated Parkinson Disease Patients and Parkinsonian Monkeys. *Neurochem. Int.* **2006**, *48*, 404–414. [CrossRef] [PubMed]
34. Schmid, S.P.; Schleicher, E.D.; Cegan, A.; Deuschle, C.; Baur, S.; Hauser, A.K.; Synofzik, M.; Srulijes, K.; Brockmann, K.; Berg, D.; et al. Cerebrospinal Fluid Fatty Acids in Glucocerebrosidase-Associated Parkinson's Disease. *Mov. Disord.* **2012**, *27*, 288–292. [CrossRef]
35. Abbott, S.K.; Jenner, A.M.; Spiro, A.S.; Batterham, M.; Halliday, G.M.; Garner, B. Fatty Acid Composition of the Anterior Cingulate Cortex Indicates a High Susceptibility to Lipid Peroxidation in Parkinson's Disease. *J. Parkinsons Dis.* **2015**, *5*, 175–185. [CrossRef] [PubMed]
36. Ben Gedalya, T.; Loeb, V.; Israeli, E.; Altschuler, Y.; Selkoe, D.J.; Sharon, R. Alpha-Synuclein and Polyunsaturated Fatty Acids Promote Clathrin-Mediated Endocytosis and Synaptic Vesicle Recycling. *Traffic* **2009**, *10*, 218–234. [CrossRef] [PubMed]
37. Sharon, R.; Bar-Joseph, I.; Frosch, M.P.; Walsh, D.M.; Hamilton, J.A.; Selkoe, D.J. The Formation of Highly Soluble Oligomers of Alpha-Synuclein is Regulated by Fatty Acids and Enhanced in Parkinson's Disease. *Neuron* **2003**, *37*, 583–595. [CrossRef]
38. Perrin, R.J.; Woods, W.S.; Clayton, D.F.; George, J.M. Exposure to Long Chain Polyunsaturated Fatty Acids Triggers Rapid Multimerization of Synucleins. *J. Biol. Chem.* **2001**, *276*, 41958–41962. [CrossRef] [PubMed]
39. Tu-Sekine, B.; Goldschmidt, H.; Raben, D.M. Diacylglycerol, Phosphatidic Acid, and Their Metabolic Enzymes in Synaptic Vesicle Recycling. *Adv. Biol. Regul.* **2015**, *57*, 147–152. [CrossRef] [PubMed]
40. Almena, M.; Merida, I. Shaping Up the Membrane: Diacylglycerol Coordinates Spatial Orientation of Signaling. *Trends Biochem. Sci.* **2011**, *36*, 593–603. [CrossRef]
41. Ahmadian, M.; Duncan, R.E.; Jaworski, K.; Sarkadi-Nagy, E.; Sul, H.S. Triacylglycerol Metabolism in Adipose Tissue. *Future Lipidol.* **2007**, *2*, 229–237. [CrossRef] [PubMed]
42. Zhang, J.; Zhang, X.; Wang, L.; Yang, C. High Performance Liquid Chromatography-Mass Spectrometry (LC-MS) Based Quantitative Lipidomics Study of Ganglioside-NANA-3 Plasma to Establish Its Association with Parkinson's Disease Patients. *Med. Sci. Monit.* **2017**, *23*, 5345–5353. [CrossRef] [PubMed]
43. Chan, R.B.; Perotte, A.J.; Zhou, B.; Liong, C.; Shorr, E.J.; Marder, K.S.; Kang, U.J.; Waters, C.H.; Levy, O.A.; Xu, Y.; et al. Elevated GM3 Plasma Concentration in Idiopathic Parkinson's Disease: A Lipidomic Analysis. *PLoS ONE* **2017**, *12*, e0172348. [CrossRef]
44. Vikdahl, M.; Backman, L.; Johansson, I.; Forsgren, L.; Haglin, L. Cardiovascular Risk Factors and the Risk of Parkinson's Disease. *Eur. J. Clin. Nutr.* **2015**, *69*, 729–733. [CrossRef]
45. He, Q.; Wang, M.; Petucci, C.; Gardell, S.J.; Han, X. Rotenone Induces Reductive Stress and Triacylglycerol Deposition in C2C12 Cells. *Int. J. Biochem. Cell Biol.* **2013**, *45*, 2749–2755. [CrossRef]
46. Sere, Y.Y.; Regnacq, M.; Colas, J.; Berges, T. A Saccharomyces Cerevisiae Strain Unable to Store Neutral Lipids is Tolerant to Oxidative Stress Induced by Alpha-Synuclein. *Free. Radic. Biol. Med.* **2010**, *49*, 1755–1764. [CrossRef]
47. Spann, N.J.; Glass, C.K. Sterols and Oxysterols in Immune Cell Function. *Nat. Immunol.* **2013**, *14*, 893–900. [CrossRef]
48. Hannich, J.T.; Umebayashi, K.; Riezman, H. Distribution and Functions of Sterols and Sphingolipids. *Cold Spring Harb. Perspect. Biol.* **2011**, *3*, a004762. [CrossRef]
49. Cheng, D.; Jenner, A.M.; Shui, G.; Cheong, W.F.; Mitchell, T.W.; Nealon, J.R.; Kim, W.S.; McCann, H.; Wenk, M.R.; Halliday, G.M.; et al. Lipid Pathway Alterations in Parkinson's Disease Primary Visual Cortex. *PLoS ONE* **2011**, *6*, e17299. [CrossRef] [PubMed]
50. Musanti, R.; Parati, E.; Lamperti, E.; Ghiselli, G. Decreased Cholesterol Biosynthesis in Fibroblasts from Patients with Parkinson Disease. *Biochem. Med. Metab. Biol.* **1993**, *49*, 133–142. [CrossRef] [PubMed]
51. Magalhaes, J.; Gegg, M.E.; Migdalska-Richards, A.; Doherty, M.K.; Whitfield, P.D.; Schapira, A.H. Autophagic Lysosome Reformation Dysfunction in Glucocerebrosidase Deficient Cells: Relevance to Parkinson Disease. *Hum. Mol. Genet.* **2016**, *25*, 3432–3445. [CrossRef]
52. Zhang, S.; Glukhova, S.A.; Caldwell, K.A.; Caldwell, G.A. NCEH-1 Modulates Cholesterol Metabolism and Protects Against Alpha-Synuclein Toxicity in a C. Elegans Model of Parkinson's Disease. *Hum. Mol. Genet.* **2017**, *26*, 3823–3836. [CrossRef]
53. Treede, I.; Braun, A.; Sparla, R.; Kuhnel, M.; Giese, T.; Turner, J.R.; Anes, E.; Kulaksiz, H.; Fullekrug, J.; Stremmel, W.; et al. Anti-Inflammatory Effects of Phosphatidylcholine. *J. Biol. Chem.* **2007**, *282*, 27155–27164. [CrossRef]
54. Lagace, T.A. Phosphatidylcholine: Greasing the Cholesterol Transport Machinery. *Lipid Insights* **2015**, *8*, 65–73. [CrossRef] [PubMed]

55. Marcucci, H.; Paoletti, L.; Jackowski, S.; Banchio, C. Phosphatidylcholine Biosynthesis during Neuronal Differentiation and Its Role in Cell Fate Determination. *J. Biol. Chem.* **2010**, *285*, 25382–25393. [CrossRef]
56. Wood, P.L.; Tippireddy, S.; Feriante, J.; Woltjer, R.L. Augmented Frontal Cortex Diacylglycerol Levels in Parkinson's Disease and Lewy Body Disease. *PLoS ONE* **2018**, *13*, e0191815. [CrossRef] [PubMed]
57. Seyfried, T.N.; Choi, H.; Chevalier, A.; Hogan, D.; Akgoc, Z.; Schneider, J.S. Sex-Related Abnormalities in Substantia Nigra Lipids in Parkinson's Disease. *ASN Neuro* **2018**, *10*, 1759091418781889. [CrossRef] [PubMed]
58. Farmer, K.; Smith, C.A.; Hayley, S.; Smith, J. Major Alterations of Phosphatidylcholine and Lysophosphotidylcholine Lipids in the Substantia Nigra Using an Early Stage Model of Parkinson's Disease. *Int. J. Mol. Sci.* **2015**, *16*, 18865–18877. [CrossRef] [PubMed]
59. Lu, Z.; Wang, J.; Li, M.; Liu, Q.; Wei, D.; Yang, M.; Kong, L. (1)H NMR-Based Metabolomics Study on a Goldfish Model of Parkinson's Disease Induced by 1-Methyl-4-Phenyl-1,2,3,6-Tetrahydropyridine (MPTP). *Chem. Biol. Interact.* **2014**, *223*, 18–26. [CrossRef] [PubMed]
60. Stockl, M.; Fischer, P.; Wanker, E.; Herrmann, A. Alpha-Synuclein Selectively Binds to Anionic Phospholipids Embedded in Liquid-Disordered Domains. *J. Mol. Biol.* **2008**, *375*, 1394–1404. [CrossRef]
61. Jiang, Z.; de Messieres, M.; Lee, J.C. Membrane Remodeling by Alpha-Synuclein and Effects on Amyloid Formation. *J. Am. Chem. Soc.* **2013**, *135*, 15970–15973. [CrossRef] [PubMed]
62. Di Pasquale, E.; Fantini, J.; Chahinian, H.; Maresca, M.; Taieb, N.; Yahi, N. Altered Ion Channel Formation by the Parkinson's-Disease-Linked E46K Mutant of Alpha-Synuclein is Corrected by GM3 but not by GM1 Gangliosides. *J. Mol. Biol.* **2010**, *397*, 202–218. [CrossRef] [PubMed]
63. O'Leary, E.I.; Jiang, Z.; Strub, M.P.; Lee, J.C. Effects of Phosphatidylcholine Membrane Fluidity on the Conformation and Aggregation of N-Terminally Acetylated Alpha-Synuclein. *J. Biol. Chem.* **2018**, *293*, 11195–11205. [CrossRef]
64. Hirsch, E.C.; Standaert, D.G. Ten Unsolved Questions About Neuroinflammation in Parkinson's Disease. *Mov. Disord.* **2021**, *36*, 16–24. [CrossRef] [PubMed]
65. Lee, J.Y.; Jin, H.K.; Bae, J.S. Sphingolipids in Neuroinflammation: A Potential Target for Diagnosis and Therapy. *BMB Rep.* **2020**, *53*, 28–34. [CrossRef] [PubMed]
66. Hannun, Y.A.; Obeid, L.M. Sphingolipids and Their Metabolism in Physiology and Disease. *Nat. Rev. Mol. Cell Biol.* **2018**, *19*, 175–191. [CrossRef]
67. Assi, E.; Cazzato, D.; De Palma, C.; Perrotta, C.; Clementi, E.; Cervia, D. Sphingolipids and Brain Resident Macrophages in Neuroinflammation: An Emerging Aspect of Nervous System Pathology. *Clin. Dev. Immunol.* **2013**, *2013*, 309302. [CrossRef]
68. Young, M.M.; Kester, M.; Wang, H.G. Sphingolipids: Regulators of Crosstalk between Apoptosis and Autophagy. *J. Lipid Res.* **2013**, *54*, 5–19. [CrossRef]
69. de Wit, N.M.; den Hoedt, S.; Martinez-Martinez, P.; Rozemuller, A.J.; Mulder, M.T.; de Vries, H.E. Astrocytic Ceramide as Possible Indicator of Neuroinflammation. *J. Neuroinflammation* **2019**, *16*, 48. [CrossRef]
70. Mielke, M.M.; Maetzler, W.; Haughey, N.J.; Bandaru, V.V.; Savica, R.; Deuschle, C.; Gasser, T.; Hauser, A.K.; Graber-Sultan, S.; Schleicher, E.; et al. Plasma Ceramide and Glucosylceramide Metabolism is Altered in Sporadic Parkinson's Disease and Associated with Cognitive Impairment: A Pilot Study. *PLoS ONE* **2013**, *8*, e73094. [CrossRef]
71. Atashrazm, F.; Hammond, D.; Perera, G.; Dobson-Stone, C.; Mueller, N.; Pickford, R.; Kim, W.S.; Kwok, J.B.; Lewis, S.J.G.; Halliday, G.M.; et al. Reduced Glucocerebrosidase Activity in Monocytes from Patients with Parkinson's Disease. *Sci. Rep.* **2018**, *8*, 15446. [CrossRef] [PubMed]
72. Lupescu, A.; Jilani, K.; Zbidah, M.; Lang, F. Induction of Apoptotic Erythrocyte Death by Rotenone. *Toxicology* **2012**, *300*, 132–137. [CrossRef] [PubMed]
73. Lin, G.; Lee, P.T.; Chen, K.; Mao, D.; Tan, K.L.; Zuo, Z.; Lin, W.W.; Wang, L.; Bellen, H.J. Phospholipase PLA2G6, a Parkinsonism-Associated Gene, Affects Vps26 and Vps35, Retromer Function, and Ceramide Levels, Similar to Alpha-Synuclein Gain. *Cell Metab.* **2018**, *28*, 605–618.e6. [CrossRef] [PubMed]
74. Ferrazza, R.; Cogo, S.; Melrose, H.; Bubacco, L.; Greggio, E.; Guella, G.; Civiero, L.; Plotegher, N. LRRK2 Deficiency Impacts Ceramide Metabolism in Brain. *Biochem. Biophys. Res. Commun.* **2016**, *478*, 1141–1146. [CrossRef] [PubMed]
75. Torres-Odio, S.; Key, J.; Hoepken, H.H.; Canet-Pons, J.; Valek, L.; Roller, B.; Walter, M.; Morales-Gordo, B.; Meierhofer, D.; Harter, P.N.; et al. Progression of Pathology in PINK1-Deficient Mouse Brain from Splicing via Ubiquitination, ER Stress, and Mitophagy Changes to Neuroinflammation. *J. Neuroinflamm.* **2017**, *14*, 154. [CrossRef] [PubMed]
76. Satoi, H.; Tomimoto, H.; Ohtani, R.; Kitano, T.; Kondo, T.; Watanabe, M.; Oka, N.; Akiguchi, I.; Furuya, S.; Hirabayashi, Y.; et al. Astroglial Expression of Ceramide in Alzheimer's Disease Brains: A Role during Neuronal Apoptosis. *Neuroscience* **2005**, *130*, 657–666. [CrossRef] [PubMed]
77. Nixon, G.F. Sphingolipids in Inflammation: Pathological Implications and Potential Therapeutic Targets. *Br. J. Pharmacol.* **2009**, *158*, 982–993. [CrossRef] [PubMed]
78. Norris, G.H.; Blesso, C.N. Dietary and Endogenous Sphingolipid Metabolism in Chronic Inflammation. *Nutrients* **2017**, *9*, 1180. [CrossRef]
79. Kiraz, Y.; Adan, A.; Kartal Yandim, M.; Baran, Y. Major Apoptotic Mechanisms and Genes Involved in Apoptosis. *Tumor Biol.* **2016**, *37*, 8471–8486. [CrossRef]

80. Tommasino, C.; Marconi, M.; Ciarlo, L.; Matarrese, P.; Malorni, W. Autophagic Fux and Autophagosome Morphogenesis Require the Participation of Sphingolipids. *Apoptosis* **2015**, *20*, 645–657. [CrossRef] [PubMed]
81. den Jager, W.A. Sphingomyelin in Lewy Inclusion Bodies in Parkinson's Disease. *Arch. Neurol.* **1969**, *21*, 615–619. [CrossRef] [PubMed]
82. Foo, J.N.; Liany, H.; Bei, J.X.; Yu, X.Q.; Liu, J.; Au, W.L.; Prakash, K.M.; Tan, L.C.; Tan, E.K. A Rare Lysosomal Enzyme Gene SMPD1 Variant (p.R591C) Associates with Parkinson's Disease. *Neurobiol. Aging* **2013**, *34*, 2890.e13–2890.e15. [CrossRef] [PubMed]
83. Mao, C.Y.; Yang, J.; Wang, H.; Zhang, S.Y.; Yang, Z.H.; Luo, H.Y.; Li, F.; Shi, M.; Liu, Y.T.; Zhuang, Z.P.; et al. SMPD1 Variants in Chinese Han Patients with Sporadic Parkinson's Disease. *Parkinsonism Relat. Disord.* **2017**, *34*, 59–61. [CrossRef] [PubMed]
84. Mattace Raso, G.; Russo, R.; Calignano, A.; Meli, R. Palmitoylethanolamide in CNS Health and Disease. *Pharmacol. Res.* **2014**, *86*, 32–41. [CrossRef] [PubMed]
85. Skaper, S.D.; Facci, L.; Barbierato, M.; Zusso, M.; Bruschetta, G.; Impellizzeri, D.; Cuzzocrea, S.; Giusti, P. N-Palmitoylethanolamine and Neuroinflammation: A Novel Therapeutic Strategy of Resolution. *Mol. Neurobiol.* **2015**, *52*, 1034–1042. [CrossRef]
86. Esposito, E.; Impellizzeri, D.; Mazzon, E.; Paterniti, I.; Cuzzocrea, S. Neuroprotective Activities of Palmitoylethanolamide in an Animal Model of Parkinson's Disease. *PLoS ONE* **2012**, *7*, e41880. [CrossRef]
87. Galan-Rodriguez, B.; Suarez, J.; Gonzalez-Aparicio, R.; Bermudez-Silva, F.J.; Maldonado, R.; Robledo, P.; Rodriguez de Fonseca, F.; Fernandez-Espejo, E. Oleoylethanolamide Exerts Partial and Dose-Dependent Neuroprotection of Substantia Nigra Dopamine Neurons. *Neuropharmacology* **2009**, *56*, 653–664. [CrossRef]
88. Farrell, E.K.; Chen, Y.; Barazanji, M.; Jeffries, K.A.; Cameroamortegui, F.; Merkler, D.J. Primary Fatty Acid Amide Metabolism: Conversion of Fatty Acids and an Ethanolamine in N18TG2 and SCP Cells. *J. Lipid Res.* **2012**, *53*, 247–256. [CrossRef]
89. Varvel, S.A.; Cravatt, B.F.; Engram, A.E.; Lichtman, A.H. Fatty Acid Amide Hydrolase (-/-) Mice Exhibit an Increased Sensitivity to the Disruptive Effects of Anandamide or Oleamide in a Working Memory Water Maze Task. *J. Pharmacol. Exp. Ther.* **2006**, *317*, 251–257. [CrossRef]
90. Huitron-Resendiz, S.; Gombart, L.; Cravatt, B.F.; Henriksen, S.J. Effect of Oleamide on Sleep and Its Relationship to Blood Pressure, Body Temperature, and Locomotor Activity in Rats. *Exp. Neurol.* **2001**, *172*, 235–243. [CrossRef]
91. Farrell, E.K.; Merkler, D.J. Biosynthesis, Degradation and Pharmacological Importance of the Fatty Acid Amides. *Drug Discov. Today* **2008**, *13*, 558–568. [CrossRef] [PubMed]
92. Kim, M.; Snowden, S.; Suvitaival, T.; Ali, A.; Merkler, D.J.; Ahmad, T.; Westwood, S.; Baird, A.; Proitsi, P.; Nevado-Holgado, A.; et al. Primary Fatty Amides in Plasma Associated with Brain Amyloid Burden, Hippocampal Volume, and Memory in the European Medical Information Framework for Alzheimer's Disease Biomarker Discovery Cohort. *Alzheimers Dement* **2019**, *15*, 817–827. [CrossRef] [PubMed]
93. Ren, S.Y.; Wang, Z.Z.; Zhang, Y.; Chen, N.H. Potential Application of Endocannabinoid System Agents in Neuropsychiatric and Neurodegenerative Diseases-Focusing on FAAH/MAGL Inhibitors. *Acta Pharmacol. Sin.* **2020**, *41*, 1263–1271. [CrossRef]
94. Alecu, I.; Bennett, S.A.L. Dysregulated Lipid Metabolism and Its Role in Alpha-Synucleinopathy in Parkinson's Disease. *Front. Neurosci.* **2019**, *13*, 328. [CrossRef] [PubMed]
95. Belarbi, K.; Cuvelier, E.; Bonte, M.A.; Desplanque, M.; Gressier, B.; Devos, D.; Chartier-Harlin, M.C. Glycosphingolipids and Neuroinflammation in Parkinson's Disease. *Mol. Neurodegener.* **2020**, *15*, 59. [CrossRef]
96. Stoessel, D.; Schulte, C.; Teixeira Dos Santos, M.C.; Scheller, D.; Rebollo-Mesa, I.; Deuschle, C.; Walther, D.; Schauer, N.; Berg, D.; Nogueira da Costa, A.; et al. Promising Metabolite Profiles in the Plasma and CSF of Early Clinical Parkinson's Disease. *Front. Aging Neurosci.* **2018**, *10*, 51. [CrossRef]
97. Kosicek, M.; Zetterberg, H.; Andreasen, N.; Peter-Katalinic, J.; Hecimovic, S. Elevated Cerebrospinal Fluid Sphingomyelin Levels in Prodromal Alzheimer's Disease. *Neurosci. Lett.* **2012**, *516*, 302–305. [CrossRef]
98. Wood, P.L.; Barnette, B.L.; Kaye, J.A.; Quinn, J.F.; Woltjer, R.L. Non-Targeted Lipidomics of CSF and Frontal Cortex Grey and White Matter in Control, Mild Cognitive Impairment, and Alzheimer's Disease Subjects. *Acta Neuropsychiatr.* **2015**, *27*, 270–278. [CrossRef]

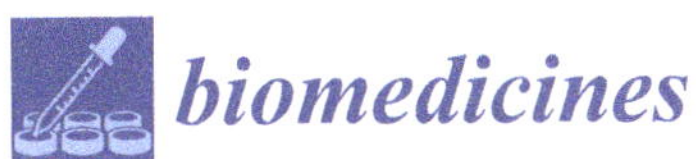 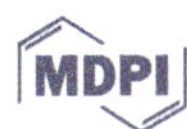

*Article*

# Foveal Avascular Zone and Choroidal Thickness Are Decreased in Subjects with Hard Drusen and without High Genetic Risk of Developing Alzheimer's Disease

Inés López-Cuenca [1,2,†], Rosa de Hoz [1,2,3,†], Celia Alcántara-Rey [1], Elena Salobrar-García [1,2,3], Lorena Elvira-Hurtado [1], José A. Fernández-Albarral [1], Ana Barabash [4,5], Federico Ramírez-Toraño [6,7], Jaisalmer de Frutos-Lucas [6,7,8,9], Juan J. Salazar [1,2,3], Ana I. Ramírez [1,2,3,*] and José M. Ramírez [1,2,10,*]

1 Instituto de Investigaciones Oftalmológicas Ramón Castroviejo, Universidad Complutense de Madrid (UCM), IdISSC, 28040 Madrid, Spain; inelopez@ucm.es (I.L.-C.); rdehoz@med.ucm.es (R.d.H.); celiaalc@ucm.es (C.A.-R.); elenasalobrar@med.ucm.es (E.S.-G.); marelvir@ucm.es (L.E.-H.); joseaf08@ucm.es (J.A.F.-A.); jjsalazar@med.ucm.es (J.J.S.)
2 OFTARED—Instituto de Salud Carlos III, 28029 Madrid, Spain
3 Departamento de Inmunología, Oftalmología y ORL, Facultad de Óptica y Optometría, Universidad Complutense de Madrid, 28037 Madrid, Spain
4 Endocrinology and Nutrition Department, Instituto de Investigación Sanitaria, Hospital Clínico Universitario San Carlos, 28040 Madrid, Spain; ana.barabash@gmail.com
5 Centro de Investigación Biomédica en Red de Diabetes y Enfermedades Metabólicas Asociadas, Instituto de Salud Carlos III, 28029 Madrid, Spain
6 Laboratory of Cognitive and Computational Neuroscience, Center for Biomedical Technology, Technical University of Madrid, 28233 Madrid, Spain; federico.ramirez@ctb.upm.es (F.R.-T.); jaisamer.defrutos@ctb.upm.es (J.d.F.-L.)
7 Department of Experimental Psychology, Universidad Complutense de Madrid, 28223 Madrid, Spain
8 Centre for Precision Health, Edith Cowan University, Joondalup, WA 6027, Australia
9 Departamento de Psicología, Facultad de Ciencias de la Vida y de la Naturaleza, Universidad Antonio de Nebrija, 28015 Madrid, Spain
10 Departamento de Inmunología, Oftalmología y ORL, Facultad de Medicina, Universidad Complutense de Madrid, 28040 Madrid, Spain
* Correspondence: airamirez@med.ucm.es (A.I.R.); ramirezs@med.ucm.es (J.M.R.)
† These authors contributed equally to this work.

**Citation:** López-Cuenca, I.; de Hoz, R.; Alcántara-Rey, C.; Salobrar-García, E.; Elvira-Hurtado, L.; Fernández-Albarral, J.A.; Barabash, A.; Ramírez-Toraño, F.; de Frutos-Lucas, J.; Salazar, J.J.; et al. Foveal Avascular Zone and Choroidal Thickness Are Decreased in Subjects with Hard Drusen and without High Genetic Risk of Developing Alzheimer's Disease. *Biomedicines* **2021**, 9, 638. https://doi.org/10.3390/biomedicines9060638

Academic Editor: Arnab Ghosh

Received: 6 May 2021
Accepted: 1 June 2021
Published: 2 June 2021



**Abstract:** A family history (FH+) of Alzheimer's disease (AD) and ε4 allele of the ApoE gene are the main genetic risk factors for developing AD, whereas ε4 allele plays a protective role in age-related macular degeneration. Ocular vascular changes have been reported in both pathologies. We analyzed the choroidal thickness using optical coherence tomography (OCT) and the foveal avascular zone (FAZ) using OCT-angiography and compared the results with ApoE gene expression, AD FH+, and the presence or absence of hard drusen (HD) in 184 cognitively healthy subjects. Choroidal thickness was statistically significantly different in the (FH−, ε4−, HD+) group compared with (i) both the (FH−, ε4−, HD−) and the (FH+, ε4+, HD+) groups in the superior and inferior points at 1500 μm, and (ii) the (FH+, ε4−, HD+) group in the superior point at 1500 μm. There were statistically significant differences in the superficial FAZ between the (FH+, ε4−, HD+) group and (i) the (FH+, ε4−, HD−) group and (ii) the (FH+, ε4+, HD−) group. In conclusion, ocular vascular changes are not yet evident in participants with a genetic risk of developing AD.

**Keywords:** Alzheimer's; family history; ApoE ε4; AMD; choroid; foveal avascular zone; hard drusen; retina; OCT; OCTA

## 1. Introduction

Alzheimer's disease (AD) is the most common cause of dementia, responsible for 60–70% of cases [1]. This neurodegenerative disease is characterized by a continuous and irreversible pathological process that begins 15–20 years before the onset of clinical symptoms [2]. The main pathological features are the hyperphosphorylation of the Tau protein and deposition of amyloid β-protein (Aβ) [3], which aggregates in the cerebral vessel walls [4], leading to cerebral amyloid angiopathy (CAA) [5]. These vascular amyloid deposits primarily consist of $A\beta_{1-40}$ and $A\beta_{1-42}$ [6], but *N*-terminal-truncated forms of Aβ and other proteins such as Apolipoprotein E (ApoE) and the α2-macroglobulin receptor/LDL receptor-related protein are also found in these deposits [7,8]. Reduced blood and lymphatic flow [9], the impairment of the gliovascular unit [10], and alterations in both vessel diameter and peripheral immune cell accessibility [11] can result in cerebral vascular deposits and lead to a series of events that result in neurodegeneration [12]. About 85% of AD patients exhibit CAA [13], and it has been reported to be an early and fundamental contributor to the development of the disease and a reliable predictor of cognitive decline [14].

There are similarities between cerebral and retinal vessels [15], and the vascular changes that occur in AD share common pathogenic mechanisms in both tissues [15–17]. For this reason, the retinal vascular changes observed in AD can be used to monitor alterations caused by this pathology in the central nervous system. Ocular vascularization has the particularity of being supplied by two different systems, which differ in their regulatory mechanisms and perfusion pressure [18]. While the inner retina is nourished by blood vessels derived from the central retinal artery (CRA), the outer retina is supplied by the choriocapillaris of the choroid [18].

Genetic factors play a critical role in the development of late-onset AD. Two of the most important risk factors are (i) having a first-degree family history of the disease [19] and (ii) being a carrier of at least one ε4 allele of ApoE [20]. Children of parents with AD have a six-fold greater risk of developing the disease compared with those without a family history [21].

ApoE is a multi-function protein; it is polymorphic and has three isoforms (ε2, ε3, and ε4). This protein is highly expressed in the liver, brain, and retina [22,23], where the retinal pigmented epithelium (RPE)/choroid complex has significant levels of ApoE mRNA [23]. The ε2, ε3, and ε4 isoforms exhibit differences in lipid binding and confer genetic risks for several diseases of aging, including atherosclerosis, AD, and age-related macular degeneration (AMD) [24]. A single ε4 allele increases the risk of developing AD [20], whereas it is associated with a protective effect against AMD [25]. In AD, the ε4 allele alters the way that neurons process the amyloid precursor protein (APP) through a cholesterol-mediated pathway [24]. Carriers of two copies of ApoE ε4 have shown reduced C-reactive protein (CRP) levels compared with non-carriers, suggesting that the ApoE isoform plays a mediating role in the inflammatory response involved in AMD etiology [26].

In addition, the role of ε2, which is protective against AD [20], has been extensively studied in AMD [24,25]. It is associated with a slightly increased risk of developing late AMD, and female ε2 carriers have a higher risk of progression compared with female ε3 carriers [27].

AMD is a degenerative disorder of the central retina. This pathology has a higher prevalence in patients over 65 years of age and is the main cause of blindness in this age group [28]. In early stages, the pathological changes are characterized by the presence of drusen and changes in the RPE. Drusen are focal deposits composed mainly of extracellular matrix deposits and inflammatory components located between the basal lamina of the RPE and the inner collagenous layer of Bruch's membrane. The formation of these deposits is due to the continuous phagocytosis and deposition of photoreceptor outer segment components, resulting in an imbalance between the production and clearance of lipid material [29]. AD and AMD share environmental risk factors and histopathological features, particularly the deposition of Aβ in ocular drusen and in senile brain plaques [30]. Analysis of the eyes of aging individuals with AMD by electron microscopy revealed that the basement membranes of retinal capillaries were considerably thicker compared with those of younger individuals. In addition, advanced cases of AMD were associated with a higher proportion of acellular capillaries, which were non-functional, predisposing these patients to ischemia in the inner retina [31]. Changes in the choroid and choroidal microcirculation have been reported in AD [32–34] and play an important role in the pathogenesis of AMD [35].

The aim of the present study was to analyze differences in choroidal thickness and the retinal foveal avascular zone (FAZ) and assess whether the findings were associated with ApoE gene expression, AD family history, and the presence or absence of hard drusen in cognitively healthy subjects.

## 2. Materials and Methods

### 2.1. Study Design

This study is part of the project "The cognitive and neurophysiological characteristics of subjects at high risk of developing dementia: a multidimensional approach" (COGDEM study) conducted by the Ramon Castroviejo Institute of Ophthalmic Research (IIORC) of the Complutense University of Madrid (UCM), the Centre for Biomedical Technology (CBT), and the Hospital Clínico San Carlos (HCSC), Madrid, among others. All participants provided written informed consent, and the research followed the tenets of the declaration of Helsinki. This study was approved by the local Ethics Committee (HCSC) with the internal code 18/422-E_BS.

The inclusion of patients is summarized in Figure 1. We analyzed two major groups:

- Group 1 is a control group, which consisted of middle-aged subjects without a first-degree family history of AD (FH−).
- Group 2 comprises subjects with a family history of AD (FH+). Subjects were middle-aged with at least one parent with sporadic AD. To verify the AD diagnoses of parents, a review of their medical records was conducted by a multidisciplinary diagnostic consensus panel. Only diagnoses that were made under internationally accepted criteria were included. Because autopsies were not performed in most AD patients, postmortem reports were welcome but were not used as the basis of inclusion. Relatives with known autosomal dominant mutations (i.e., preseniline-1 or 2) were not included.

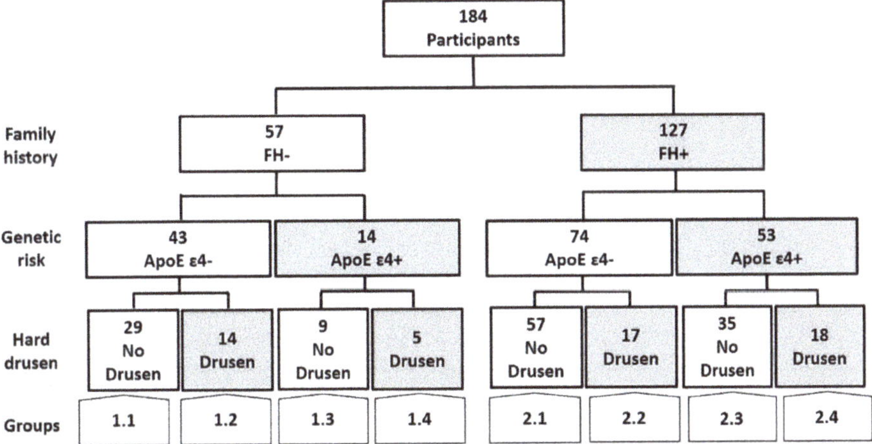


**Figure 1.** Flow diagram of the patients included in the present work. FH+: subjects with a family history of Alzheimer's disease (AD); FH−: Subjects without a family history of AD.

Both groups were matched in terms of age, socioeconomic status, and other demographic characteristics and had no history of neurological or psychiatric disorders or serious medical conditions. Both groups had normal scores on the Mini-Mental State Examination (MMSE) (above 26) and normal MRIs, with no evidence of brain lesions or pathology.

The two main groups were each subdivided into four subgroups. First, carriers and non-carriers of ApoE ε4 were assigned to different groups, which were then subdivided into groups with and without hard drusen in the retina.

The groups are represented as follows:

1.1. FH−; ApoE ε4−; No Drusen (FH−, ε4−, HD−).
1.2. FH−; ApoE ε4−; Drusen (FH−, ε4−, HD+).
1.3. FH−; ApoE ε4+; No Drusen (FH−, ε4+, HD−).
1.4. FH−; ApoE ε4+; Drusen (FH−, ε4+, HD+).
2.1. FH+; ApoE ε4−; No Drusen (FH+, ε4−, HD−).
2.2. FH+; ApoE ε4−; Drusen (FH+, ε4−, HD+).
2.3. FH+; ApoE ε4+; No Drusen (FH+, ε4+, HD−).
2.4. FH+; ApoE ε4+; Drusen (FH+, ε4+, HD+).

### 2.2. *Subjects*

In this prospective study, we included participants from COGDEM's Database, which consists of 251 subjects. The participants had to be free of ophthalmological pathology, which we confirmed through phone screening.

The participants were examined in the clinic of IIORC. The phone screening questions, visual exams, and inclusion criteria are described in Table 1.

**Table 1.** Ophthalmological evaluation of COGDEM participants.

| Ophthalmological Evaluation | | |
|---|---|---|
| **Screening Questions** | **Visual Exam** | **Inclusion Criteria** |
| Do you use glasses? Yes/no<br>Do you know if you have myopia, hypermetropy, or astigmatism? Yes/no<br>Do you know your diopter measurements? Yes/no<br>Do you have any ocular pathologies? Yes/no<br>Do you receive any type of ocular treatment? Yes/no<br>Have you undergone any type of ocular surgery? Yes/no | Refraction<br>Visual acuity<br>Biomicroscopy<br>Intraocular pressure<br>OCT/OCTA | ±5 Spherocylindrical refractive<br>>0.5 dec<br><21 mmHg<br>Free of ocular disease<br>Free of congenital malformation<br>Free of known or suspected glaucoma |

OCT: optical coherence tomography; OCTA: OCT angiography; dec: decimal scale.

We included 57 and 127 participants with and without a family history of AD, respectively. In addition, we classified participants on the basis of whether they carried the ApoE ε4 allele and whether they had hard drusen.

Figure 1 shows a flow diagram that illustrates the different study groups included in the present work.

### 2.3. *ApoE Genotyping*

Genomic DNA was extracted from whole blood in EDTA using standard DNA isolation methods (DNAzol®; Molecular Research Center, Inc., Cincinnati, OH, USA) from FH+ and FH− subjects. Two single-nucleotide polymorphisms (SNPs), rs7412 and rs429358, were genotyped using TaqMan Genotyping Assays on an Applied Biosystems 7500 Fast Real-Time PCR instrument (Applied Biosystems, Forster City, CA, USA). APOE haplotypes were accordingly established. Sample controls for each genotype and negative sample controls were included in each assay. Several intra- and interplate duplicates of DNA samples were included.

### 2.4. Spectral-Domain Optical Coherence Tomography (OCT) Imaging: Choroidal Thickness and FAZ Measurement

The choroidal thickness and the foveal avascular zone (FAZ) were measured by OCT Spectralis (Heidelberg Engineering, Heidelberg, Germany). High-quality scans were defined by a minimum signal-to-noise ratio of 25 and an average of 16 B-scans. The choroidal thickness was delimited manually and perpendicularly to the retina by the same examiner using the measurement function in Heidelberg software (Heidelberg, Germany, version 1.10.4.0). The choroidal thickness was measured from the outer hyper-reflective line to the sclerochoroidal interface of the RPE. These measurements were made in the subfoveal choroid and superior, inferior, nasal, and temporal sectors at 500, 1000, and 1500 μm from the center of the fovea (Figure 2A,B).

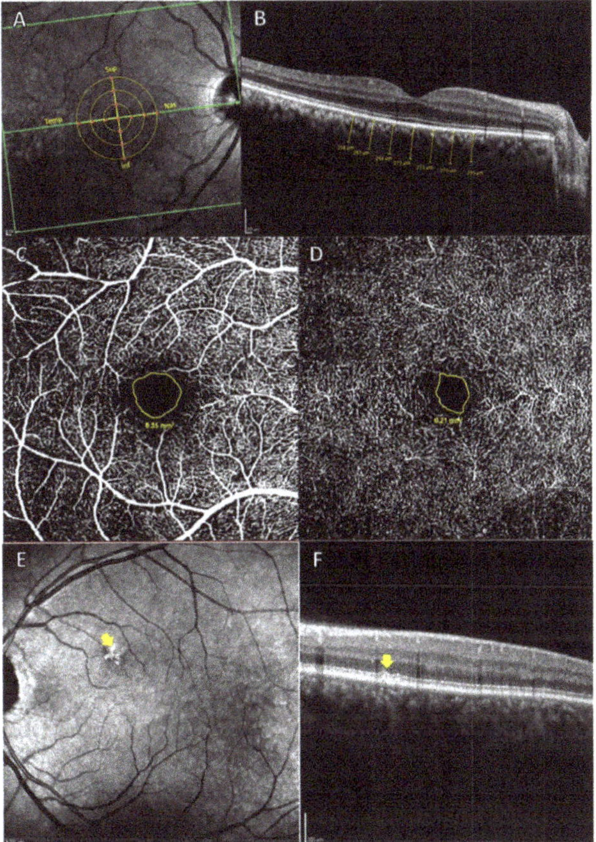


**Figure 2.** (**A**,**B**) measurement of the choroidal thickness. (**A**) Retinal zone analyzed. The 13 red points indicate where the choroidal thickness measurements were carried out. Sup: superior; Nas: Nasal; Inf: Inferior; Temp: Temporal. (**B**) Choroidal thickness measur measurements (μm). (**C**,**D**), measurement of FAZ. (**C**) OCTA of superficial vascular plexus, with the avascular area outlined in yellow. (**D**) OCTA of deep vascular plexus, with the avascular area outlined in yellow and, (**E**) and (**F**), hard drusen analysis by OCT. (**E**) The yellow arrow shows hyper-reflective shapes in the HRA fundus image. (**F**) Cross-Sectional OCT. The yellow arrow indicates hard drusen localized between the basal lamina of the RPE and the inner collagen layer of Bruch's membrane.

The Spectralis OCT angiography (OCTA) module was used to measure the superficial and deep FAZ. The avascular area of each plexus was delimited manually with the area measurement tool in Heidelberg software (Figure 2C,D).

Hard drusen were identified as hyper-reflective shapes on high-reflectance acquisition (HRA) fundus images and as hyper-reflective material located between the basal lamina of the RPE and the inner collagen layer of Bruch's membrane on cross-sectional OCT scans (Figure 2E,F). All OCT scans were analyzed by the same ophthalmologist who determined the type of deposit.

Both the measurements that were performed manually and the classification of the deposits were carried out blindly to avoid the possibility that the information from the participants could influence the measurements carried out by the professionals.

### 2.5. Statistical Analysis

SPSS 25.0 (SPSS Inc., Inc., Chicago, IL, USA) was used to perform the statistical analysis. The differences between study groups were analyzed using the Mann–Whitney test. Data are reported as the median (interquartile range). The chi-square test was used for the analysis of qualitative variables. A $p$-value < 0.05 was considered statistically significant.

## 3. Results

### 3.1. Demographic Data

Eight study groups were included in this work. The demographic data are shown in Table 2.

**Table 2.** Demographic data on the participants in the different study groups.

| Demographic/ MMSE Data | FH− | | | | FH+ | | | |
|---|---|---|---|---|---|---|---|---|
| | ApoE ε4− | | ApoE ε4+ | | ApoE ε4− | | ApoE ε4+ | |
| | No HD | HD | No HD | HD | No HD | HD | No HD | HD |
| | Group 1.1 | Group 1.2 | Group 1.3 | Group 1.4 | Group 2.1 | Group 2.2 | Group 2.3 | Group 2.4 |
| N | 29 | 14 | 9 | 5 | 57 | 17 | 35 | 18 |
| Age | 59.0 (54.0–65.0) | 62.5 (56.0–69.0) | 63.0 (54.0–70.0) | 63.0 (58.0–76.5) | 58.0 (53.0–62,0) | 63.0 (56.5–58.5) | 57.0 (57.0–65.0) | 55.5 (51.0–63.0) |
| Sex Male/Female | 12/17 | 6/8 | 3/6 | 0/5 | 22/35 | 6/11 | 11/24 | 9/9 |
| MMSE | 29.0 (28.0–29.0) | 29.0 (29.0–29.0) | 29.0 (28.0–30.0) | 29.0 (29.0–30.0) | 29.0 (28.5–29.0) | 29.0 (28.0–29.0) | 29.0 (29.0–29.0) | 29.0 (28.0–30.0) |

Median (interquartile range); FH+, subjects with a family history of Alzheimer's disease (AD); FH−, subjects without a family history of AD; ApoE, Apolipoprotein E.

Groups 1.1, 1.2, 1.3, and 1.4 consisted of individuals without a family history of AD. Group 1.1 (FH−, ε4−, HD−) was formed by 29 subjects (12 males) with a mean age of 59.0 (54.0–65.0) and mean MMSE score of 29.0 (28.0–29.0). Group 1.2 (FH−, ε4−, HD+) was formed by 14 participants (6 males) with a mean age of 62.5 (56.0–69.0) and mean MMSE score of 29.0 (29.0–29.0). Group 1.3 (FH−, ε4+, HD−) had 9 subjects (3 males) with a mean age of 63.0 (54.0–70.0) and mean MMSE score of 29.0 (28.0–30.0), and Group 1.4 (FH−, ε4+, HD+) had 5 participants (0 males) with a mean age of 63.0 (58.0–76.5) and mean MMSE score of 29.0 (29.0–30.0).

Groups 2.1, 2.2, 2.3, and 2.4 included individuals with a family history of AD. Group 2.1 (FH+, ε4−, HD−) comprised 57 participants (22 males) with a mean age of 58.0 (53.0–62.0) and mean MMSE of 29.0 (28.5–29.0). Group 2.2 (FH+, ε4−, HD+) had 17 subjects (6 males) with a mean age of 63.0 (56.5–68.5) and mean MMSE score of 29.0 (28.0–29.0). Group 2.3 (FH+, ε4+, HD−) included 35 subjects (11 males) with a mean age of 57.0 (57.0–65.0) and mean MMSE score of 29.0 (29.0–29.0), and Group 2.4 (FH+, ε4+, HD+) had 18 subjects (9 males) with a mean age of 55.5 (51.0–63.0) and mean MMSE score of 29.0 (28.0–30.0).

### 3.2. Choroidal Thickness

The choroidal thickness of Group 1.2 (FH−, ε4−, HD+) was statistically different ($p < 0.05$) from that of (i) Group 1.1 (FH−, ε4−, HD−) in the superior and inferior points at 1500 µm, (ii) Group 2.2 (FH+, ε4−, HD+) in the superior point at 1500 µm, and (iii) Group 2.4 (FH+, ε4+, HD+) in the superior and inferior points at 1500 µm (Tables 3 and 4).

**Table 3.** Median and interquartile range of the FAZ and choroidal thickness in the study groups.

| Vascular Areas Analyzed | | | FH− | | | | FH+ | | | |
|---|---|---|---|---|---|---|---|---|---|---|
| | | | ApoE ε4− | | ApoE ε4+ | | ApoE ε4− | | ApoE ε4+ | |
| | | | No HD | HD | No HD | HD | No HD | HD | No HD | HD |
| | | | Group 1.1 | Group 1.2 | Group 1.3 | Group 1.4 | Group 2.1 | Group 2.2 | Group 2.3 | Group 2.4 |
| FAZ | Superficial | | 0.47 (0.39–0.62) | 0.45 (0.42–0.68) | 0.47(0.37–0.84) | 0.47 (0.37–0.82) | 0.51 (0.39–0.62) | 0.67 (0.62–0.80) | 0.54 (0.44–0.68) | 0.59 (0.43–0.83) |
| | Deep | | 0.23 (0.18–0.31) | 0.22 (0.16–0.34) | 0.24 (0.2–0.359) | 0.23 (0.12–0.34) | 0.26 (0.39–0.33) | 0.29 (0.24–0.38) | 0.28 (0.23–0.33) | 0.29 (0.21–0.41) |
| Choroidal Thickness | Subfoveal | | 268.0 (213.5–307.5) | 249.5 (176.8–268.0) | 257.0 (234.0–318.0) | 252.5 (164.5–279.8) | 273.0 (231.0–309.5) | 255.0 (215.5–287.0) | 263.0 (212.0–302.0) | 241.0 (224.5–296.5) |
| | Temporal | 500 µm | 260.0 (210.5–325.0) | 234.0 (159.8–259.0) | 266.0 (231.5–316.0) | 256.5 (173.3–296.3) | 263.0 (220.5–302.0) | 252.0 (199.5–292.0) | 256.0 (228.0–295.0) | 252.0 (222.8–297.3) |
| | | 1000 µm | 248.0 (207.5–316.0) | 219.5 (161.8–267.50) | 276.0 (202.5–300.0) | 256.5 (176.5–310.3) | 263.0 (218.5–288.5) | 248.0 (195.5–292.0) | 253.0 (219.0–287.0) | 247.5 (217.5–282.0) |
| | | 1500 µm | 232.0 (202.0–296.0) | 222.5 (157.5–255.3) | 254,0 (186.5–343.0) | 255.0 (189.8–292.5) | 255.0 (216.0–288.5) | 251.0 (202.5–282.0) | 250.0 (215.0–280.0) | 265.0 (214.5–291.0) |
| | Nasal | 500 µm | 261.0 (204.5–313.5) | 230.5 (177.0–252.5) | 238.0 (228.0–302.5) | 256.5 (180.3–292.3) | 267.0 (220.5–295.0) | 234.0 (198.5–285.5) | 249.0 (199.0–297.0) | 244.0 (224.0–286.2) |
| | | 1000 µm | 233.0 (195.5–303.5) | 206.0 (150.8–282.0) | 223.0 (204.5–291.5) | 257.0 (173.3–295.8) | 255.0 (190.5–299.0) | 225.0 (191.0–274.5) | 240.0 (182.0–281.0) | 248.5 (198.8–268.0) |
| | | 1500 µm | 221 (175.50–278.5) | 182.5 (140.5–269.3) | 217.0 (171.0–278.0) | 271.0 (134.0–300.0) | 228.0 (183.5–274.5) | 205.0 (170.5–242.0) | 218.0 (174.0–265.0) | 252.0 (179.8–263.0) |
| | Superior | 500 µm | 262.0 (218.0–301.0) | 222.0 (170.8–273.5) | 260.0 (228.5–311.5) | 265.5 (182.8–292.8) | 265.0 (228.0–299−0) | 262.0 (219.5–282.5) | 257.0 (209.0–309.0) | 252.5 (222.0–284.0) |
| | | 1000 µm | 255.0 (218.5 297.0) | 227.0 (170.8–263.8) | 256.0 (227.5–308.5) | 272.5 (180.8–281.8) | 271.0 (228.5–302.0) | 259.0 (217.5–289.0) | 267.0 (223.0–299.0) | 252.5 (234.3–288.0) |
| | | 1500 µm | 259.0 (209.5–306.5) | 223.0 (147.0–253.3) | 250.0 (225.5–319.0) | 269.0 (174.0–298.0) | 261.0 (224.5–305.5) | 261.0 (206.0–286.0) | 262.0 (226.0–300.0) | 257.5 (233.3–290.3) |
| | Inferior | 500 µm | 262.0 (209.5–311.5) | 222.5 (172.8–274.3) | 256.0 (222.0–308.5) | 272.0 (179.5–284.3) | 270.0 (231.5–304.0) | 252.0 (208.5–276.5) | 265.0 (216.0–310.0) | 251.5 (216,3–301,3) |
| | | 1000 µm | 266.0 (217.0–306.5) | 219.0 (165.0–270.8) | 267.0 (229.5–308.5) | 267.5 (171.0–296.5) | 271.0 (227.5–295.5) | 252.0 (211.5–268.0) | 270.0 (216.0–322.0) | 243.0 (219.8–287.3) |
| | | 1500 µm | 264.0 (213.5–312.0) | 217.0 (169.0–257.25) | 262.0 (218.5–300.5) | 271.5 (183.0–276.0) | 268.0 (224.0–304.0) | 257.0 (211.0–266.5) | 250.0 (214.0–317.0) | 269.0 (216.0–309.5) |

Median (interquartile range); FH+, subjects with a family history of Alzheimer's disease (AD); FH, subjects without a family history of AD; HD, hard drusen; ApoE, Apolipoprotein E; FAZ, Foveal avascular zone.

**Table 4.** Significant $p-$values for differences between groups in the FAZ and choroidal thickness. $p-$values are in parentheses.

| Study Groups | | | | FH− | | | | FH+ | | | |
|---|---|---|---|---|---|---|---|---|---|---|---|
| | | | | ApoE ε4− | | ApoE ε4+ | | ApoE ε4− | | ApoE ε4+ | |
| | | | | No HD | HD | No HD | HD | No HD | HD | No HD | HD |
| | | | | Group 1.1 | Group 1.2 | Group 1.3 | Group 1.4 | Group 2.1 | Group 2.2 | Group 2.3 | Group 2.4 |
| FH− | ApoE ε4− | No HD | 1.1 | | Choroid: Sup 1500 (0.030), Inf 1500 (0.028) | | | | | | |
| | | HD | 1.2 | | | | | | Choroid: Sup 1500 (0.039) | | Choroid: Sup 1500 (0.019), Inf 1500 (0.040) |
| | ApoE ε4+ | No HD | 1.3 | | | | | | | | |
| | | HD | 1.4 | | | | | | | | |
| FH+ | ApoE ε4− | No HD | 2.1 | | | | | | Superficial FAZ (<0.001) | | |
| | | HD | 2.2 | | | | | | | Superficial FAZ (0.013) | |
| | ApoE ε4+ | No HD | 2.3 | | | | | | | | |
| | | HD | 2.4 | | | | | | | | |

$p$-values are in parentheses. FH+, subjects with a family history of Alzheimer's disease (AD); FH−, subjects without a family history of AD; HD, hard drusen; ApoE, Apolipoprotein E; FAZ, Foveal avascular zone.

### 3.3. Foveal Avascular Zone (FAZ)

There were statistically significant differences in the superficial FAZ between Group 2.1 (FH+, ε4−, HD−) (0.51 (0.39–0.62)) and Group 2.2 (FH+, ε4−, HD+) (0.67 (0.62–0.80)) (Tables 3 and 4). In addition, there were significant differences ($p < 0.05$) in the superficial FAZ between Group 2.2 (FH+, ε4−, HD+) (0.67 (0.62–0.80)) and Group 2.3 (FH+, ε4+, HD−) (0.54 (0.44–0.68)) (Tables 3 and 4).

## 4. Discussion

The present study demonstrates that ocular vascular changes are not yet evident in participants with a genetic risk of developing AD, while in participants without genetic risk for developing AD who have HD, changes in choroidal thickness are presented. In addition, superficial FAZ also showed small changes between the (FH+, ε4−, HD+) group and the (FH+, ε4−, HD−) and the (FH+, ε4+, HD−) groups.

Changes in the retinal vasculature have been identified as potential biomarkers of AD [36–38]. One of the most important ocular vascular layers is the choroid, whose flow is supplied by the posterior ciliary arteries, which are branches of the ophthalmic artery [39]. The choroid has one of the highest blood flows of any tissue in the body, and its primary function is to provide nutrients and oxygen to the outer retina, including the RPE and photoreceptors [40,41]. The choroidal circulation is controlled mainly by autonomic and sensory innervation and not by a self-regulatory mechanism [39,42]. Nerve fibers that regulate choroidal vascularization are predominantly located in the submacular region, where most NPY+ and TH+ ganglion cells are also concentrated [43]. This neuronal distribution in the submacular region suggests the possibility that vascular conditions of certain eye diseases, such as diabetic macular edema or AMD, may be related to the dysfunction of these cells [44]. Some authors have correlated AD with AMD, so it is not surprising that choroidal vascular changes appear before retinal changes in AD [30].

A decrease in choroidal thickness has been reported in patients with AD compared with healthy older subjects [15,33,34,45–49]. These changes have also been observed in early stages of the disease [32], including in patients with preclinical and prodromal AD [49] and those with mild cognitive impairment (MCI) [41]. Choroidal thinning may indicate abnormal choroidal blood supply associated with hypoperfusion or atrophic changes related to various pathological events, with cerebral Aβ accumulation being the main trigger [33]. Capillary occlusion detected in imaging studies provides a possible explanation for hypoperfusion in AD brains [50,51].

In the present study, no differences were observed between groups with a high genetic risk of developing AD (subjects with a family history and carriers of ApoE ε4) and control groups (participants without a family history and non-carriers of ApoE ε4). One possible explanation is that our participants are cognitively healthy people, and it is unknown whether they will develop the disease in the future. Although genetic factors play an important role in determining a person's risk of developing the disease [52], there are other contributing factors, such as the influence of the environment or modifiable risk factors, including physical activity, diet, and alcohol consumption, all of which can modify the course or even the onset of the disease [53].

The statistically significant differences found in our study are in groups that have hard drusen. In addition, the thinnest choroids correspond to subjects who have no family history of the disease and are non-carriers of ApoE ε4 (Group 1.2; FH−, ε4−, HD+). ApoE ε4 is known to be a protective factor for AMD, and the risk of late (end-stage) AMD in individuals of Caucasian descent is 20–50% lower than that of carriers of the ε3 allele [54,55], while the ε2 allele is associated with increased disease progression in women [27]. However, the association between ApoE ε4 and protection is stronger than that between ε2 and risk [25].

The allelic variants of the ApoE gene represent one of the most important genetic risk factors for developing AMD [55]. ApoE plays a role in cell-membrane remodeling and is essential for the normal function and maintenance of the retina [54]. Lipid transport across Bruch's membrane is easier in carriers of the ε4 allele compared with ε2 and ε3 allele carriers. The positive charges in proteins coded by ε4 alleles account for their improved ability to clear debris because they interact with the hydrophobic barrier generated by the accumulation of neutral lipids [56].

The formation of drusen is not random but is influenced by the anatomy of the choroid, and the mechanisms leading to the formation of these deposits in intercapillary areas or areas devoid of capillary lumens are unknown [57]. Drusen are associated with decreased choriocapillaris density and decreased choroid flow [57–59]. Similarly, reduced blood flow to the choriocapillaris can lead to dysfunction of the RPE, promoting further accumulation of debris in the form of drusen or basal lamellar deposits [58]. In early AMD, choroidal thickness already tends to be thinner than in normal eyes [60]. The exact cause of this thinning is unknown; it may be a response to choroidal atrophy or hypoxia, or it may be a secondary response to the accumulation of deposits or damage to the RPE [60].

Numerous studies with different imaging techniques have shown choroidal changes in AMD, but no consensus has been reached. Previous studies with fluorescein angiography have reported abnormalities in choroidal perfusion, such as decreased blood flow, increased fluorescein blockage [61,62], and areas of delayed choroidal perfusion, which were associated with decreased visual function [63]. In another study, slow choroidal filling on fluorescein angiography was reported to be a significant risk factor for developing geographic RPE atrophy, suggesting the importance of ischemia in this etiology [64]. In addition, in another study in subjects with dry AMD, an increase in arterial filling time was found, suggesting a decrease in choroidal blood flow [65].

In a recent study using color Doppler imaging, AMD patients showed decreased blood velocity and increased pulsatility in the central retinal artery and posterior short ciliary arteries [66]. In other neurodegenerative diseases, such as AD or previous stages such as MCI, the accumulation of vascular deposits in the retina ($A\beta_{40}$ and $A\beta_{42}$) is also associated with vascular changes [67]. The accumulation of Aβ was shown to reduce the expression of LDL receptor-related protein-1 (LRPG), leading to a decrease in the expression of vascular platelet-derived growth factor receptor-β (PDGFRβ) and an increase in pericyte death by apoptosis [12]. Brain pericytes and vascular smooth muscle cells are critical in regulating blood flow and the integrity of the blood–brain barrier [68]. Because of its similarity to the blood-retinal barrier, damage at this level is implicated in pathologies such as AMD and diabetic retinopathy [12]. Although drusen are one of the first signs to appear in AMD, the subjects in our study do not have AMD, so we cannot claim that the changes in choroidal thickness are comparable to those found in patients with AMD. The vascular changes in the choroid in our patients may be a very early sign secondary to altered blood flow.

On the other hand, retinal circulation is characterized by low blood flow, high perfusion pressure [39], and three distinct structures: radial peripapillary capillaries, superficial vascular, and deep vascular plexus [15]. In the foveal zone, in both the deep and superficial plexus, there is a capillary-free zone called the FAZ [69]. The enlargement of the FAZ is a sign of ischemia and is detected in cases of diabetic retinopathy and macular vein branch occlusion [70]. This parameter has received interest as a biomarker for the monitoring and follow-up of pathologies such as AD [15]. For this reason, the FAZ has been studied at different stages of the disease using OCTA.

In our study, among the participants without drusen, we found no statistically significant differences between those with a high genetic risk of AD (group 2.3) and those without a genetic risk of AD (group 1.1). Our results are similar to those of a previous study in preclinical AD, in which no differences in the FAZ were found between Aβ+ patients and controls (Aβ−), who had lower vascular density [71]. However, in a previous study, the FAZ of cognitively healthy individuals who had preclinical AD and positive biomarkers for AD, such as PET scanning for PiB or $^{18}$F-AV-45 and $A\beta_{42}$+ levels in the cerebrospinal fluid (CSF), was increased in comparison with participants without these biomarkers. However, information about the family histories of the participants and results of genetic testing (ApoE ε4 status) were not collected [72]. In our analysis of the FAZ, the only statistically significant differences were in the superficial FAZ in Group 2.2 (FH+, ε4−, HD+) in comparison with both Groups 2.1 (FH+, ε4−, HD−) and 2.3 (FH+, ε4+, HD−). These changes are consistent with those found in studies of patients with MCI, who showed a decrease in vascular density and, therefore, an increase in the FAZ area [38,73,74]. In a recent study in patients with MCI, an increased deep FAZ was observed compared with controls. The same study analyzed the influence of ApoE ε4 on vascularization in people with and without MCI and found no significant differences [75].

The results obtained in FAZ analyses in AD patients are quite diverse. Some studies have found no statistically significant differences between the FAZ of AD patients and healthy controls [32,76]. However, others have found differences in both the superficial [15,77] and deep FAZ [78] compared with controls. An increased FAZ is attributed to reduced angiogenesis, a consequence of decreased vascular endothelial growth factor (VEGF), which binds to Aβ protein plaques [15], as well as the competitive binding of Aβ to the VEGF-2 receptor [79,80].

These discrepancies in the results of different studies may be explained by the degree of cognitive impairment of the participants. However, our participants were cognitively healthy, so the increased area of the superficial FAZ could reflect compromised blood perfusion, which may trigger the deposition of drusenoid material.

One of the strengths of this study is the strict selection of participants. Only young, cognitively healthy participants with a family history of Alzheimer's disease were included in the study. Another strength is the knowledge of the genetic characterization of the subjects. However, among the main limitations of the study are the small sample size in some of the study groups (there are groups with only 9 and 5 participants) and its retrospective character. Longitudinal studies will be necessary to know the evolution of all participants.

## 5. Conclusions

In conclusion, in this study, ocular vascular changes are not yet evident in healthy cognitive participants at high genetic risk of developing AD. The statistically significant differences in our study are in subjects who have hard drusen who should be evaluated periodically. In addition, the thinnest choroids correspond to subjects who have no family history of AD and are non-carriers of ApoE ε4.

**Author Contributions:** Conceptualization, I.L.-C., R.d.H., E.S.-G., J.J.S., A.I.R. and J.M.R.; data curation, I.L.-C., C.A.-R., E.S.-G., L.E.-H., J.A.F.-A., A.B., F.R.-T. and J.d.F.-L.; formal analysis, I.L.-C., R.d.H., C.A.-R., E.S.-G., L.E.-H., J.A.F.-A., F.R.-T. and J.d.F.-L.; funding acquisition, R.d.H., J.J.S., A.I.R. and J.M.R.; investigation, I.L.-C., R.d.H., C.A.-R., E.S.-G., L.E.-H., J.A.F.-A. and J.M.R.; methodology, I.L.-C., E.S.-G., L.E.-H., A.B., F.R.-T., J.d.F.-L. and A.I.R.; project administration, R.d.H., J.J.S., A.I.R. and J.M.R.; resources, R.d.H.; supervision, R.d.H., J.J.S. and J.M.R.; validation, I.L.-C., E.S.-G., A.B., J.J.S., A.I.R. and J.M.R.; visualization, I.L.-C., R.d.H., E.S.-G., J.A.F.-A., J.J.S., A.I.R. and J.M.R.; writing—original draft, I.L.-C., R.d.H., E.S.-G., A.I.R. and J.M.R.; writing—review and editing, I.L.-C., R.d.H., C.A.-R., E.S.-G., L.E.-H., J.A.F.-A., A.B., F.R.-T., J.d.F.-L., J.J.S., A.I.R. and J.M.R. All authors have read and agreed to the published version of the manuscript.

**Funding:** This research was funded by the Ophthalmological Network OFTARED (RD16/0008/0005) of the Institute of Health of Carlos III of the Spanish Ministry of Science and Innovation; the Research Network RETIBRAIN (RED2018-102499-T) of the Spanish Ministry of Science and Innovation; and the Spanish Ministry of Economy and Competitiveness (Grant PSI2015-68793-C3-1-R). I.L.-C. is currently supported by a Predoctoral Fellowship (CT42/18-CT43/18) from the Complutense University of Madrid. J.A.F.-A. is currently supported by a Predoctoral Fellowship (FPU17/01023) from the Spanish Ministry of Science, Innovation, and Universities. The sponsor or funding organization had no role in the design or conduct of this research. Approval date: 17 December 2018.

**Institutional Review Board Statement:** This study was approved by the local ethics committee (HCSC) with the internal code 18/422-E_BS (accepted 17 December 2018).

**Informed Consent Statement:** Informed consent was obtained from all subjects involved in the study.

**Data Availability Statement:** The data supporting the findings of this study are available from the corresponding author upon request.

**Conflicts of Interest:** The authors declare no conflict of interest. The funders had no role in the design of the study; in the collection, analyses, or interpretation of data; in the writing of the manuscript; or in the decision to publish the results.

## References

1. Savva, G.M.; Wharton, S.B.; Ince, P.G.; Forster, G.; Matthews, F.E.; Brayne, C. Age, Neuropathology, and Dementia. *N. Engl. J. Med.* **2009**, *360*, 2302–2309. [CrossRef] [PubMed]
2. Sperling, R.A.; Aisen, P.S.; Beckett, L.A.; Bennett, D.A.; Craft, S.; Fagan, A.M.; Iwatsubo, T.; Jack, C.R.; Kaye, J.; Montine, T.J.; et al. Toward defining the preclinical stages of Alzheimer's disease: Recommendations from the National Institute on Aging-Alzheimer's Association workgroups on diagnostic guidelines for Alzheimer's disease. *Alzheimer's Dement.* **2011**, *7*, 280–292. [CrossRef]
3. Perl, D.P. Neuropathology of Alzheimer's Disease. *Mt. Sinai J. Med. A J. Transl. Pers. Med.* **2010**, *77*, 32–42. [CrossRef] [PubMed]
4. Glenner, G.G.; Wong, C.W. Alzheimer's disease: Initial report of the purification and characterization of a novel cerebrovascular amyloid protein. *Biochem. Biophys. Res. Commun.* **1984**, *120*, 885–890. [CrossRef]
5. Thal, D.R.; Griffin, W.S.T.; de Vos, R.A.I.; Ghebremedhin, E. Cerebral amyloid angiopathy and its relationship to Alzheimer's disease. *Acta Neuropathol.* **2008**, *115*, 599–609. [CrossRef] [PubMed]

6. Roher, A.E.; Lowenson, J.D.; Clarke, S.; Woods, A.S.; Cotter, R.J.; Gowing, E.; Ball, M.J. β-amyloid-(1-42) is a major component of cerebrovascular amyloid deposits: Implications for the pathology of Alzheimer disease. *Proc. Natl. Acad. Sci. USA* **1993**, *90*, 10836–10840. [CrossRef] [PubMed]
7. Namba, Y.; Tomonaga, M.; Kawasaki, H.; Otomo, E.; Ikeda, K. Apolipoprotein E immunoreactivity in cerebral amyloid deposits and neurofibrillary tangles in Alzheimer's disease and kuru plaque amyloid in Creutzfeldt-Jakob disease. *Brain Res.* **1991**, *541*, 163–166. [CrossRef]
8. Tekirian, T.L.; Saido, T.C.; Markesbery, W.R.; Russell, M.J.; Wekstein, D.R.; Patel, E.; Geddes, J.W. N-terminal heterogeneity of parenchymal and cerebrovascular aβ deposits. *J. Neuropathol. Exp. Neurol.* **1998**, *57*, 76–94. [CrossRef] [PubMed]
9. Louveau, A.; Plog, B.A.; Antila, S.; Alitalo, K.; Nedergaard, M.; Kipnis, J. Understanding the functions and relationships of the glymphatic system and meningeal lymphatics. *J. Clin. Investig.* **2017**, *127*, 3210–3219. [CrossRef]
10. Kimbrough, I.F.; Robel, S.; Roberson, E.D.; Sontheimer, H. Vascular amyloidosis impairs the gliovascular unit in a mouse model of Alzheimer's disease. *Brain* **2015**, *138*, 3716–3733. [CrossRef]
11. Koronyo, Y.; Salumbides, B.C.; Sheyn, J.; Pelissier, L.; Li, S.; Ljubimov, V.; Moyseyev, M.; Daley, D.; Fuchs, D.T.; Pham, M.; et al. Therapeutic effects of glatiramer acetate and grafted CD115+ monocytes in a mouse model of Alzheimer's disease. *Brain* **2015**, *138*, 2399–2422. [CrossRef] [PubMed]
12. Shi, H.; Koronyo, Y.; Rentsendorj, A.; Regis, G.C.; Sheyn, J.; Fuchs, D.T.; Kramerov, A.A.; Ljubimov, A.V.; Dumitrascu, O.M.; Rodriguez, A.R.; et al. Identification of early pericyte loss and vascular amyloidosis in Alzheimer's disease retina. *Acta Neuropathol.* **2020**, *139*, 813–836. [CrossRef] [PubMed]
13. Arvanitakis, Z.; Leurgans, S.E.; Wang, Z.; Wilson, R.S.; Bennett, D.A.; Schneider, J.A. Cerebral amyloid angiopathy pathology and cognitive domains in older persons. *Ann. Neurol.* **2011**, *69*, 320–327. [CrossRef]
14. Boyle, P.A.; Yu, L.; Nag, S.; Leurgans, S.; Wilson, R.S.; Bennett, D.A.; Schneider, J.A. Cerebral amyloid angiopathy and cognitive outcomes in community-based older persons. *Neurology* **2015**, *85*, 1930–1936. [CrossRef]
15. Bulut, M.; Kurtuluş, F.; Gözkaya, O.; Erol, M.K.; Cengiz, A.; Akldan, M.; Yaman, A. Evaluation of optical coherence tomography angiographic findings in Alzheimer's type dementia. *Br. J. Ophthalmol.* **2018**, *102*, 233–237. [CrossRef]
16. Williams, M.A.; McGowan, A.J.; Cardwell, C.R.; Cheung, C.Y.; Craig, D.; Passmore, P.; Silvestri, G.; Maxwell, A.P.; McKay, G.J. Retinal microvascular network attenuation in Alzheimer's disease. *Alzheimer's Dement. Diagn. Assess. Dis. Monit.* **2015**, *1*, 229–235. [CrossRef]
17. Frost, S.; Kanagasingam, Y.; Sohrabi, H.; Vignarajan, J.; Bourgeat, P.; Salvado, O.; Villemagne, V.; Rowe, C.C.; Lance MacAulay, S.; Szoeke, C.; et al. Retinal vascular biomarkers for early detection and monitoring of Alzheimer's disease. *Transl. Psychiatry* **2013**, *3*, e233. [CrossRef] [PubMed]
18. Ramírez, J.M.; Rojas, B.; Gallego, B.I.; García-Martín, E.S.; Triviño, A.; Ramírez, A.I.; Salazar, J.J.; de Hoz, R. Glia and blood retinal barrier: Effects of ocular hypertension. In *Cardiovascular Disease II*; iConcept Press Ltd.: Hong Kong, China, 2014; pp. 123–162.
19. Donix, M.; Small, G.W.; Bookheimer, S.Y. Family history and APOE-4 genetic risk in Alzheimer's disease. *Neuropsychol. Rev.* **2012**, *22*, 298–309. [CrossRef]
20. Bendlin, B.B.; Carlsson, C.M.; Gleason, C.E.; Johnson, S.C.; Sodhi, A.; Gallagher, C.L.; Puglielli, L.; Engelman, C.D.; Ries, M.L.; Xu, G.; et al. Midlife predictors of Alzheimer's disease. *Maturitas* **2010**, *65*, 131–137. [CrossRef]
21. Jayadev, S.; Steinbart, E.J.; Chi, Y.Y.; Kukull, W.A.; Schellenberg, G.D.; Bird, T.D. Conjugal Alzheimer disease: Risk in children when both parents have Alzheimer disease. *Arch. Neurol.* **2008**, *65*, 373–378. [CrossRef]
22. Ribalta, J.; Vallvé, J.C.; Girona, J.; Masana, L. Apolipoprotein and apolipoprotein receptor genes, blood lipids and disease. *Curr. Opin. Clin. Nutr. Metab. Care* **2003**, *6*, 177–187. [CrossRef] [PubMed]
23. Anderson, D.H.; Ozaki, S.; Nealon, M.; Neitz, J.; Mullins, R.F.; Hageman, G.S.; Johnson, L.V. Local cellular sources of apolipoprotein E in the human retina and retinal pigmented epithelium: Implications for the process of drusen formation. *Am. J. Ophthalmol.* **2001**, *131*, 767–781. [CrossRef]
24. Toops, K.A.; Tan, L.X.; Lakkaraju, A. Apolipoprotein E isoforms and AMD. *Adv. Exp. Med. Biol.* **2016**, *854*, 3–9. [PubMed]
25. McKay, G.J.; Patterson, C.C.; Chakravarthy, U.; Dasari, S.; Klaver, C.C.; Vingerling, J.R.; Ho, L.; de Jong, P.T.V.M.; Fletcher, A.E.; Young, I.S.; et al. Evidence of association of *APOE* with age-related macular degeneration—A pooled analysis of 15 studies. *Hum. Mutat.* **2011**, *32*, 1407–1416. [CrossRef] [PubMed]
26. März, W.; Scharnagl, H.; Hoffmann, M.M.; Boehm, B.O.; Winkelmann, B.R. The apolipoprotein E polymorphism is associated with circulating C-reactive protein (the Ludwigshafen risk and cardiovascular health study). *Eur. Heart J.* **2004**, *25*, 2109–2119. [CrossRef]
27. Baird, P.N.; Richardson, A.J.; Robman, L.D.; Dimitrov, P.N.; Tikellis, G.; McCarty, C.A.; Guymer, R.H. Apolipoprotein (APOE) gene is associated with progression of age-related macular degeneration (AMD). *Hum. Mutat.* **2006**, *27*, 337–342. [CrossRef]
28. De Jong, P.T.V.M. Age-Related Macular Degeneration. *N. Engl. J. Med.* **2006**, *355*, 1474–1485. [CrossRef] [PubMed]
29. Boon, C.J.F.; van de Ven, J.P.H.; Hoyng, C.B.; den Hollander, A.I.; Klevering, B.J. Cuticular drusen: Stars in the sky. *Prog. Retin. Eye Res.* **2013**, *37*, 90–113. [CrossRef] [PubMed]
30. Kaarniranta, K.; Salminen, A.; Haapasalo, A.; Soininen, H.; Hiltunen, M. Age-related macular degeneration (AMD): Alzheimer's disease in the eye? *J. Alzheimer's Dis.* **2011**, *24*, 615–631. [CrossRef] [PubMed]

31. Ramírez, J.M.; Ramírez, A.I.; Salazar, J.J.; de Hoz, R.; Triviño, A. Changes of astrocytes in retinal ageing and age-related macular degeneration. *Exp. Eye Res.* **2001**, *73*, 601–615. [CrossRef]
32. Salobrar-Garcia, E.; Méndez-Hernández, C.; de Hoz, R.; Ramírez, A.I.; López-Cuenca, I.; Fernández-Albarral, J.A.; Rojas, P.; Wang, S.; García-Feijoo, J.; Gil, P.; et al. Ocular Vascular Changes in Mild Alzheimer's Disease Patients: Foveal Avascular Zone, Choroidal Thickness, and ONH Hemoglobin Analysis. *J. Pers. Med.* **2020**, *10*, 231. [CrossRef]
33. Gharbiya, M.; Trebbastoni, A.; Parisi, F.; Manganiello, S.; Cruciani, F.; D'Antonio, F.; De Vico, U.; Imbriano, L.; Campanelli, A.; De Lena, C. Choroidal thinning as a new finding in Alzheimer's Disease: Evidence from enhanced depth imaging spectral domain Optical Coherence Tomography. *J. Alzheimer's Dis.* **2014**, *40*, 907–917. [CrossRef] [PubMed]
34. Cheung, C.Y.; Chan, V.T.T.; Mok, V.C.; Chen, C.; Wong, T.Y. Potential retinal biomarkers for dementia: What is new? *Curr. Opin. Neurol.* **2019**, *32*, 82–91. [CrossRef] [PubMed]
35. Koh, L.H.L.; Agrawal, R.; Khandelwal, N.; Sai Charan, L.; Chhablani, J. Choroidal vascular changes in age-related macular degeneration. *Acta Ophthalmol.* **2017**, *95*, e597–e601. [CrossRef] [PubMed]
36. Feke, G.T.; Hyman, B.T.; Stern, R.A.; Pasquale, L.R. Retinal blood flow in mild cognitive impairment and Alzheimer's disease. *Alzheimer's Dement. Diagn. Assess. Dis. Monit.* **2015**, *1*, 144–151. [CrossRef] [PubMed]
37. Teja, K.V.R.; Berendschot, T.J.M.T.; Steinbusch, H.; Webers, A.B.C.; Murthy, R.P.; Mathuranath, P.S. Cerebral and Retinal Neurovascular Changes: A Biomarker for Alzheimer's Disease. *J. Gerontol. Geriatr. Res.* **2017**, *6*, 447.
38. Jiang, H.; Liu, Y.; Wei, Y.; Shi, Y.; Wright, C.B.; Sun, X.; Rundek, T.; Baumel, B.S.; Landman, J.; Wang, J. Impaired retinal microcirculation in patients with Alzheimer's disease. *PLoS ONE* **2018**, *13*, e0192154.
39. Delaey, C.; Van de Voorde, J. Regulatory mechanisms in the retinal and choroidal circulation. *Ophthalmic Res.* **2000**, *32*, 249–256. [CrossRef] [PubMed]
40. Nickla, D.L.; Wallman, J. The multifunctional choroid. *Prog. Retin. Eye Res.* **2010**, *29*, 144–168. [CrossRef]
41. Bulut, M.; Yaman, A.; Erol, M.K.; Kurtulus, F.; Toslak, D.; Dogan, B.; Turgut Coban, D.; Kaya Basar, E. Choroidal thickness in patients with mild cognitive impairment and Alzheimer's type dementia. *J. Ophthalmol.* **2016**, *2016*, 7291257. [CrossRef]
42. Triviño, A.; de Hoz, R.; Salazar, J.J.; Ramírez, A.I.; Rojas, B.; Ramírez, J.M. Distribution and organization of the nerve fiber and ganglion cells of the human choroid. *Anat. Embryol.* **2002**, *205*, 417–430. [CrossRef]
43. Triviño, A.; de Hoz, R.; Rojas, B.; Salazar, J.J.; Ramirez, A.I.; Ramirez, J.M. NPY and TH innervation in human choroidal whole-mounts. *Histol. Histopathol.* **2005**, *20*, 393–402. [PubMed]
44. Ramírez, J.M.; Ramírez, A.I.; Salazar, J.J.; de Hoz, R.; Rojas, B.; Triviño, A. Anatomofisiología de la úvea posterior: Coroides. In *Degeneracion Macular Asociada a la Edad*; Mones, J., Gómez-Ulla, F., Eds.; Probus Science: Barcelona, Spain, 2005; pp. 1–28.
45. Bayhan, H.A.; Aslan Bayhan, S.; Celikbilek, A.; Tanik, N.; Gürdal, C. Evaluation of the chorioretinal thickness changes in Alzheimer's disease using spectral-domain optical coherence tomography. *Clin. Exp. Ophthalmol.* **2015**, *43*, 145–151. [CrossRef]
46. Cunha, J.P.J.P.; Proença, R.; Dias-Santos, A.; Melancia, D.; Almeida, R.; Águas, H.; Santos, B.O.; Alves, M.; Ferreira, J.; Papoila, A.L.L.; et al. Choroidal thinning: Alzheimer's disease and aging. *Alzheimer's Dement. Diagn. Assess. Dis. Monit.* **2017**, *8*, 11–17. [CrossRef] [PubMed]
47. Trebbastoni, A.; Marcelli, M.; Mallone, F.; D'Antonio, F.; Imbriano, L.; Campanelli, A.; de Lena, C.; Gharbiya, M. Attenuation of choroidal thickness in patients with Alzheimer Disease: Evidence from an Italian Prospective Study. *Alzheimer Dis. Assoc. Disord.* **2016**, *31*, 128–134. [CrossRef] [PubMed]
48. Wylęgała, A. Principles of OCTA and Applications in Clinical Neurology. *Curr. Neurol. Neurosci. Rep.* **2018**, *18*, 96. [CrossRef]
49. López-de-Eguileta, A.; Lage, C.; López-García, S.; Pozueta, A.; García-Martínez, M.; Kazimierczak, M.; Bravo, M.; de Arcocha-Torres, M.; Banzo, I.; Jimenez-Bonilla, J.; et al. Evaluation of choroidal thickness in prodromal Alzheimer's disease defined by amyloid PET. *PLoS ONE* **2020**, *15*, e0239484. [CrossRef]
50. Foster, N.L.; Chase, T.N.; Mansi, L.; Brooks, R.; Fedio, P.; Patronas, N.J.; Di Chiro, G. Cortical abnormalities in Alzheimer's disease. *Ann. Neurol.* **1984**, *16*, 649–654. [CrossRef] [PubMed]
51. Johnson, N.A.; Jahng, G.H.; Weiner, M.W.; Miller, B.L.; Chui, H.C.; Jagust, W.J.; Gorno-Tempini, M.L.; Schuff, N. Pattern of cerebral hypoperfusion in Alzheimer disease and mild cognitive impairment measured with arterial spin-labeling MR imaging: Initial experience. *Radiology* **2005**, *234*, 851–859. [CrossRef]
52. Bertram, L.; Lill, C.M.; Tanzi, R.E. The genetics of alzheimer disease: Back to the future. *Neuron* **2010**, *68*, 270–281. [CrossRef]
53. Edwards, G.A.; Gamez, N.; Escobedo, G.; Calderon, O.; Moreno-Gonzalez, I. Modifiable risk factors for Alzheimer's disease. *Front. Aging Neurosci.* **2019**, *11*, 146. [CrossRef]
54. Klaver, C.C.W.; Kliffen, M.; Van Duijn, C.M.; Hofman, A.; Cruts, M.; Grobbee, D.E.; Van Broeckhoven, C.; De Jong, P.T.V.M. Genetic association of apolipoprotein E with age-related macular degeneration. *Am. J. Hum. Genet.* **1998**, *63*, 200–206. [CrossRef]
55. Zareparsi, S.; Reddick, A.C.; Branham, K.E.H.; Moore, K.B.; Jessup, L.; Thoms, S.; Smith-Wheelock, M.; Yashar, B.M.; Swaroop, A. Association of apolipoprotein E alleles with susceptibility to age-related macular degeneration in a large cohort from a single center. *Investig. Ophthalmol. Vis. Sci.* **2004**, *45*, 1306–1310. [CrossRef] [PubMed]
56. Souied, E.H.; Benlian, P.; Amouyel, P.; Feingold, J.; Lagarde, J.P.; Munnich, A.; Kaplan, J.; Coscas, G.; Soubrane, G. The ε4 allele of the Apolipoprotein E gene as a potential protective factor for exudative age-related macular degeneration. *Am. J. Ophthalmol.* **1998**, *125*, 353–359. [CrossRef]

57. Mullins, R.F.; Johnson, M.N.; Faidley, E.A.; Skeie, J.M.; Huang, J. Choriocapillaris vascular dropout related to density of drusen in human eyes with early age-related macular degeneration. *Investig. Ophthalmol. Vis. Sci.* **2011**, *52*, 1606–1612. [CrossRef] [PubMed]
58. Lutty, G.A.; McLeod, D.S.; Bhutto, I.A.; Edwards, M.M.; Seddon, J.M. Choriocapillaris dropout in early age-related macular degeneration. *Exp. Eye Res.* **2020**, *192*, 107939. [CrossRef]
59. Berenberg, T.L.; Metelitsina, T.I.; Madow, B.; Dai, Y.; Ying, G.S.; Dupont, J.C.; Grunwald, L.; Brucker, A.J.; Grunwald, J.E. The association between drusen extent and foveolar choroidal blood flow in age-related macular degeneration. *Retina* **2012**, *32*, 25–31. [CrossRef]
60. Chung, S.E.; Kang, S.W.; Lee, J.H.; Kim, Y.T. Choroidal thickness in polypoidal choroidal vasculopathy and exudative age-related macular degeneration. *Ophthalmology* **2011**, *118*, 840–845. [CrossRef]
61. Pauleikhoff, D.; Chen, J.C.; Chisholm, I.H.; Bird, A.C. Choroidal perfusion abnormality with age-related Bruch's membrane change. *Am. J. Ophthalmol.* **1990**, *109*, 211–217. [CrossRef]
62. Böker, T.; Fang, T.; Steinmetz, R. Refractive error and choroidal perfusion characteristics in patients with choroidal neovascularization and age-related macular degeneration. *Ger. J. Ophthalmol.* **1993**, *2*, 10–13.
63. Chen, J.C.; Fitzke, F.W.; Pauleikhoff, D.; Bird, A.C. Functional loss in age-related Bruch's membrane change with choroidal perfusion defect. *Investig. Ophthalmol. Vis. Sci.* **1992**, *33*, 334–340.
64. Holz, F.G.; Wolfensberger, T.J.; Piguet, B.; Gross-Jendroska, M.; Wells, J.A.; Minassian, D.C.; Chisholm, I.H.; Bird, A.C. Bilateral Macular Drusen in Age-related Macular Degeneration: Prognosis and Risk Factors. *Ophthalmology* **1994**, *101*, 1522–1528. [CrossRef]
65. Prünte, C.; Niesel, P. Quantification of choroidal blood-flow parameters using indocyanine green video-fluorescence angiography and statistical picture analysis. *Graefe's Arch. Clin. Exp. Ophthalmol.* **1988**, *226*, 55–58. [CrossRef]
66. Friedman, E.; Ivry, M.; Ebert, E.; Glynn, R.; Gragoudas, E.; Seddon, J. Increased Scleral Rigidity and Age-related Macular Degeneration. *Ophthalmology* **1989**, *96*, 104–108. [CrossRef]
67. Schultz, N.; Byman, E.; Wennström, M. Levels of Retinal Amyloid-β Correlate with Levels of Retinal IAPP and Hippocampal Amyloid-β in Neuropathologically Evaluated Individuals. *J. Alzheimer's Dis.* **2020**, *73*, 1201–1209. [CrossRef] [PubMed]
68. Smyth, L.C.D.; Rustenhoven, J.; Scotter, E.L.; Schweder, P.; Faull, R.L.M.; Park, T.I.H.; Dragunow, M. Markers for human brain pericytes and smooth muscle cells. *J. Chem. Neuroanat.* **2018**, *92*, 48–60. [CrossRef]
69. Snodderly, D.M.; Weinhaus, R.S.; Choi, J.C. Neural-vascular relationships in central retina of macaque monkeys (Macaca fascicularis). *J. Neurosci.* **1992**, *12*, 1169–1193. [CrossRef] [PubMed]
70. Conrath, J.; Giorgi, R.; Raccah, D.; Ridings, B. Foveal avascular zone in diabetic retinopathy: Quantitative vs. qualitative assessment. *Eye* **2005**, *19*, 322–326. [CrossRef]
71. Van De Kreeke, J.A.; Nguyen, H.T.; Konijnenberg, E.; Tomassen, J.; Den Braber, A.; Ten Kate, M.; Yaqub, M.; Van Berckel, B.; Lammertsma, A.A.; Boomsma, D.I.; et al. Optical coherence tomography angiography in preclinical Alzheimer's disease. *Br. J. Ophthalmol.* **2019**, *104*, 157–161. [CrossRef]
72. O'bryhim, B.; Apte, R.; Kung, N.; Coble, D.; Van Starven, G.P. Association of preclinical Alzheimer disease with optical coherence tomographic angiography findings. *JAMA Ophthalmol.* **2018**, *136*, 1242–1248. [CrossRef] [PubMed]
73. Chua, J.; Hu, Q.; Ke, M.; Tan, B.; Hong, J.; Yao, X.; Hilal, S.; Venketasubramanian, N.; Garhöfer, G.; Cheung, C.; et al. Retinal Microvascular Alterations in Alzheimer's Disease and Mild Cognitive Impairment. *Alzheimers. Res. Ther.* **2020**, *12*, 161. [CrossRef]
74. Zhang, Y.S.; Zhou, N.; Knoll, B.M.; Samra, S.; Ward, M.R.; Weintraub, S.; Fawzi, A.A. Parafoveal vessel loss and correlation between peripapillary vessel density and cognitive performance in amnestic mild cognitive impairment and early Alzheimer's Disease on optical coherence tomography angiography. *PLoS ONE* **2019**, *14*, e0214685. [CrossRef] [PubMed]
75. Shin, J.Y.; Choi, E.Y.; Kim, M.; Lee, H.K.; Byeon, S.H. Changes in retinal microvasculature and retinal layer thickness in association with apolipoprotein E genotype in Alzheimer's disease. *Sci. Rep.* **2021**, *11*, 1847. [CrossRef] [PubMed]
76. Wang, X.; Zhao, Q.; Tao, R.; Lu, H.; Xiao, Z.; Zheng, L.; Ding, D.; Ding, S.; Ma, Y.; Lu, Z.; et al. Decreased Retinal Vascular Density in Alzheimer's Disease (AD) and Mild Cognitive Impairment (MCI): An Optical Coherence Tomography Angiography (OCTA) Study. *Front. Aging Neurosci.* **2021**, *12*, 295. [CrossRef] [PubMed]
77. Grewal, D.S.; Polascik, B.W.; Hoffmeyer, G.C.; Fekrat, S. Assessment of differences in retinal microvasculature using OCT angiography in Alzheimer's disease: A twin discordance report. *Ophthalmic Surg. Lasers Imaging Retin.* **2018**, *49*, 440–444. [CrossRef] [PubMed]
78. Zabel, P.; Kaluzny, J.J.; Wilkosc-Debczynska, M.; Gebska-Toloczko, M.; Suwala, K.; Zabel, K.; Zaron, A.; Kucharski, R.; Araszkiewicz, A. Comparison of Retinal Microvasculature in Patients with Alzheimer's Disease and Primary Open-Angle Glaucoma by Optical Coherence Tomography Angiography. *Investig. Ophthalmol. Vis. Sci.* **2019**, *60*, 3447. [CrossRef]
79. Yoon, S.P.; Grewal, D.S.; Thompson, A.C.; Polascik, B.W.; Dunn, C.; Burke, J.R.; Fekrat, S. Retinal Microvascular and Neurodegenerative Changes in Alzheimer's Disease and Mild Cognitive Impairment Compared with Control Participants. *Ophthalmol. Retin.* **2019**, *3*, 489–499. [CrossRef] [PubMed]
80. Brown, W.R.; Thore, C.R. Review: Cerebral microvascular pathology in ageing and neurodegeneration. *Neuropathol. Appl. Neurobiol.* **2011**, *37*, 56–74. [CrossRef]

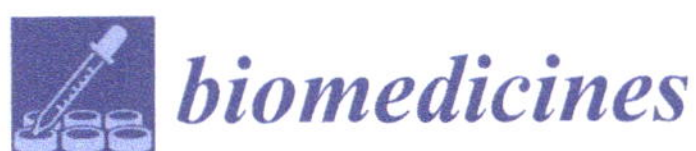 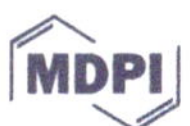

*Article*

# Antibody Protection against Long-Term Memory Loss Induced by Monomeric C-Reactive Protein in a Mouse Model of Dementia

**Elisa García-Lara [1], Samuel Aguirre [1], Núria Clotet [1], Xenia Sawkulycz [2], Clara Bartra [1], Lidia Almenara-Fuentes [1], Cristina Suñol [1], Rubén Corpas [1], Peter Olah [3], Florin Tripon [3], Andrei Crauciuc [3], Mark Slevin [2,3,*] and Coral Sanfeliu [1,*]**

1 Institut d'Investigacions Biomèdiques de Barcelona (IIBB), CSIC and IDIBAPS, 08036 Barcelona, Spain; elisaglara21@gmail.com (E.G.-L.); samuelaguirreinfantes@gmail.com (S.A.); nuria.cg07@gmail.com (N.C.); clara.bartra@iibb.csic.es (C.B.); almenara.lidia.22@gmail.com (L.A.-F.); cristina.sunol@iibb.csic.es (C.S.); rubencorpas@gmail.com (R.C.)

2 School of Life Sciences, John Dalton Building, Manchester Metropolitan University, Manchester M15 6BH, UK; XENIA.SAWKULYCZ@stu.mmu.ac.uk

3 Genetics Department, George Emil Palade University of Medicine, Pharmacy, Science and Technology of Targu Mures, 540142 Targu Mures, Romania; olah_peter@yahoo.com (P.O.); tripon.florin.2010@gmail.com (F.T.); andrei.crauciuc@gmail.com (A.C.)

* Correspondence: M.A.Slevin@mmu.ac.uk (M.S.); coral.sanfeliu@iibb.csic.es (C.S.); Tel.: +44-(0)-161-247-1172 (M.S.); +34-93-363-8338 (C.S.)

**Citation:** García-Lara, E.; Aguirre, S.; Clotet, N.; Sawkulycz, X.; Bartra, C.; Almenara-Fuentes, L.; Suñol, C.; Corpas, R.; Olah, P.; Tripon, F.; et al. Antibody Protection against Long-Term Memory Loss Induced by Monomeric C-Reactive Protein in a Mouse Model of Dementia. *Biomedicines* **2021**, *9*, 828. https://doi.org/10.3390/biomedicines9070828

Academic Editors: Arnab Ghosh and Masaru Tanaka

Received: 6 May 2021
Accepted: 12 July 2021
Published: 16 July 2021



**Abstract:** Monomeric C-reactive protein (mCRP), the activated isoform of CRP, induces tissue damage in a range of inflammatory pathologies. Its detection in infarcted human brain tissue and its experimentally proven ability to promote dementia with Alzheimer's disease (AD) traits at 4 weeks after intrahippocampal injection in mice have suggested that it may contribute to the development of AD after cerebrovascular injury. Here, we showed that a single hippocampal administration of mCRP in mice induced memory loss, lasting at least 6 months, along with neurodegenerative changes detected by increased levels of hyperphosphorylated tau protein and a decrease of the neuroplasticity marker *Egr1*. Furthermore, co-treatment with the monoclonal antibody 8C10 specific for mCRP showed that long-term memory loss and tau pathology were entirely avoided by early blockade of mCRP. Notably, 8C10 mitigated *Egr1* decrease in the mouse hippocampus. 8C10 also protected against mCRP-induced inflammatory pathways in a microglial cell line, as shown by the prevention of increased generation of nitric oxide. Additional in vivo and in vitro neuroprotective testing with the anti-inflammatory agent TPPU, an inhibitor of the soluble epoxide hydrolase enzyme, confirmed the predominant involvement of neuroinflammatory processes in the dementia induced by mCRP. Therefore, locally deposited mCRP in the infarcted brain may be a novel biomarker for AD prognosis, and its antibody blockade opens up therapeutic opportunities for reducing post-stroke AD risk.

**Keywords:** monomeric C-reactive protein (mCRP); biomarker; Alzheimer's disease; mouse model of mCRP dementia

## 1. Introduction

Sustained neuroinflammation is a risk factor for age-related diseases, including cerebrovascular injuries and Alzheimer's disease (AD) [1,2]. Systemic inflammatory conditions may trigger or aggravate a range of cardiovascular and metabolic diseases that also contribute to brain dysfunction and dementia [3,4]. Indeed, inflammatory processes are increasingly being considered the culprits of frailty and disease in the elderly. As a result, the search for reliable inflammatory biomarkers and intervention targets to combat dementia and other disabling conditions has intensified.

C-reactive protein (CRP) is a widely used peripheral marker of inflammatory processes. It was identified by Tillet and Francis in 1930 in the blood of patients with pneumococcal infection [5], and its synthesis in the liver is stimulated by circulating pro-inflammatory cytokines during the acute phase of infection [6]. Chronic moderately elevated expression of CRP is associated with an increased risk of a wide range of diseases [7–9], and CRP has been proposed as a biomarker for several inflammatory-associated ailments [10,11]. High-sensitivity CRP (hsCRP) testing, able to detect values under 3 mg/L, is a sensitive test of low-grade inflammation, whereby the normal population presents mean hsCRP levels of 2 mg/L, but desirable values are less than 1 mg/L [8]. CRP molecules that circulate in blood have the structure of a pentamer with five identical monomers in a β-jelly roll characteristic of the pentraxin superfamily of proteins. Pentraxins are evolutionary conserved proteins involved in immunological responses. Interestingly, native pentameric CRP may suffer conformational changes into the isoforms, termed pCRP*, or dissociate into modified or monomeric CRP (mCRP), where pCRP* and mCRP expose functionally active neoepitopes that carry out highly pro-inflammatory functions [12]. Molecular studies ex vivo have shown that CRP activation occurs in damaged vessels and other tissues, where pro-inflammatory forms may activate immune cells and complement reactions [13]. Deposition of mCRP, which has a much lower aqueous solubility than CRP, has been shown in the brain in infarcted areas of AD patients [14] and in regions with amyloid burden [15], in atherosclerotic plaques in vascular disease [16] and in other foci of inflammatory tissue injuries [17,18]. An unbound fraction of mCRP has also recently been reported in serum of patients with high levels of circulating native CRP (>100 mg/L, in the range of acute inflammatory response), although the dissociation site of origin is unclear [19]. Furthermore, mCRP has been detected in U937-derived macrophages [20] and exosomes derived from monocytes of patients with coronary artery disease [21]. Additionally, other cell types such as neurons in the AD brain may produce CRP, albeit in lower amounts than hepatocytes [22]. New specific antibodies and upcoming analytical tools for quantifying the different forms of CRP will help to understand the functionality of the complex CRP system [23]. However, whereas CRP is essential in host defense and clearance of apoptotic cells, mCRP seems to exert severe pro-inflammatory and tissue damaging effects and is emerging as a target for anti-inflammatory therapies in chronic diseases [24,25].

Specific targeting of mCRP can be a therapeutic approach in areas in which rapid increases in its local generation are expected, such as stroke-affected brain areas, in order to halt subsequent neurodegeneration and dementia. The prevalence of dementia in stroke survivors is about 30%, and a high proportion of these patients suffer AD (in addition to those with either vascular or mixed AD plus vascular dementia) [26]. Furthermore, cerebrovascular pathological findings are common in post-mortem AD brain [27]. Inflammatory damage spreading from small blood vessels and linked dysregulation of amyloid β metabolism in the neurons have been implicated in the origin of AD [28]. It is known that mCRP accumulates in brain micro-vessels after ischemic stroke [14], where it promotes aberrant angiogenesis [29], accumulation of amyloid β [30] and probably de novo synthesis of amyloid β [31]. Therefore, mCRP may cause both vascular and neuronal degeneration and underlie the processes leading to poststroke dementia [14,28]. Furthermore, in a previous experimental study, we demonstrated that mCRP injected into the hippocampus of mice induces memory loss after 4 weeks, as well as other traits of AD such as mild amyloid and tau pathology in neurons of the hippocampus and cortical areas [30]. We have also shown that intrahippocampal mCRP may partially spread through the microvasculature to the cortical and hypothalamic areas [32]. Neurotransmission dysfunction in cortical-limbic areas causes behavioral alterations, known as 'behavioral and psychological symptoms of dementia' (BPSDs), that are common in patients of AD and other dementia [33]. Anxiety, depression and apathy are some of these behaviors that may be reproduced in AD mouse models [34].

We hypothesize that mCRP is a biomarker of AD prognosis in the infarcted brain and probably also in other inflammatory brain pathologies that increase the risk of AD.

In this study, we wished to further characterize the mCRP mouse model of poststroke dementia to investigate whether memory loss, the concomitant presence of BPSDs and pathological pro-neurodegenerative processes are maintained in the long term, up to 6 months after intrahippocampal injection of mCRP. We also used a specific antibody against mCRP, the monoclonal 8C10 antibody [29], to test whether blockade of mCRP may halt subsequent damaging mechanisms and confer long-term neuroprotection in this proposed model of neurodegeneration. We aimed to prove that mCRP can be therapeutically inhibited once injected into the mouse hippocampus. We also aimed to analyze the inflammatory mechanisms in mCRP-induced dementia by using 1-trifluoromethoxyphenyl-3-(1-propionylpiperidin-4-yl)-urea (TPPU), an inhibitor of the epoxide hydrolase enzyme, since inhibition of this enzyme has recently been proposed as a protective mechanism against neuroinflammation [35]. Finally, we wished to characterize the modulation of the well-known inflammatory pathways of nitric oxide by mCRP, 8C10 and TPPU in an in vitro setting using the BV2 microglial cell line.

## 2. Material and Methods

### 2.1. Experimental Agents

Monomeric C-reactive protein (mCRP) was generated from a commercial source of recombinant human native CRP using the Potempa method [32]. Briefly, 1 mL commercial CRP protein was chelated in a 1:1 ratio with EDTA/urea buffer (10 mM EDTA, 8M urea) and incubated at 37 °C for 2 h and further dialyzed (20 kDa MWCO) in buffer (25 mM Tris–HCl, 50 mM NaCl; pH 8.3) for 24 h to recover a solution of pure monomers of mCRP. Native CRP was obtained from YO Proteins (Ronninge, Sweden); all other reagents were from Sigma (St. Louis, MO, USA) where not otherwise indicated.

Mouse monoclonal antibody against human mCRP clone 8C10 was obtained from Dr L.A. Potempa by hybridoma technology and fully characterized, as described previously [29,36]. The non-purified hybridoma culture supernatant was directly used as an experimental 8C10 solution. We have shown its ability to block mCRP, preventing the activation of U937 monocytes [13].

The soluble epoxide hydrolase inhibitor TPPU was used as a reference anti-inflammatory agent. TPPU was purchased from MedChemExpress (Monmouth Junction, NJ, USA).

### 2.2. Animals and Experimental Design

One hundred and fifty-two C57BL/6J male mice were used in this study. Mice bred by Janvier Labs (France) were purchased from Novaintermed (Pipera, Romania) and maintained for the study in the Animal Unit of the University of Barcelona (UB), Spain. Animals were individually housed in Makrolon cages (Techniplast, Buguggiatte, Italy) with free access to food and water in a temperature-controlled room (22 ± 2 °C) with a 12 h light/12 h dark cycle. All the animal procedures, including surgery, behavioral testing and necropsies, were performed at the UB animal facilities. The study design and protocols were approved by the UB Ethics Committee for Animal Experimentation (Comitè Ètic d'Experimentació Animal, CEEA-UB) under the guidelines of the Animal Experimentation Commission of the Autonomous Government of Catalonia (Comissió d'Experimentació Animal, Generalitat de Catalunya) (Approval references: #6991 and #10921). All procedures were carried out in accordance with the Directive 214/97 of the Generalitat de Catalunya, Spanish legislation (Real Decreto 1386/2018), and the European Union (EU) Directive 2010/63/EU for animal experiments.

We performed 3 independent studies with intrahippocampal mCRP treatment over periods of 1 month, 3 months and 6 months respectively, to test neuroprotection by 8C10. Animals received a single bilateral intrahippocampal injection (see Section 2.3 for details) of 1 μL mCRP at 3.5 μg/μL and/or 1 μL 8C10 antibody solution. Dosage was selected in a preliminary study. Volume in the mice dosed with either solution was completed to 2 μL, with 1 μL of artificial solution of CSF (NaCl 148 mM, KCl 3 mM, $CaCl_2$ 1 mM, $MgCl_2$ 0.8 mM, $Na_2HPO_4$ 0.8 mM, $NaH_2PO_4$ 0.2 mM). Mice in the control group received a bilateral injection of 2 μL CSF. Therefore, for each study, the experimental groups were as follows: control (CSF), mCRP, mCRP plus anti-mCRP antibody (mCRP + 8C10) and anti-mCRP antibody (8C10). Experimental procedures were established in a previous 1-month study with the mCRP mouse model of dementia [30]. An additional study was performed with the same intrahippocampal mCRP treatment for 1 month to test neuroprotection by oral TPPU dosing. TPPU was administered orally beginning 2 days before a single bilateral mCRP or CSF injection, and throughout the study in the drinking water, mixed with cyclodextrin 3% to improve its solubility. The control group received the same dose of cyclodextrin in the drinking water. TPPU was added to the drinking water at a concentration that yielded a daily dose of 5 mg/kg body weight. The initial concentration of TPPU was established in a preliminary study of water consumption per mouse. Thereafter, the water consumption and body weight of the mice were measured twice a week and the TPPU concentration was adjusted accordingly in a freshly prepared drinking solution. This treatment regimen was found to be neuroprotective in AD mouse models [37]. The experimental groups were: control (CSF), mCRP and mCRP plus TPPU (mCRP + TPPU). A schematic drawing of the experimental design is shown in Figure 1a. The number of animals per group was as follows: (i) 1-month mCRP/8C10 study, CSF N = 6, mCRP N = 9, mCRP + 8C10 N = 12 and 8C10 N = 6; (ii) 3-month mCRP/8C10 study, CSF N = 13, mCRP N = 12, mCRP + 8C10 N = 12 and 8C10 N = 11; (iii) 6-month mCRP/8C10 study, CSF N = 11, mCRP N = 11, mCRP + 8C10 N = 12 and 8C10 N = 10; (iv) 1-month mCRP/TPPU study, CSF N = 9, mCRP N = 9 and mCRP + TPPU N = 9. Mice were visually inspected and weighed on a regular basis throughout the studies in order to control their general health status. All animals survived to termination.

Heterozygous transgenic AD mice of the strain 5XFAD [38] and their wild-type siblings (WT), 7-month-old males, were used for a selected analysis (see Section 2.6). All mice, N = 8 per group, were bred from first progenitors obtained from Jackson Laboratory (Bar Harbor, ME, United States) and maintained in the same housing conditions as described for the C57BL/6J mice.

### 2.3. *Hippocampal Surgery and Treatment Administration*

Treatments of mCRP and 8C10 were administered in the CA1 region of the mouse hippocampus by stereotactic surgery procedures, as previously performed [30]. Three-month-old C57BL/6J mice were anesthetized with 100 mg/kg ketamine (Ketolar 50 mg/mL, Pfizer, Alcobendas, Madrid, Spain) and 10 mg/kg xylazine (Rompun 2%, Bayer, Leverkusen, Germany) mixture i.p., and immobilized in a stereotactic apparatus (David Kopf Instruments, Tujunga, CA, USA). The experimental agent solutions were infused bilaterally into the CA1 area of the hippocampus. Injections were performed at a rate of $5 \times 10^{-4}$ mL/min at coordinates relative to Bregma of −2 mm A/P, ±1.3 mm M/L, −1.6 mm V/D. Two microliters of each solution were delivered to the application point with a 2 μL 25-gauge 7000 series Neuros Syringe (Hamilton Central Europe S.R.L., Giarmata, Romania). The syringe was attached to a micro-infusion pump (Bioanalytical systems Inc., West Lafayette, IN, USA) and left in position for 5 min after delivery in order to prevent the solution from surging back.

### 2.4. *Behavioral Testing*

All animals were tested for behavioral changes induced by the specific treatments. Age at testing was 4, 6 and 9 months for the 1-, 3- and 6-month mCRP exposure studies, respectively. A battery of tests was applied in daily consecutive sessions, as was performed in previous studies [39,40]. After a handling habituation, animals were analyzed for sensorimotor changes and BPSD-like behaviors, such as neophobia, apathy to exploration, anxiety and depression. Learning and memory were analyzed with tests focused on recognition memory and spatial memory.

Handling habituation was performed to minimize animal stress during subsequent testing. In the handling procedure, the mouse was picked up by its tail and held in the hand for 2 min, and mice were allowed to move along the experimenter's arm before being returned to their home cage. This procedure was repeated twice a day for 3 days with all mice. Gloves and cover sleeves were cleaned with 70° ethanol to eliminate olfactory cues between the mice.

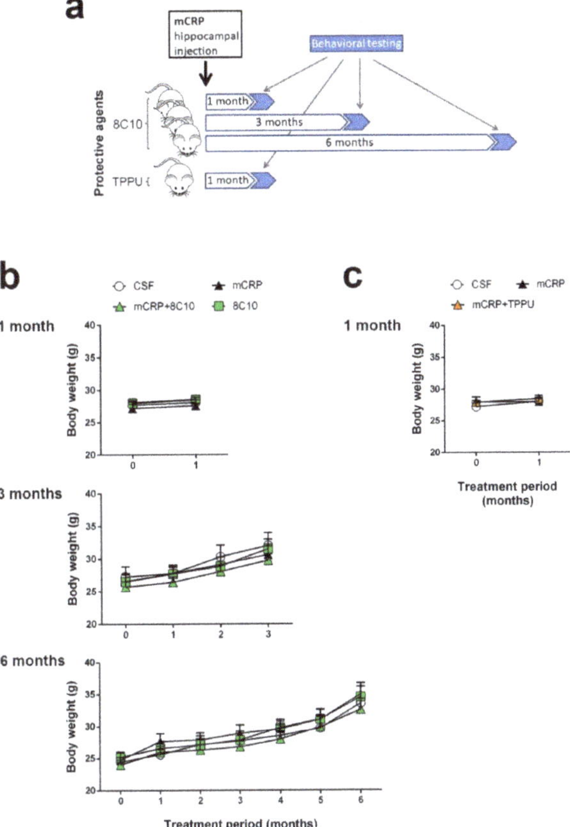


**Figure 1.** Monomeric C-reactive protein (mCRP) treatment in C57BL/6J male mice. (**a**) Scheme of the experimental design (see Methods Section for details). (**b**) Body weight control for the 1-, 3- and 6-month studies assaying a protective treatment with the anti-mCRP antibody 8C10 and (**c**) for the 1-month study assaying a protective treatment with Trifluoromethoxyphenyl-3-(1-propionylpiperidin-4-yl)-urea (TPPU). Progression of body weight confirmed the absence of unwanted systemic effects. Values are mean ± SEM ((**b**) 1-month graph: CSF N = 6, mCRP N = 9, mCRP + 8C10 N = 12 and 8C10 N = 6; 3-month graph: CSF N = 13, mCRP N = 12, mCRP + 8C10 N = 12 and 8C10 N = 11; 6-month graph; CSF N = 11, mCRP N = 11, mCRP + 8C10 N = 12, 8C10 N = 10. (**c**) CSF N = 9, mCRP N = 9 and mCRP + TPP N = 9).

The following specific tests were applied to all mice except for the two alternative spatial memory tests, as indicated.

Sensorimotor responses. Visual reflex and posterior leg extension reflex were measured by holding the animal by its tail and slowly lowering it toward a black surface. Motor coordination and equilibrium were assessed with a 20 s trial by the distance covered and the latency to fall off a horizontal wooden rod and a metal wire rod. Each trial was performed twice. Prehensility and motor coordination were measured as the distance covered on the wire hang test, in which the animal was allowed to cling from the middle of a horizontal wire (2 mm diameter × 40 cm length) with its forepaws for two trials of 5 s and a third trial of 60 s.

Open-field test. This test analyzes general behavior and activity. Mice were placed in the center of the apparatus (home-made, wooden, white, 55 × 55 cm surface and 25 cm high walls) and observed for 5 min. Patterns of horizontal locomotor activity (distance covered and thigmotaxis) and vertical movement (rearings) were analyzed throughout the test. Initial freezing, self-grooming behavior and the number of urine spots and defecation boli were also recorded. A computerized tracking system (SMART v3.0, Panlab S.A., Barcelona, Spain) was used to measure the distance covered, along with the ambulatory pattern.

Corner test. Neophobia to a new home-cage was assessed by introducing the animal into the center of a standard square cage (Makrolon cage 35 × 35 × 25 cm) with fresh bedding, and counting the number of corners visited and rearings during a period of 30 s. The latency of the first rearing was also recorded.

Boissier's four-hole-board test. Exploratory and apathy-like behavior were measured as the number of head dips and time spent head-dipping on each of the four holes (3 cm diameter) equally spaced in the floor of the hole-board (woodwork white box of 32 × 32 × 32 cm). The latencies of movement, first dipping and four holes dipping were also recorded.

Dark and light box test. Anxiety-like behavior was measured in a dark–light box. The apparatus consisted of two compartments (black: 27 × 18 × 27 cm with a red light; white: 27 × 27 × 27 cm with white lighting intensity of 600 lux) connected by an opening (7 × 7 cm). The mice were introduced into the black compartment and observed for 5 min. The latency to enter the lit compartment, the time spent in the lit compartment, the number of crossings to each compartment and the vertical movement (number of rearings) were recorded.

Tail suspension test. To assess depression-like behavior, mice were suspended by the tail 30 cm above the surface. The tail was fixed with adhesive tape at 1 cm from its tip. The duration of immobility (defined as the absence of all movements except for those required for respiration) was scored over a 6 min period.

Novel object recognition test (NORT). This test assesses recognition memory. It is based on the spontaneous tendency of rodents to spend more time exploring a novel object than a familiar one. Animals were placed in the middle of a black rectangular box (30 × 40 × 30.5 cm) with a lighting intensity of 100 lux. The objects to be discriminated were made of plastic (6–10 cm high). After three days of habituation, the animals were submitted to a 10 min acquisition trial (first trial), during which they were placed in the cage in the presence of two identical novel objects (A + A) placed equidistant from each other. A 10 min retention trial (second trial) was performed 2 h later, replacing object A in the cage with object B. Another 10 min retention trial (third trial) was performed 24 h later, replacing object A in the box with object C. The trials were recorded using a camera mounted above the testing box; later, the time that the animal explored the new and the old objects was analyzed. The ratio between the time taken to explore the new object and the time spent on both objects provides an index of recognition memory in the short (2 h) and long term (24 h). In order to avoid object preference biases, the sequence of presentation of the different objects was counter-balanced in each experimental group. The cage and the objects were cleaned with 70° ethanol between different animals to eliminate olfactory cues.

Object location test (OLT). The OLT assesses cognition, specifically spatial memory and discrimination. This test is based on the ability of rodents to recognize when an object has been moved from its previous position and their spontaneous tendency to spend more time exploring the relocated object than the one in a familiar position. Testing was performed in a black box (30 × 40 × 30.5 cm), where the animals are first habituated for 10 min. The next day, two identical objects were introduced in the dark box. Objects were placed equidistant from each other with space around them so that the mice could explore them (A1 + A2). Each mouse was allowed to explore the objects for 5 min. Object exploration was defined as the orientation of the nose to the object at a distance of less than 2 cm. In the second trial conducted 2 h later, the animal again encountered the two objects, but one of them had changed position (A1 + A3). The trials were also video recorded, and for each mouse, the amount of time spent exploring each object was scored. The object location discrimination index was calculated as the ratio between the time spent exploring the relocated object and the total time spent on both objects, in order to evaluate spatial memory. This test was used in the 1-month mCRP exposure study.

Morris water maze test (MWM). The MWM was used to test animals for spatial learning and memory. The test consisted of one day of training and six days of place task learning for spatial reference memory, followed by one probe trial. Mice were trained to locate a hidden platform, 10 cm in diameter, located 20 cm from the wall and 0.5 cm below the water surface. The platform was placed in a circular pool 100 cm in diameter, 40 cm high, with 22–24 °C opaque water, surrounded by black curtains. The animals learned to find the platform using 4 distinctive landmarks as visual cues attached to the pool wall and placed equidistant from each other. The platform was placed between two of these landmarks. Five trial sessions of 60 s per day were performed. In each trial, the mouse was gently released (facing the wall) from one randomly selected starting point (N, S, E or W) and allowed to swim until it escaped onto the platform. Mice that failed to find the platform within 60 s were placed on it for 20 s, the same period as was allowed for the successful animals. On day 7, the platform was removed, and the mice performed a probe trial of 60 s to test learning retention. The computerized tracking system (SMART) was used to measure the distance covered during the learning tasks, along with the time spent in each quadrant of the pool after the removal of the platform in the probe test. The MWM test was used in the 3- and 6-month mCRP exposure studies instead of the OLT test, for a more potent analysis of spatial memory.

### 2.5. Western Blot Analysis of Hippocampus Tissue

After completion of the behavioral tests, mice were sacrificed by dislocation and the brains were dissected on ice to obtain the hippocampus. The tissue was frozen with liquid nitrogen and stored at −80 °C until protein analysis by Western blot, as previously described [41], with some modifications. Hippocampi (right hippocampus samples) were suspended in 15 volumes of ice-cold RIPA buffer (1% IGEPAL, 0.5% sodium deoxycholate, 0.1% SDS in PBS) supplemented with 1 mM orthovanadate, 5 mM sodium fluoride and Complete Protease Inhibitor Cocktail (#11697498001; Roche, Mannheim, Germany). Samples were sonicated and, after centrifuging (13,000× $g$, 10 min, 4 °C), supernatants were collected. The protein concentration of cell lysates was determined using the Bradford protein assay (#5000002; Bio-Rad, Munich, Germany), and equal quantities of proteins (20 µg) were denatured by boiling at 95 °C for 5 min in loading buffer (2% SDS, 10% glycerol, 0.05% bromophenol blue and 50 mM DTT in 50 mM Tris-HCl buffer pH 6.8) and separated by SDS PAGE at 100 V for 2 h. Polyacrylamide gels were prepared with 30% Acrylamide/Bis Solution 29:1 (#1610156, Bio-Rad) at 10% or 15% according to the target protein size, Tris-HCl/SDS, 10% ($w/v$) ammonium persulfate and TEMED [42]. Electrophoresed proteins in the gels were transferred to 0.45 µm PVDF membranes (Immobilon-P, Millipore, Burlington, MA, USA) at 200 mA for 1 h 30 min. The different membranes were blocked for 1 h at room temperature with TBS-T buffer containing 5% Blotting-Grade Blocker (#170-6404; Bio-Rad). Subsequently, the membranes were incubated overnight at 4 °C with primary antibodies diluted 1:1000. Total tau clone HT7 mouse monoclonal antibody (#MN1000; Pierce Endogen, ThermoFisher Scientific, Waltham, MA, USA), p-tau clone AT8 mouse monoclonal antibody (#MN1020; ThermoFisher Scientific), and p-tau Ser396 rabbit polyclonal antibody (#44752G; Life Technologies, Carlsbad, CA, USA) were used for immunodetection of tau-related changes. Mouse monoclonal antibody against amyloid β clone 4G8 (SIG-39220; BioLegend, San Diego, CA, USA) were used to detect increased amyloid pathology. Ionized calcium-binding adapter molecule 1 (Iba1) (#019-19741; Wako; Richmond, VA, Canada) were used to immunodetect activated microglia. Furthermore, monoclonal 8C10 antibody obtained as described above was used to detect mCRP. However, the Western blot technique will not discern between CRP isoforms because the pentameric form will dissociate to monomers in the presence of reducing and denaturing reagents of the blotting buffers [29]. After washing, the corresponding secondary antibody (1:2000) was prepared for 1.5 h incubation at room temperature. Antibodies used for loading control were rabbit polyclonal actin (20–33) (#A5060; Sigma-Aldrich) and monoclonal β-tubulin (#T4026; Sigma-Aldrich) at 1:10,000. Secondary antibodies were peroxidase-conjugated. Antibodies were diluted in the West Vision Block and Diluent SP-7000 (Vector Labs Inc., Burlingame, CA, USA). Proteins were visualized using enhanced chemiluminescence (ECL) detection (Chemidoc™ Imaging System, Bio-Rad, Hercules, CA, USA) and the semi-quantitative fold differences were identified using Image Lab software (v3.0.1; Bio-Rad). Proteins were normalized to actin, to β-tubulin or to the total form for phosphorylated proteins, always analyzed in the same membrane. When p-tau and total tau could not be analyzed in the same membrane, both proteins were previously normalized to actin or to β-tubulin. All membranes contained samples from the control group and the other experimental groups. Normalized densitometry value for each sample was calculated relative to the mean of the values of the control sample in each membrane. To increase the reliability of the results in the mouse Western blots, we analyzed some of the samples in duplicate membranes. In this case, we used the mean value obtained from each hippocampus sample as a value for statistical analysis. Cell culture samples were more readily available, and each well extract was analyzed once.

### 2.6. Quantitative PCR Analysis of Hippocampus Tissue

We determined the transcription levels of the gene Early growth response protein 1 (*Egr1*), as an indicator of hippocampal plasticity underlying neuron dysfunction and memory loss, by real-time quantitative PCR (qPCR). Analysis was performed in the hippocampus of mice submitted to the diverse treatments for 6 months. As a reference for the severity of any decrease found after mCRP treatment, *Egr1* activation was also analyzed in the hippocampus of 5XFAD mice with advanced AD pathology. RNA was extracted from hippocampus samples (left hippocampus) using mirVana miRNA Isolation Kits (#AM156; Life Technologies), following the manufacturer's instructions, to obtain RNA, including small RNA. The quantity and quality of the RNA samples were determined using a ND-1000 spectrophotometer (NanoDrop Technologies, Wilmington, DE, USA). Random-primed cDNA synthesis was performed using high-capacity cDNA Reverse Transcription Kits (#4368814; Life Technologies). Gene expression of *Egr1* and the reference gene TATA-box binding protein (*Tbp*) was determined using TaqMan Fluorescein amidite (FAM)-labeled specific probes (*Egr1*, #Mm00656724_m1 and Tbp, #Mm00446971_m1; Applied Biosystems) and Quantimix Easy Probe kits (#10.601-4149; Biotools, Madrid, Spain) in an RFX96TM real-time system (Bio-Rad). qPCR assay was run with cDNA obtained from 3.75 ng of RNA. Samples were analyzed in duplicate. Data were normalized to *Tbp* gene expression using the Comparative Cycle Threshold method (ΔΔCT).

The transcription level of the *Crp* gene was also analyzed by qPCR in the hippocampus tissue to discern any contribution of endogenous CRP throughout the 6-month treatment time. For this purpose, we analyzed mouse tissue at 1 month, 3 months and 6 months after CSF or mCRP injection. *Crp* expression was very low in the hippocampus, as expected for brain tissue, and the analysis required a preamplification step. Specific preamplification of *Crp* and *Tbp* cDNA was simultaneously performed using TaqMan Preamp Master Mix (#4391128; Applied Biosystems, Foster City, CA, USA) according to the manufacturer's instructions. Next, gene expression of *Crp* was determined using TaqMan Fluorescein amidite (FAM)-labeled specific probes (*Crp*, #Mm00432680_g1; Applied Biosystems). qPCR assay was run with cDNA obtained from 10 ng of RNA and submitted to 14 cycles of preamplification. Samples were analyzed in duplicate. Data were normalized to *Tbp* expression after simultaneous preamplification, using the $\Delta\Delta C_T$ method. Two samples of liver cDNA from the same strain of mice were used as a positive control.

### 2.7. Assays in the Microglial BV2 Cell Line

We analyzed inflammatory changes in an in vitro experimental setting by the determination of nitric oxide generation in the mouse microglial cell line BV2 (#ATL03001, ICLC, Banca Biologica e Cell Factory, Genova, Italy). BV2 cells were grown in T25 flasks (NuncTM, ThermoFisher Scientific) with culture medium composed of RPMI 1640 with L-glutamine 2 mM, gentamycin 50 μM and 10% heat-inactivated fetal bovine serum (FBS), at 37 °C in a humidified incubator with 5% $CO_2$. Cells were sub-cultured at a 1:10 ratio when they reached 80–90% of confluence. Each set of experiments was performed with cells of at least 3 independent passages. For experiments, cells were seeded in 96- or 12-well plates at 2–3 × $10^5$ cells/mL (1.42 × $10^5$ cells/$cm^2$). After 24 h, the medium was replaced with fresh culture medium without FBS containing vehicle or anti-inflammatory agents. Anti-inflammatory treatments were TPPU at 50 or 100 μM and 8C10 monoclonal antibody at 1:20 dilution. DMSO 0.1% was used as a vehicle in the TPPU treatment experiments. After 1 h of incubation, the cells were treated with the proinflammatory chemicals lipopolysaccharide (LPS; 0.1 μg/mL) or mCRP (100 μg/mL), and further incubated for 24 h. Native pentameric CRP at 100 μg/mL was also assayed as an additional control.

Nitric oxide generation by activated BV2 was measured by the colorimetric Griess reaction [43] that detects nitrite ($NO_2^-$), a stable reaction product of nitric oxide and molecular oxygen. Briefly, 50 μL of conditioned medium was incubated with 50 μL of Griess reagent for 10 min at room temperature. Optical density was measured at 540 nm using a microplate reader (iEMS Reader MF; Labsystems, Vantaa, Finland). Nitrite concentration was determined from a sodium nitrite standard curve and was then expressed as a percentage of the average maximal values given by the pro-inflammatory agent for each experiment.

Level of inducible nitric oxide synthase (iNOS), the enzyme that catalyzes nitric oxide generation, was analyzed in cell extracts. After incubation, cells were washed with cold PBS and immediately homogenized in ice-cold RIPA buffer supplemented with protease and phosphatase inhibitors. Cell extracts were processed for Western blot analysis following the procedures described for hippocampus tissue extracts. For iNOS immunotesting, membranes were incubated overnight with purified mouse anti-mouse iNOS clone 54/iNOS (#610431; BD Transduction Laboratories, BD, San José, CA, USA) at the concentration of 1:500.

### 2.8. Statistical Analysis

Results are shown as mean ± SEM. The distribution of the data was checked with the Shapiro–Wilk normality test. Data were analyzed by ANOVA, where not stated otherwise. Results were considered significant when $p < 0.05$. Post-hoc Fisher's LSD test was performed to compare the means between groups. Statistical analysis was performed using GraphPad Prism v6 (GraphPad Software, San Diego, CA, USA) and IBM SPSS Statistics v23 (IBM Corp., Armonk, NY, USA). Exact N value per group is provided in the figure legends.

## 3. Results

### 3.1. General Indicators of Body Health Were Not Modified by mCRP

Several experimental groups of 3-month-old male C57BL/6J mice were used to analyze the neuroprotection of the antibody 8C10 against mCRP-induced dementia at 1, 3 and 6 months and of TPPU at 1 month, as described in the experimental design (Figure 1a). Body weight did not change significantly in any of the treatment groups in either 1-month study and progressed similarly over time for all the treated groups in the 3- and 6-month studies of mCRP treatment to assay 8C10 protection (Figure 1b) or the 1-month study to assay TPPU protection (Figure 1c) (two-way ANOVA, main effect of age: $F(3, 116) = 9.959$, $p < 0.001$ and $F(6, 203) = 17.79$, $p < 0.001$ for 3 and 6 months with 8C10, respectively). The statistical analysis did not show alterations in vertical and horizontal activities or in the pattern of movement evaluated in the open-field test, or in the Sensorimotor tests for motor coordination studies (Supplementary Figure S1). Furthermore, all animals in all experimental groups had preserved vision, as indicated by the presence of visual reflex and posterior leg extension reflex. Body weight, sensorimotor abilities and mobility were recorded as general indicators of the systemic condition of the mice. Visual inspection throughout the study did not reveal any abnormal appearance of the mice or their behavior in the home-cage. Thus, no gross body health alterations were induced by intrahippocampal mCRP treatment or by the neuroprotective treatments with the anti-mCRP antibody 8C10 or the reference anti-inflammatory drug TPPU.

### *3.2. Anti-mCRP Antibody 8C10 Protected Against Anxiety Induced by mCRP at 6 Months of Treatment*

Tests used to detect BPSD-like behaviors did not show significant effects in the mice treated with mCRP for 1 month or 3 months of exposure. In contrast, mCRP hippocampal injection induced symptoms of anxiety after 6 months of treatment, observed as the trend toward an increased latency to enter the lit area during the dark and light box test (Figure 2a) (one-way ANOVA, F (3, 40) = 2.566, $p = 0.068$; Control vs. mCRP by two-tailed Student's *t*-test, $t$ (20) = 2.381, $p = 0.027$). A similar trend was observed for the increase in grooming time in the open-field test, which is considered an indicator of stress (Figure 2b) (F (3, 40) = 2.701, $p = 0.058$; Control vs. mCRP, $t$ (20) = 2.350, $p = 0.029$). These anxiety symptoms at 6 months of treatment were not present with the joint injection of mCRP and the 8C10 antibody, indicating a neuroprotective effect of 8C10. No changes in other BPSD-like behaviors tested, such as neophobia, apathy and depression, were detected in any of the experimental groups, as analyzed in the Corner test, Boissier's four-hole-board test and Tail suspension test, respectively (Supplementary Figure S2).

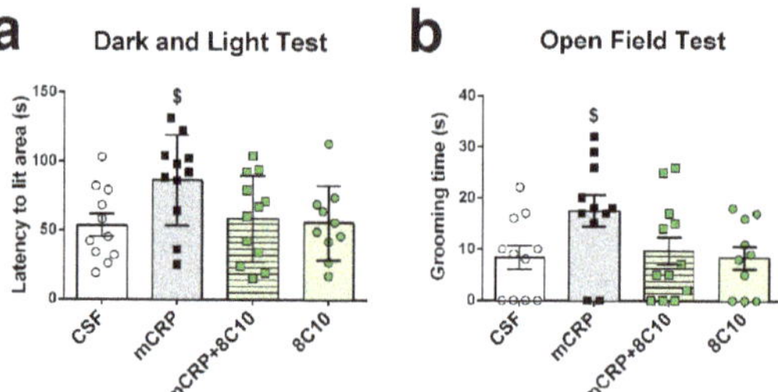


**Figure 2.** Anxiety induced by mCRP treatment was not evident in the co-treatment with 8C10 antibody. Six months of exposure to mCRP induced traits of anxiety, as shown by increased latency to enter to the lit area in the dark and light test (**a**) and increased grooming time in the open-field test (**b**). 8C10 showed a clear trend toward protecting against anxiety. Values are mean ± SEM (CSF N = 11, mCRP N = 11, mCRP + 8C10 N = 12 and 8C10 N = 10). Statistics: one-way ANOVA showed a trend to significance (**a**) $p = 0.068$, (**b**) $p = 0.058$; $^{\$}$ $p < 0.05$ compared to control by Student's $t$ test.

### *3.3. Anti-mCRP Antibody 8C10 Protected against Loss of Recognition Memory Induced by mCRP at 1, 3 and 6 Months of Treatment*

The results of the NORT analysis showed a total loss of recognition memory at 1, 3 and 6 months after infusion of mCRP in the mouse hippocampus, but also showed that injection of mCRP with 8C10 monoclonal antibody protected against this loss (Figure 3a) (one-way ANOVA 1-month study, F (3, 29) = 5.081, $p = 0.006$ and F (3, 29) = 4.087, $p = 0.016$, at 2 and 24 h of testing, respectively; 3-month study, F (3, 44) = 6.009, $p = 0.002$, F (3, 44) = 4.680, $p = 0.006$, at 2 and 24 h of testing, respectively; 6-month study, F (3, 40) = 8.755, $p < 0.001$, F (3, 40) = 10.76, $p < 0.001$, at 2 and 24 h of testing, respectively). NORT showed that all mice explored two identical objects for a similar time. However, the mCRP group of mice did not recognize the novel versus the familiar object in the test after a time interval of 2 h or in the retest after a time interval of 24 h. In contrast, the experimental group treated with mCRP plus 8C10 performed the test at the same level as the control group, with similar discrimination indexes (around 0.2 and above), indicating a significantly longer time spent exploring the novel object than the familiar one (see Figure 3a legend for graph details). Therefore, anti-mCRP antibody 8C10 showed neuroprotective effects against mCRP cognitive loss in both short and long time-intervals.

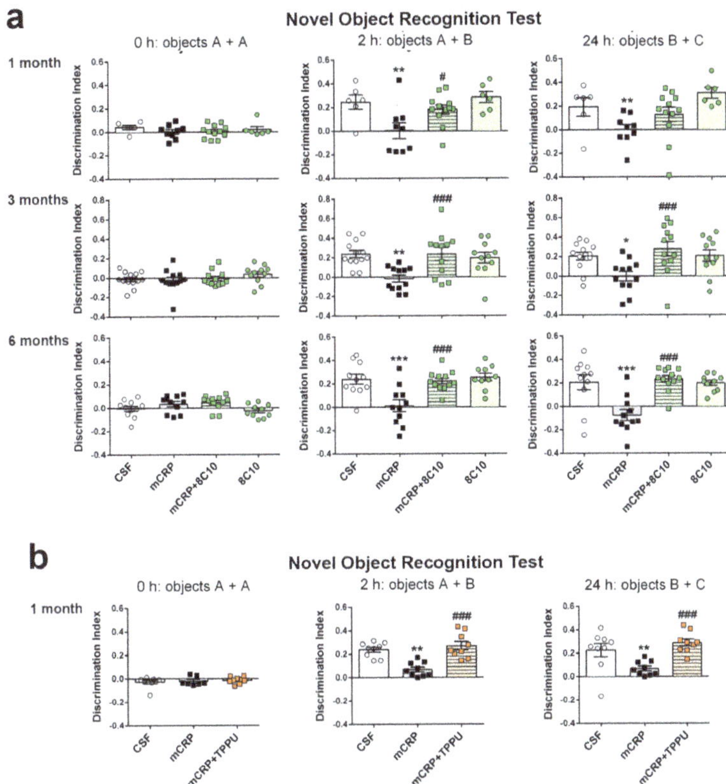


**Figure 3.** Long-term loss of recognition memory induced by mCRP was prevented by 8C10 antibody. (**a**) 1, 3 and 6 months of exposure to mCRP induced total memory loss shown at 2 and 24 h after an assay of recognition learning in the Novel object recognition test. 8C10 totally prevented memory loss for all the assayed periods. (**b**) TTPU similarly protected against loss of recognition memory after 1 month of exposure to mCRP. Values are mean ± SEM ((**a**) 1 month: CSF N = 6, mCRP N = 9, mCRP + 8C10 N = 12 and 8C10 N = 6; 3 months: CSF N = 13, mCRP N = 12, mCRP + 8C10 N = 12 and 8C10 N = 11; 6 months: CSF N = 11, mCRP N = 11, mCRP + 8C10 N = 12, 8C10 N = 10. (**b**) CSF N = 9, mCRP N = 9 and mCRP + TPP N = 9). Statistics: * $p < 0.05$, ** $p < 0.01$, *** $p < 0.001$, compared to Control group; # $p < 0.05$, ### $p < 0.001$ compared to mCRP group.

### *3.4. TPPU Protected Against Loss of Recognition Memory Induced by mCRP at 1 Month of Treatment*

The reference anti-inflammatory compound TPPU showed a protective effect against the mCRP-induced loss of recognition memory assayed by NORT 1 month after treatment (Figure 3b) (one-way ANOVA, F (2, 24) = 16.48, $p < 0.0001$ and F (2, 24) = 8.613, $p = 0.0015$, at 2 and 24 h of testing, respectively). One animal of the mCRP group was discarded from the basal values because it did not reach a minimum exploration time at 0 h, but showed exploratory activity at 2 and 24 h. Similar to the protective treatment with 8C10, TPPU administered orally to mice injected with mCRP blocked the memory loss that appeared in the mCRP group (see Figure 3b legend for details). Cognitive protection was present at the test time of 2 h and also at the longer test time of 24 h.

### 3.5. Anti-mCRP Antibody 8C10 Protected Against Loss of Spatial Memory Induced by mCRP at 1, 3 and 6 Months of Treatment

The results of the OLT showed a loss of spatial memory response in mCRP-injected mice, but not in the mice also treated with 8C10 antibody (Figure 4a) (one-way ANOVA, F (3, 29) = 4.139, $p$ = 0.015 in the study at 1 month). Mice treated with mCRP did not discern between an object that was maintained in the same position and one that had been relocated to a new position at 2 h after previous exploration. In contrast, the experimental group treated with mCRP plus 8C10 performed the test at the level of the control group. These results on spatial memory confirmed the previous protective effects on cognition through recognition memory preservation by 8C10.

For the confirmation of the protective effects of 8C10 after 3 and 6 months of treatment with mCRP, spatial memory was analyzed using the widely known test of MWM instead of OLT. Results of the MWM for the 3- and 6-month studies showed a loss of spatial memory in the mCRP group and total preservation in the mCRP + 8C10 group (Figure 4b) (two-way ANOVA, effect of the percentage of time spent in each quadrant of the pool during the probe test, F (3, 149) = 3.779 $p$ = 0.0119 and F (3, 164) = 9.596, $p < 0.001$ for 3- and 6-month treatments, respectively). A few mice that floated instead of actively swimming, as detected in the videotape examination, were not included in the analysis, where discarded animals were: N = 1 in mCRP 3-month group, N = 2 in mCRP + 8C10 3-month group, N = 2 in CSF 6-month group and N = 1 in mCRP 6-month group. Mice in the mCRP groups spent a random amount of time (around 25%) swimming in the pool quadrant where the escape platform was located during the previous acquisition training; however, mice treated with mCRP + 8C10 showed a distinct preference for swimming into the area of the target quadrant, suggesting a preserved spatial memory after 24 h. Otherwise, the acquisition curves, either latency time or swimming distance to the scape platform, did not reach statistical differences between groups, as analyzed by repeated measures ANOVA (Supplementary Figure S3). Therefore, there was some preservation in the learning capacity under our intense protocol of 5 trials per day over 6 days, but memory was totally abolished by mCRP. The group treated with 8C10 alone behaved similarly to the control group treated with vehicle (CSF) in this and all the previous behavioral and cognitive tests.

### 3.6. TPPU Protected against Loss of Spatial Memory Induced by mCRP at 1 Month of Treatment

The protective effect of TPPU against loss of spatial memory induced by mCRP was demonstrated by OLT (Figure 4c) (one-way ANOVA, F (2, 24) = 28.14, $p < 0.001$). Mice injected with mCRP and dosed with TPPU for 1 month were able to recognize the relocated object from the one whose position was maintained 2 h after the previous exploration. Their OLT discrimination index was significantly higher than that of the mCRP-injected mice, which were unable to discriminate between the different spatial positions of the object.

### 3.7. Anti-mCRP Antibody 8C10 Inhibited Tau Hyperphosphorylation Induced by mCRP at 6 Months of Treatment

Western blot analysis of tau protein of the hippocampus extracts revealed changes in phosphorylation levels in the 6-month study (Figure 5a,b and Supplementary Figures S4 and S5). Mice treated with mCRP showed significant hyperphosphorylation by two antibodies directed to different tau epitopes that detect pathological tau in AD. Antibodies presented an approximately two-fold increase of p-tau Ser202/Thr305 (clone AT8) (Figure 5a and Supplementary Figure S4) and p-tau Ser396 (Figure 5b and Supplementary Figure S5) by mCRP after normalization for tau content (clone HT7) (one-way ANOVA, F (3, 22) = 3.667, $p$ = 0.028 and F (3, 26) = 4.816, $p$ = 0.008 for the ratios AT8/HT7 and S396/HT7, respectively). Notably, the hippocampus of mice treated with mCRP and 8C10 showed normalized levels of p-tau as compared to controls. In this group, we discarded an outlier sample that showed very high levels of both AT8 and HT7. Treatment with 8C10 alone did not interfere with the p-tau levels. No changes were detected in the shorter time studies. However, no significant increase of amyloid β in the hippocampus was detected by Western blot after mCRP treatment (Supplementary Figure S6). Therefore, increased p-tau may reflect long-term changes of cognitive loss and neurodegeneration caused by mCRP. Finally, treatment with mCRP or 8C10 antibody did not induce changes in the protein levels of Iba1 (Supplementary Figure S7). Iba1 is a pan-microglial marker, but its expression increases with microglial activation [44]. Therefore, treatments did not cause a generalized activation of microglia to a reactive phenotype, indicating absence of a major inflammatory response.

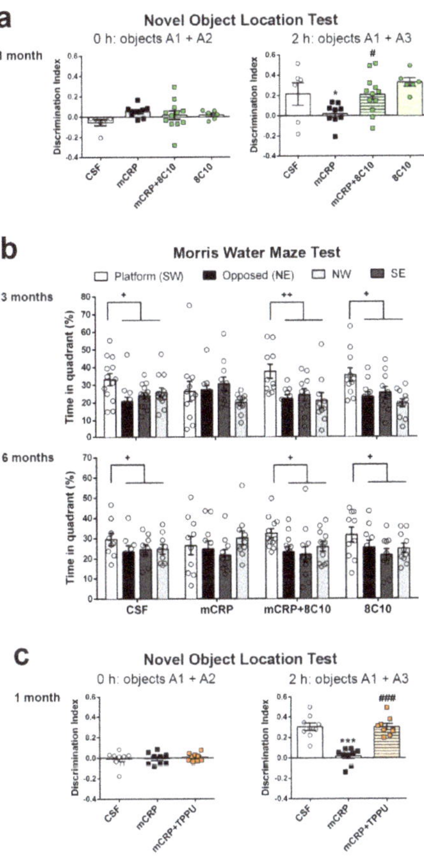


**Figure 4.** Long-term loss of spatial memory induced by mCRP was prevented by 8C10 antibody. Exposure to mCRP induced total loss of spatial memory, which was prevented by 8C10, as shown by the Novel object location test in the 1-month assessment (**a**) and by the Morris water maze test in the 3 and 6-month assessments (**b**). (**c**) TTPU similarly protected against loss of spatial memory after 1 month of exposure to mCRP, as shown by the Novel object location test. Values are mean ± SEM ((**a**) CSF N = 6, mCRP N = 9, mCRP + 8C10 N = 12 and 8C10 N = 6; (**b**) 3 months, CSF N = 13, mCRP N = 11, mCRP + 8C10 N = 10 and 8C10 N = 11; 6 months, CSF N = 9, mCRP N = 10, mCRP + 8C10 N = 12 and 8C10 N = 10. (**c**) CSF N = 9, mCRP N = 9 and mCRP + TPP N = 9). Statistics: * $p < 0.05$, *** $p < 0.001$, compared to Control group; # $p < 0.05$, ### $p < 0.001$ compared to mCRP group; + $p < 0.05$, ++ $p < 0.01$, Platform quadrant compared to the average of the other quadrants.

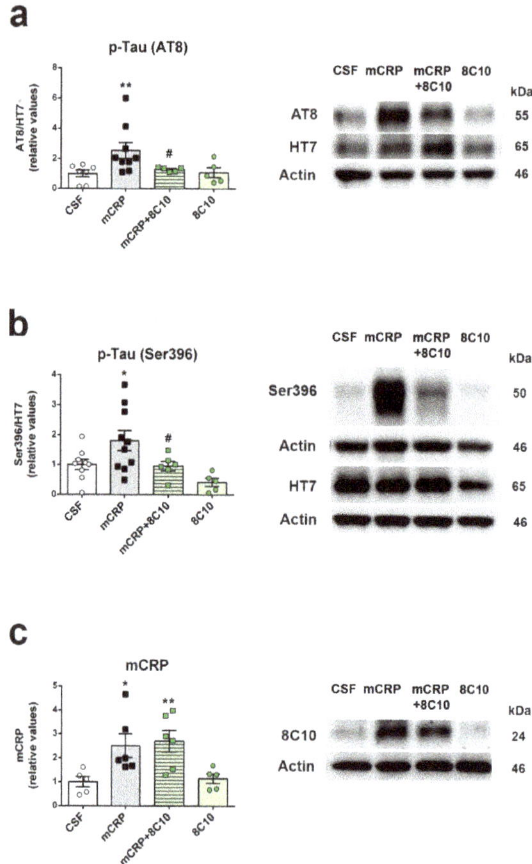


**Figure 5.** Tau pathology induced by mCRP was prevented by 8C10 antibody. Protein extracts of the whole hippocampus tissue showed higher levels of hyperphosphorylated tau (p-tau) after 6 months of mCRP treatment, but 8C10 prevented this pro-neurodegenerative change. Protein levels detected by p-tau antibodies AT8 (**a**) and Ser396 (**b**) were calculated as a ratio of the levels detected by total tau antibody HT7. (**c**) Protein levels of mCRP detected by 8C10 antibody in the hippocampus 6 months after the intrahippocampal injection were not decreased by co-treatment with 8C10. Representative blots of each experimental group are shown in the same order as the densitometric analysis values in the histograms. The images presented in this figure reproduce the cropped gels, while full-length gels are presented in Supplementary Figures S4, S5 and S8, respectively. Values are mean ± SEM ((**a**) CSF N = 7, mCRP N = 9, mCRP + 8C10 N = 5 and 8C10 N = 5; (**b**) CSF N = 9, mCRP N = 10, mCRP + 8C10 N = 6 and 8C10 N = 5; (**c**) CSF N = 5, mCRP N = 6, mCRP + 8C10 N = 6 and 8C10 N = 6). Statistics: * $p < 0.05$, ** $p < 0.01$ compared to Control group; # $p < 0.05$ compared to mCRP group.

Increased levels of mCRP protein were found in the hippocampus of mice 6 months after the injection (Figure 5c and Supplementary Figure S8) (one-way ANOVA, $F(3, 18) = 5.137$, $p = 0.010$). Interestingly, mCRP was detected at similar rates in mice receiving treatment with mCRP + 8C10. Proteins are denaturized during the Western blot procedure; therefore, the previous binding of mCRP with 8C10 was destroyed, allowing for fresh 8C10 antibody detection. Pentameric CRP is also disassembled and only mCRP can be detected, as indicated in the Methods Section. However, the 8C10 antibody, although generated against human mCRP, showed immunodetection of mCRP in all the mice and did not discern endogenous from injected mCRP. Nevertheless, transcriptomic analysis showed that *Crp* mRNA levels did not increase significantly in hippocampal tissue after mCRP injection compared to CSF injection (Figure 6) (two-way ANOVA, factors age and treatment, and interaction age x treatment, all $p > 0.05$). Although the specific cDNA preamplification step required for near-undetectable *Crp* expression by standard procedures increased data dispersion, qPCR results ruled out a significant contribution of endogenous CRP or mCRP.

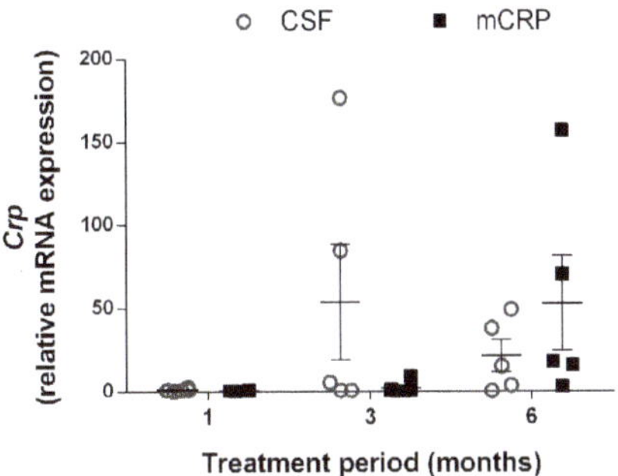


**Figure 6.** Exposure to mCRP did not induce a significantly increased expression of endogenous *Crp* gene at different times after its injection into the mouse hippocampus. Expression of *Crp* was normalized to the corresponding expression of *Tbp* gene and calculated as fold change of the 1-month CSF group. Values are mean ± SEM (1 month, CSF N = 6, mCRP N = 6; 3 months, CSF N = 5, mCRP N = 6; 6 months, CSF N = 5, mCRP N = 5).

### 3.8. Anti-mCRP Antibody 8C10 Palliated the Decrease of a Neural Plasticity Marker by mCRP at 6 Months of Treatment

The injection of mCRP significantly decreased the levels of *Egr1* mRNA in the hippocampus, as detected at 6 months of treatment, and 8C10 showed a trend to avoid loss of this plasticity marker by maintaining *Egr1* levels in the same range as that of control-treated mice (Figure 7a) (one-way ANOVA, $F(3, 17) = 3.525$, $p = 0.037$). The protective effect of antibody treatment did not reach statistical significance according to the post hoc analysis (mCRP + 8C10 did not differ from any other group). Therefore, results indicated only a partial prevention of *Egr1* expression loss by 8C10 treatment. In addition, 8C10 may have some unexpected effect that prevented maximum *Egr* expression, as the 8C10 group showed levels similar to the CRP + 8C10 group. Untreated AD transgenic 5XFAD mice showed a similarly reduced level of *Egr1* gene expression as compared to WT mice (Figure 7b) ($t(14) = 3.590$, $p = 0.0030$).

### 3.9. Anti mCRP Antibody 8C10 and TPPU Reduced Inflammatory Activation of BV2 Cells by mCRP

The generation of nitric oxide by BV2 microglial cells was analyzed in order to evaluate the pro-inflammatory effects of mCRP and the protective effects of the 8C10 monoclonal antibody and the anti-inflammatory compound TPPU. First, the anti-inflammatory properties of TPPU in this cell system were demonstrated against a pro-inflammatory stimulus of LPS (Figure 8a) (two-way ANOVA, effect of TPPU $F(2, 87) = 18.80$, $p < 0.001$, effects of LPS and interaction between the two factors also $p < 0.001$). A significant increase in generation was observed when treating BV2 with LPS 0.1 μg/mL for 24 h in comparison to the basal values in control-treated cells. However, the LPS increase was significantly diminished by TPPU at 50 and 100 μM concentrations.

Next, we evaluated the reaction of microglial BV2 cells to mCRP. In a preliminary assay, we established that the concentration of 100 μg/mL of mCRP showed significant pro-inflammatory effects (Supplementary Figure S9). Nitrite assay demonstrated that mCRP, but not native pentameric CRP, had pro-inflammatory effects on BV2 cells incubated for

24 h, which were protected by both 8C10 (1:20) and TPPU at 100 μM (Figure 8b) (one-way ANOVA, F (4, 35) = 62.62, $p < 0.001$). Therefore, mCRP showed a major pro-inflammatory effect that was inhibited by 8C10 when simultaneously added to the culture medium of BV2 cells. Analysis of iNOS protein levels in the BV2 cell extracts confirmed that mCRP activated the iNOS pathway, and this effect was abolished by 8C10 and partially inhibited by TPPU (Figure 8c and Supplementary Figure S10) (one-way ANOVA, F (3, 47) = 4.555, $p = 0.004$).

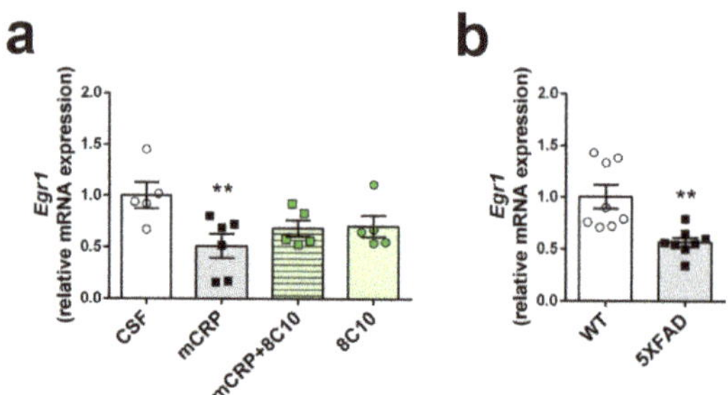


**Figure 7.** Decreased expression of the neural plasticity marker *Egr1* induced by mCRP was partially prevented by 8C10 antibody. RNA extracts of the whole hippocampus tissue showed reduced levels of expression of the *Egr1* gene after 6 months of mCRP treatment, but 8C10 showed a trend to palliate this decline (**a**). *Egr1* expression was decreased in the hippocampus of 5XFAD mice to a level similar to mCRP-injected mice (**b**). Expression of *Egr1* was normalized to the corresponding expression of *Tbp* gene. Values are mean ± SEM ((**a**) CSF N = 5, mCRP N = 6, mCRP + 8C10 N = 5 and 8C10 N = 5, and (**b**) WT N = 8 and 5XFAD N = 8). Statistics: ** $p < 0.01$ compared to Control group.

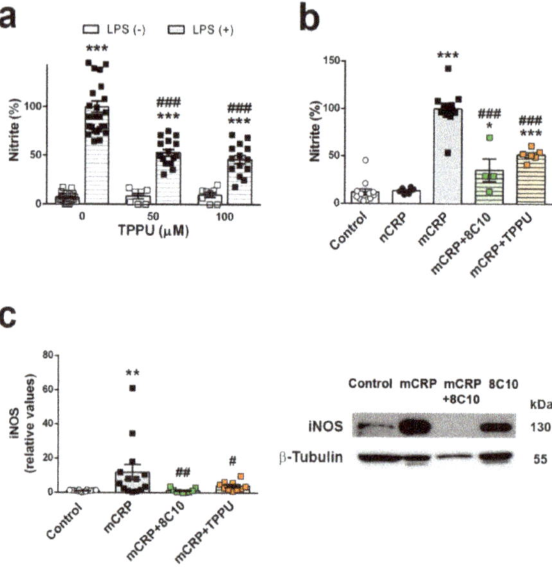


**Figure 8.** Nitric oxide generation by mCRP in BV2 microglial cells was inhibited by 8C10 and TPPU. (**a**) TPPU decreased the generation of nitric oxide induced by lipopolysaccharide (LPS), as shown by nitrite detection in the culture media of BV2 cells after 24 h of incubation. (**b**) Increased nitric oxide generation by 24 h exposure to mCRP was decreased by both the antibody 8C10 and the anti-inflammatory agent TPPU, while pentameric native CRP (nCRP) had no effect. (**c**) Levels of iNOS

protein increased in BV2 cells treated with mCRP, and the increase was inhibited by 8C10 and TPPU. Representative blots of each experimental group are shown in the same order as the densitometric analysis values in the histogram, the blot images reproduce a cropped gel, and full-length gel is presented in Supplementary Figure S10. Values are mean ± SEM ((**a**) TPPU 0 μM Control N = 22, LPS N = 26; TPPU 50 μM Control N = 7, LPS N = 16; TPPU 100 μM Control N = 8, LPS N = 14. (**b**) Control N = 12, CRP N = 6, mCRP N = 12, mCRP + 8C10 N = 4 and mCRP + TPPU N = 6. (**c**) Control N = 18, mCRP N = 14, +TPPU N = 10). Statistics: *** $p < 0.001$ compared to the corresponding Control group, +++ $p < 0.001$ compared to the LPS (+) group without TPPU in (**a**); * $p < 0.05$, *** $p < 0.001$ compared to the Control group, ### $p < 0.001$ compared to mCRP group in (**b**); ** $p < 0.01$ compared to the Control group, # $p < 0.05$ and ## $p < 0.001$ compared to mCRP group in (**c**).

## 4. Discussion

Intrahippocampal treatment of mCRP in young adult, 3-month-old mice, induced total memory loss that was detected up to 6 months later when the mice were assessed at 9 months. Here, we extended previous results obtained after 4 weeks of mCRP exposure in this mouse model of dementia [30]. Our results suggest that a single lesion may produce long-lasting cognitive impairment and late anxiety. Mice showed impairment in paradigms for assessing recognition memory and spatial memory at all age points tested. Anxiety behavior shown after 6 months of mCRP exposure is a common BPSD in AD mouse models with advanced pathology [39]. In order to avoid the effects of senescence, we used young animals; however, we may speculate that the dementia induced will be maintained as age advances. Equivalent timing in humans would mean that a single cerebrovascular episode inducing mCRP local deposition [15,30] would cause injuries lasting for a period of more than 20 years [45], and probably for the remainder of the lifetime. The mCRP molecules self-aggregate into diffuse matrix-like structures, reducing aqueous solubility [36]. Indeed, we found significant levels of the injected mCRP remaining inside the hippocampus, and some mCRP molecules were previously detected by immunostaining in blood vessels and neurons of surrounding brain areas in this experimental model [30]. Furthermore, mCRP is mostly associated with human tissue, indicating that it is a tissue-based rather than a serum-based form of this protein [46]. The hippocampus has a central role in learning and memory, and specifically, the targeted CA1 area is a very sensitive region to AD neurodegeneration [47]. Interestingly, long-term potentiation at CA1–CA3 hippocampal synapses is considered the major reflection of synaptic plasticity [48], and we found that injection of mCRP into CA1 reduced both memory responses and gene expression of the transcription factor *Egr1*. *Egr1* regulates many synaptic functions and is specifically involved in long-term potentiation and memory consolidation in the hippocampus [49,50]. It is remarkable that *Egr1* expression decreased to a similar level in mCRP-treated mice as in the 5XFAD transgenic mouse model of AD [38]. 5XFAD mice suffer from early memory loss [51], as we showed here for mCRP mice. Overall, then, these factors validate our model of mCRP-induced dementia. Considering mCRP as a significant contributor to the triggering of AD after stroke [14,30] and to the progression of neuroinflammation and loss of synaptic function in AD [14], effective treatments against it may be able to decrease poststroke AD cases and other diseases involving CRP activation.

The antibody against mCRP, 8C10, protected against the memory loss induced by mCRP at the three treatment periods assayed up to a maximum of 6 months of exposure. Both spatial memory and recognition memory were preserved by 8C10 in mice, which showed the same level of test performance as control mice despite mCRP dosing. However, we did not find significant protection against the decrease in the *Egr1* neuroplasticity marker by 8C10. Although an upward trend in *Egr1* may have caused some improvements in neuroplasticity, other pathways may be involved, and future studies to discern specific neuroprotective mechanisms are warranted. A trend toward higher anxiety in mCRP mice was also prevented by 8C10, indicating protection against the spread of damage from the hippocampus to connected brain areas. Indeed, the mCRP protein was detected in the hippocampus of the mice injected with mCRP, but also in those injected with mCRP and the 8C10 antibody. Therefore, it is likely that the antibody blocks the active region of the mCRP molecule and that this is enough to protect against any damage inflicted to the hippocampal tissue. It is known that 8C10 binds to the N-terminal part of human mCRP through aa 22–45, and that this may not allow mCRP binding to cholesterol through aa 35–47, thus preventing mCRP anchorage to the lipid rafts microdomains, which is considered its mechanism of cell interaction [13,52]. Protection by 8C10 was maintained throughout the 6-month period, and therefore it is not anticipated that mild aggregation changes of deposited mCRP molecules [36] may diminish their affinity for the antibody.

Tau pathology in the hippocampus of mCRP-injected mice was avoided with 8C10. Increases in immunostaining of p-tau have been found in neurons of brain tissue one month after mCRP intrahippocampal injection, and a double immunofluorescence analysis has demonstrated neuronal co-localization of mCRP and p-tau [30]. Here, the high levels of p-tau reached at several pathological sites after 6 months of mCRP damage were readily detected by Western blot. The high levels of p-tau were paralleled by mCRP deposits also detected by Western blot. These results are supported by previous histological demonstration of mCRP in the brain one month after its experimental injection [30,32]. Furthermore, we can speculate on an exogenous origin of the mCRP deposits according to the lack of increased gene expression of *Crp* at any of the analyzed time points of 1 month, 3 months and 6 months after surgery. If this were the case, the long-term neuroprotection attained with 8C10 despite the maintained presence of exogenous mCRP into the mouse brain is intriguing and warrants further analysis of the mCRP-antibody dynamics. Interestingly, in vitro experiments with cultured neurons and bovine aortic endothelial cells incubated with mCRP have also shown increased p-tau levels, which may be protected by 8C10 [30]. Therefore, our overall in vivo and previous in vitro results suggest that the prevention of mCRP interaction with the cell membrane by the antibody avoids the subsequent activation of cellular cascade systems, leading to a neurodegeneration stage reflected by tau pathology and loss of synaptic function. Tau pathology is a hallmark of AD and other dementia types and its progression correlates with AD stages and dementia severity [53]. It is also involved in the chain of poststroke neurodegenerative changes leading to dementia; specifically, increased p-tau was found in tissue from infarcted patients [14] and also in experimental models of cerebral hypoperfusion [54] and ischemia [55]. Protection of tau pathology by 8C10 in vivo confirms the potential of the antibody against the potential development of neurodegeneration by mCRP. Increase of pathological tau phosphorylation by mCRP is in agreement with the activation of the p38 MAPK pathway as a cytotoxicity effector of mCRP, that has been identified in human coronary artery endothelial cells [56–58] and human U937 macrophages [13]. Activation of p38 MAPK is involved in tau phosphorylation and in the pathological changes in AD [59], and would support tau pathology and AD traits of the mCRP mouse model.

Microglia cells are the first-line immune defense in the brain and are key players in neuroinflammatory processes. Activated microglia increase their phagocytic activity and release oxygen species and inflammatory molecules, as do macrophages. The direct activation of microglia by mCRP has not been demonstrated, although mCRP can be detected in microglia cells alongside neurons in areas surrounding the peri-infarcted regions of ischemic stroke tissue [30]. The absence of significant microgliosis in the mCRP mouse model, as indicated by unaltered Iba1 levels in the whole hippocampus extracts, may be due to a local effect on microglia cells next to mCRP deposition sites, and this would need confirmation in future studies. Here, we demonstrated that mCRP, but not CRP, activated the mouse microglial cell line BV2, as shown by the increased generation of nitric oxide. Notably, 8C10 blocked this effect, therefore preventing the activation of the inducible nitric oxide synthase (iNOS) pathway by mCRP. mCRP has also been shown to increase iNOS levels and NO generation in the human macrophage-like cell line U937 [60]. Overactivated iNOS has been implicated in many inflammatory pathologies, including AD [61]. It is plausible that a vicious or sustained activation of microglia by mCRP may induce a spiral of neuroinflammation and neurodegeneration [62]. In addition, microglia perform a wide range of physiological functions in normal conditions, contributing to brain homeostasis and neuron functionality [63]; therefore, we may speculate that microglia activation by mCRP makes a key contribution to the poststroke dementia and AD.

The pro-inflammatory mechanisms of mCRP are not fully known, but it is known to cause the activation of platelets, leukocytes and endothelial cells, and also of complement via C1q binding [12], all of which may potentially lead to a cascade of inflammatory damage in the cerebral microvasculature. For instance, high levels of mCRP have been detected in the AD microvasculature positive for the neovascularization marker CD105, suggesting activation and possible potential for aberrant angiogenesis [30]. Furthermore, the blood–brain barrier may be damaged in infarcted areas, facilitating the infiltration of activated leukocytes and mCRP and thus promoting poststroke AD. Finally, a sustained interaction between mCRP-induced brain pathology and AD pathology itself would further activate neuroinflammation and associated neurodegeneration [10]. For instance, mCRP is also generated by CRP interaction with amyloid β plaques in AD brain [15].

TPPU-induced neuroprotection against memory loss in mCRP-injected animals confirms the presence of neuroinflammation and related neurodegenerative processes underlying this mouse model of dementia. TPPU is a well-characterized soluble epoxide-hydrolase inhibitor that can readily cross the blood–brain barrier. Inhibition of this enzyme in order to halt the hydrolysis of beneficial epoxyeicosatrienoic acids to their corresponding metabolites is a novel approach against neuroinflammatory pathologies [35]. TPPU has been found to be neuroprotective in experimental models of chronic hypoperfusion [64], reperfusion after focal ischemia [65] and AD [37]. Soluble epoxide hydrolase blockade by another experimental drug has proven to reduce microglia activation in vivo, induced by experimental traumatic brain injury, and in vitro, proven in BV2 cells injured with LPS [66]. In line with these findings, we showed that TPPU is protective against the increase of nitric oxide by LPS in BV2 microglial cells. We also demonstrated that TPPU reduced the activation of the pro-inflammatory pathway of nitric oxide activation induced by mCRP incubation. Finally, we showed a differential effect of mCRP and native CRP in the iNOS activation, suggesting that this pathway is a target effector of mCRP neuroinflammation.

## 5. Conclusions and Future Directions

In conclusion, in this study, we provided proof of the long-term deleterious effects of mCRP after its deposition in the hippocampus of mice. The induction of processes promoting neurodegeneration as shown by increased p-tau in vivo and nitric oxide in BV2 microglial cells can be blocked by the 8C10 antibody, which is specific for the monomeric CRP but does not associate with the pentameric CRP. Furthermore, using TPPU confirmed that the proinflammatory pathways are the main inducers of neuronal damage by mCRP. The induction of dementia with AD traits by mCRP confirms the link between cerebrovascular injury and AD and identifies mCRP as a druggable therapeutic target.

Specific blockade of mCRP is a promising therapy for reducing the neurodegeneration after a cerebrovascular injury and the development of AD, the most common form of dementia in the elderly population. Furthermore, mCRP can be a useful biomarker of the prognosis of neurodegenerative processes associated with neuroinflammation, when it could be detected by non-invasive techniques. Advances in mCRP detection and therapeutic approaches open up new avenues in the fight against all the pathological conditions affected by the damaging interaction between mCRP and cells and tissues.

## 6. Limitations

The simultaneous injection of 8C10 antibody with mCRP demonstrated the beneficial effects of mCRP blockade that happen most probably before it can enter into the cells, but cannot be used as an antibody therapy test. Subsequent in vivo assays for immunotherapy require independent administration of the neutralizing monoclonal antibody 8C10 at different times after mCRP injury, using a peripheral dosing regimen tailored to its hitherto unknown bioavailability and pharmacokinetic properties. Furthermore, intracellular delivery of the antibody to directly block mCRP in the cytoplasm of neurons will require the development of a specific carrier system across cell membranes [67].

Additional control groups were not considered at this point, so as to use the minimum number of animals. However, the inclusion of control antibody groups with a scrambled 8C10 protein injected together with CSF and with mCRP, or the assay of other potential candidate antibodies, would be required to fully characterize the effects of mCRP blockade. Furthermore, a control TPPU group would be desirable, although this agent is known not to cause harmful effects in mice at the dose used [37].

Here, we did not trace the injected mCRP throughout the timeline. Assessment of the exact localization and stability of mCRP deposits in both mCRP- and mCRP + 8C10-injected hippocampus and the weight of partial spreading to other brain areas [32] would be convenient for a comprehensive characterization of the model of mCRP dementia in mice.

**Supplementary Materials:** The following are available online at https://www.mdpi.com/article/10.3390/biomedicines9070828/s1, Figure S1: Sensorimotor ability and patterns of mobility after 6 months of mCRP and 8C10 treatments, Figure S2: Behaviors of neophobia, depression and apathy after 6 months of mCRP and 8C10 treatments, Figure S3: Acquisition of learning in the Morris Water Maze Test after 3 and 6 months of mCRP and 8C10 treatments, Figure S4: Blots of the cropped image shown in Figure 5a, Figure S5: Blots of the cropped image shown in Figure 5b, Figure S6: Protein levels of amyloid β in the hippocampus tissue after 6 months of mCRP and 8C10 treatments, Figure S7: Protein levels of Iba1 in the hippocampus tissue after 6 months of mCRP and 8C10 treatments, Figure S8: Blots of the cropped image shown in Figure 5c, Figure S9: Nitric oxide generation by mCRP in BV2 microglial cells, Figure S10: Blots of the cropped image shown in Figure 7c.

**Author Contributions:** Conceptualization, M.S. and C.S. (Coral Sanfeliu); methodology, C.S. (Cristina Suñol) and C.S. (Coral Sanfeliu); validation, C.S. (Coral Sanfeliu); formal analysis, E.G.-L.; investigation, E.G.-L., S.A., N.C., X.S., C.B., L.A.-F., R.C., P.O., F.T. and A.C.; project administration, P.O.; data curation, E.G.-L., C.S. (Cristina Suñol) and C.S. (Coral Sanfeliu); writing—original draft preparation, E.G.-L. and C.S. (Coral Sanfeliu); writing—review and editing, C.S. (Coral Sanfeliu); funding acquisition, M.S. and C.S. (Coral Sanfeliu). All authors have read and agreed to the published version of the manuscript.

**Funding:** This research was funded by the European Competitiveness Operational Programme 2014–2020, C-Reactive protein therapy for stroke-associated dementia, ID P_37_674, MySMIS code: 103432, contract 51/05.09.2016; Spanish MINECO and European Regional Development Fund, grant number SAF2016-77703; Spanish MCINN, grant number PID2019-106285RB; Catalan Autonomous Government AGAUR, grant number 2017-SGR-106; the CERCA Programme/Generalitat de Catalunya. R.C was supported by a post-doctoral research contract of the Centro de Investigación Biomédica en Red de Epidemiología y Salud Pública (CIBERESP), Instituto de Salud Carlos III, Madrid, Spain.

**Institutional Review Board Statement:** The study was conducted according to the guidelines of the Declaration of Helsinki, and approved by the Institutional Ethics Committee for Animal Experimentation of the University of Barcelona (CEEA-UB) (protocol codes #6991 and #10921, approved on 19 March 2013 and 7 October 2020, respectively).

**Data Availability Statement:** Data supporting the conclusions of this article are contained in the corresponding figures and supplementary materials; full raw data will be made available by the authors without undue reservation.

**Acknowledgments:** We thank Anna Tutusaus for providing C57BL6 mouse liver mRNA for use as a positive control in our *Crp* assays. This work has been carried out within the framework of the doctoral program of Biomedicine of the University of Barcelona.

**Conflicts of Interest:** The authors declare no conflict of interest. The funders had no role in the design of the study; in the collection, analyses, or interpretation of data; in the writing of the manuscript, or in the decision to publish the results.

## References


1. Spychala, M.S.; Honarpisheh, P.; McCullough, L.D. Sex differences in neuroinflammation and neuroprotection in ischemic stroke. *J. Neurosci. Res.* **2017**, *95*, 462–471. [CrossRef] [PubMed]
2. Bolós, M.; Perea, J.R.; Avila, J. Alzheimer's disease as an inflammatory disease. *Biomol. Concepts* **2017**, *8*, 37–43. [CrossRef] [PubMed]
3. Furman, D.; Campisi, J.; Verdin, E.; Carrera-Bastos, P.; Targ, S.; Franceschi, C.; Ferrucci, L.; Gilroy, D.W.; Fasano, A.; Miller, G.W.; et al. Chronic inflammation in the etiology of disease across the life span. *Nat. Med.* **2019**, *25*, 1822–1832. [CrossRef]
4. Lénárt, N.; Brough, D.; Dénes, Á. Inflammasomes link vascular disease with neuroinflammation and brain disorders. *J. Cereb. Blood Flow Metab.* **2016**, *36*, 1668–1685. [CrossRef] [PubMed]
5. Tillett, W.S.; Francis, T. Serological reactions in pneumonia with a non-protein somatic fraction of pneumoccus. *J. Exp. Med.* **1930**, *52*, 561–571. [CrossRef]
6. Nehring, S.M.; Goyal, A.; Bansal, P.; Patel, B.C. C Reactive Protein (CRP). In *StatPearls*; StatPearls Publishing: Treasure Island, FL, USA, 2020.
7. Evers, A.K.; Veeh, J.; McNeill, R.; Reif, A.; Kittel-Schneider, S. C-reactive protein concentration in bipolar disorder: Association with genetic variants. *Int. J. Bipolar Disord.* **2019**, *7*, 26. [CrossRef] [PubMed]
8. Johns, I.; Moschonas, K.E.; Medina, J.; Ossei-Gerning, N.; Kassianos, G.; Halcox, J.P. Risk classification in primary prevention of CVD according to QRISK2 and JBS3 'heart age', and prevalence of elevated high-sensitivity C reactive protein in the UK cohort of the EURIKA study. *Open Heart* **2018**, *5*, e000849. [CrossRef]
9. Cheng, L.; Zhuang, H.; Yang, S.; Jiang, H.; Wang, S.; Zhang, J. Exposing the Causal Effect of C-Reactive Protein on the Risk of Type 2 Diabetes Mellitus: A Mendelian Randomization Study. *Front. Genet.* **2018**, *9*, 657. [CrossRef]
10. Aarstad, H.H.; Moe, S.E.E.; Bruserud, Ø.; Lybak, S.; Aarstad, H.J.; Tvedt, T.H.A. The Acute Phase Reaction and Its Prognostic Impact in Patients with Head and Neck Squamous Cell Carcinoma: Single Biomarkers Including C-Reactive Protein Versus Biomarker Profiles. *Biomedicines* **2020**, *8*, 418. [CrossRef]
11. Hung, S.K.; Lan, H.M.; Han, S.T.; Wu, C.C.; Chen, K.F. Current Evidence and Limitation of Biomarkers for Detecting Sepsis and Systemic Infection. *Biomedicines* **2020**, *8*, 494. [CrossRef]
12. McFadyen, J.D.; Zeller, J.; Potempa, L.A.; Pietersz, G.A.; Eisenhardt, S.U.; Peter, K. C-Reactive Protein and Its Structural Isoforms: An Evolutionary Conserved Marker and Central Player in Inflammatory Diseases and Beyond. *Subcell. Biochem.* **2020**, *94*, 499–520.
13. Slevin, M.; Iemma, R.S.; Zeinolabediny, Y.; Liu, D.; Ferris, G.R.; Caprio, V.; Phillips, N.; Di Napoli, M.; Guo, B.; Zeng, X.; et al. Acetylcholine Inhibits Monomeric C-Reactive Protein Induced Inflammation, Endothelial Cell Adhesion, and Platelet Aggregation; A Potential Therapeutic? *Front. Immunol.* **2018**, *9*, 2124. [CrossRef]
14. Slevin, M.; Liu, D.; Ferris, G.; Al-Hsinawi, M.; Al-Baradie, R.; Krupinski, J. Expression of Monomeric C-Reactive Protein in Infarcted Brain Tissue from Patients with Alzheimer's Disease. *Turk. Patoloji Derg.* **2017**, *33*, 25–29. [PubMed]
15. Strang, F.; Scheichl, A.; Chen, Y.C.; Wang, X.; Htun, N.M.; Bassler, N.; Eisenhardt, S.U.; Habersberger, J.; Peter, K. Amyloid plaques dissociate pentameric to monomeric C-reactive protein: A novel pathomechanism driving cortical inflammation in Alzheimer's disease? *Brain Pathol.* **2012**, *22*, 337–346. [CrossRef]
16. Slevin, M.; Krupinski, J. A role for monomeric C-reactive protein in regulation of angiogenesis, endothelial cell inflammation and thrombus formation in cardiovascular/cerebrovascular disease? *Histol. Histopathol.* **2009**, *24*, 1473–1478.
17. Luan, Y.Y.; Yao, Y.M. The Clinical Significance and Potential Role of C-Reactive Protein in Chronic Inflammatory and Neurodegenerative Diseases. *Front. Immunol.* **2018**, *9*, 1302. [CrossRef] [PubMed]
18. Rajab, I.M.; Hart, P.C.; Potempa, L.A. How C-Reactive Protein Structural Isoforms with Distinctive Bioactivities Affect Disease Progression. *Front. Immunol.* **2020**, *11*, 2126. [CrossRef] [PubMed]
19. Williams, R.D.; Moran, J.A.; Fryer, A.A.; Littlejohn, J.R.; Williams, H.M.; Greenhough, T.J.; Shrive, A.K. Monomeric C-Reactive Protein in Serum with Markedly Elevated CRP Levels Shares Common Calcium Dependent Ligand Binding Properties with an in vitro Dissociated Form of C-Reactive Protein. *Front. Immunol.* **2020**, *11*, 115. [CrossRef] [PubMed]
20. Ciubotaru, I.; Potempa, L.A.; Wander, R.C. Production of modified C-reactive protein in U937-derived macrophages. *Exp. Biol. Med.* **2005**, *230*, 762–770. [CrossRef] [PubMed]
21. Melnikov, I.; Kozlov, S.; Saburova, O.; Zubkova, E.; Guseva, O.; Domogatsky, S.; Arefieva, T.; Radyukhina, N.; Zvereva, M.; Avtaeva, Y.; et al. CRP Is Transported by Monocytes and Monocyte-Derived Exosomes in the Blood of Patients with Coronary Artery Disease. *Biomedicines* **2020**, *8*, 435. [CrossRef]
22. Yasojima, K.; Schwab, C.; McGeer, E.G.; McGeer, P.L. Human neurons generate C-reactive protein and amyloid P: Upregulation in Alzheimer's disease. *Brain Res.* **2000**, *887*, 80–89. [CrossRef]
23. Yao, Z.; Zhang, Y.; Potempa, L.A.; Rajab, I.; Ji, L.; Lv, J.; Liu, S.; Zhang, L.; Wu, H. A redox sensitivity-based method to quantify both pentameric and monomeric C-reactive protein in a single assay. *J. Immunol. Methods* **2019**, *470*, 40–45. [CrossRef]
24. Yao, Z.; Zhang, Y.; Wu, H. Regulation of C-reactive protein conformation in inflammation. *Inflamm. Res.* **2019**, *68*, 815–823. [CrossRef] [PubMed]
25. Molins, B.; Romero-Vázquez, S.; Fuentes-Prior, P.; Adan, A.; Dick, A.D. C-Reactive Protein as a Therapeutic Target in Age-Related Macular Degeneration. *Front. Immunol.* **2018**, *9*, 808. [CrossRef] [PubMed]
26. Leys, D.; Hénon, H.; Mackowiak-Cordoliani, M.A.; Pasquier, F. Poststroke dementia. *Lancet Neurol.* **2005**, *4*, 752–759. [CrossRef]

27. Toledo, J.B.; Arnold, S.E.; Raible, K.; Brettschneider, J.; Xie, S.X.; Grossman, M.; Monsell, S.E.; Kukull, W.A.; Trojanowski, J.Q. Contribution of cerebrovascular disease in autopsy confirmed neurodegenerative disease cases in the National Alzheimer's Coordinating Centre. *Brain* **2013**, *136*, 2697–2706. [CrossRef]
28. Marchesi, V.T. Alzheimer's dementia begins as a disease of small blood vessels, damaged by oxidative-induced inflammation and dysregulated amyloid metabolism: Implications for early detection and therapy. *FASEB J.* **2011**, *25*, 5–13. [CrossRef]
29. Slevin, M.; Matou-Nasri, S.; Turu, M.; Luque, A.; Rovira, N.; Badimon, L.; Boluda, S.; Potempa, L.; Sanfeliu, C.; de Vera, N.; et al. Modified C-reactive protein is expressed by stroke neovessels and is a potent activator of angiogenesis in vitro. *Brain Pathol.* **2010**, *20*, 151–165. [CrossRef]
30. Slevin, M.; Matou, S.; Zeinolabediny, Y.; Corpas, R.; Weston, R.; Liu, D.; Boras, E.; Di Napoli, M.; Petcu, E.; Sarroca, S.; et al. Monomeric C-reactive protein—A key molecule driving development of Alzheimer's disease associated with brain ischaemia? *Sci. Rep.* **2015**, *5*, 13281. [CrossRef] [PubMed]
31. Bulbarelli, A.; Lonati, E.; Brambilla, A.; Orlando, A.; Cazzaniga, E.; Piazza, F.; Ferrarese, C.; Masserini, M.; Sancini, G. Aβ42 production in brain capillary endothelial cells after oxygen and glucose deprivation. *Mol. Cell. Neurosci.* **2012**, *49*, 415–422. [CrossRef]
32. Slevin, M.; García-Lara, E.; Capitanescu, B.; Sanfeliu, C.; Zeinolabediny, Y.; AlBaradie, R.; Olah, P.; Guo, B.; Pirici, D.; Napoli, M.D.; et al. Monomeric C-Reactive Protein Aggravates Secondary Degeneration after Intracerebral Haemorrhagic Stroke and May Function as a Sensor for Systemic Inflammation. *J. Clin. Med.* **2020**, *9*, 3053. [CrossRef] [PubMed]
33. Lanari, A.; Amenta, F.; Silvestrelli, G.; Tomassoni, D.; Parnetti, L. Neurotransmitter deficits in behavioural and psychological symptoms of Alzheimer's disease. *Mech. Ageing Dev.* **2006**, *127*, 158–165. [CrossRef] [PubMed]
34. Kosel, F.; Pelley, J.M.S.; Franklin, T.B. Behavioural and psychological symptoms of dementia in mouse models of Alzheimer's disease-related pathology. *Neurosci. Biobehav. Rev.* **2020**, *112*, 634–647. [CrossRef]
35. Kodani, S.D.; Morisseau, C. Role of epoxy-fatty acids and epoxide hydrolases in the pathology of neuro-inflammation. *Biochimie* **2019**, *159*, 59–65. [CrossRef]
36. Potempa, L.A.; Yao, Z.Y.; Ji, S.R.; Filep, J.G.; Wu, Y. Solubilization and purification of recombinant modified C-reactive protein from inclusion bodies using reversible anhydride modification. *Biophys. Rep.* **2015**, *1*, 18–33. [CrossRef]
37. Griñán-Ferré, C.; Codony, S.; Pujol, E.; Yang, J.; Leiva, R.; Escolano, C.; Puigoriol-Illamola, D.; Companys-Alemany, J.; Corpas, R.; Sanfeliu, C.; et al. Pharmacological inhibition of soluble epoxide hydrolase as a new therapy for Alzheimer's Disease. *Neurotherapeutics* **2020**, *17*, 1825–1835. [CrossRef] [PubMed]
38. Oakley, H.; Cole, S.L.; Logan, S.; Maus, E.; Shao, P.; Craft, J.; Guillozet-Bongaarts, A.; Ohno, M.; Disterhoft, J.; Van Eldik, L.; et al. Intraneuronal beta-amyloid aggregates, neurodegeneration, and neuron loss in transgenic mice with five familial Alzheimer's disease mutations: Potential factors in amyloid plaque formation. *J. Neurosci.* **2006**, *26*, 10129–10140. [CrossRef]
39. García-Mesa, Y.; López-Ramos, J.C.; Giménez-Llort, L.; Revilla, S.; Guerra, R.; Gruart, A.; LaFerla, F.M.; Cristòfol, R.; Delgado-García, J.M.; Sanfeliu, C. Physical exercise protects against Alzheimer's disease in 3xTg-AD mice. *J. Alzheimers Dis.* **2011**, *24*, 421–454. [CrossRef]
40. Corpas, R.; Hernández-Pinto, A.M.; Porquet, D.; Hernández-Sánchez, C.; Bosch, F.; Ortega-Aznar, A.; Comellas, F.; de la Rosa, E.J.; Sanfeliu, C. Proinsulin protects against age-related cognitive loss through anti-inflammatory convergent pathways. *Neuropharmacology* **2017**, *123*, 221–232. [CrossRef]
41. Revilla, S.; Suñol, C.; García-Mesa, Y.; Giménez-Llort, L.; Sanfeliu, C.; Cristòfol, R. Physical exercise improves synaptic dysfunction and recovers the loss of survival factors in 3xTg-AD mouse brain. *Neuropharmacology* **2014**, *81*, 55–63. [CrossRef]
42. Gallagher, S.R. One-dimensional SDS gel electrophoresis of proteins. In *Current Protocols in Molecular Biology*; Chapter 10, Section II, Unit 10.2A; John Wiley & Sons, Inc.: Hoboken, NY, USA, 2006.
43. Green, L.C.; Wagner, D.A.; Glogowski, J.; Skipper, P.L.; Wishnok, J.S.; Tannenbaum, S.R. Analysis of nitrate, nitrite, and [15N]nitrate in biological fluids. *Anal. Biochem.* **1982**, *126*, 131–138. [CrossRef]
44. Ito, D.; Imai, Y.; Ohsawa, K.; Nakajima, K.; Fukuuchi, Y.; Kohsaka, S. Microglia-specific localisation of a novel calcium binding protein, Iba1. *Brain Res. Mol. Brain Res.* **1998**, *57*, 1–9. [CrossRef]
45. Dutta, S.; Sengupta, P. Men and mice: Relating their ages. *Life Sci.* **2016**, *152*, 244–248. [CrossRef] [PubMed]
46. Diehl, E.E.; Haines, G.K., 3rd; Radosevich, J.A.; Potempa, L.A. Immunohistochemical localization of modified C-reactive protein antigen in normal vascular tissue. *Am. J. Med. Sci.* **2000**, *319*, 79–83. [CrossRef] [PubMed]
47. Furcila, D.; DeFelipe, J.; Alonso-Nanclares, L.A. Study of Amyloid-β and Phosphotau in Plaques and Neurons in the Hippocampus of Alzheimer's Disease Patients. *J. Alzheimers Dis.* **2018**, *64*, 417–435. [CrossRef]
48. Kumar, A. Long-Term Potentiation at CA3-CA1 Hippocampal Synapses with Special Emphasis on Aging, Disease, and Stress. *Front. Aging Neurosci.* **2011**, *3*, 7. [CrossRef]
49. Duclot, F.; Kabbaj, M. The Role of Early Growth Response 1 (EGR1) in Brain Plasticity and Neuropsychiatric Disorders. *Front. Behav. Neurosci.* **2017**, *11*, 35. [CrossRef]
50. Zhou, G.; Xiong, W.; Zhang, X.; Ge, S. Retrieval of Consolidated Spatial Memory in the Water Maze Is Correlated with Expression of pCREB and Egr1 in the Hippocampus of Aged Mice. *Dement. Geriatr. Cogn. Dis. Extra* **2013**, *3*, 39–47. [CrossRef] [PubMed]

51. Griñán-Ferré, C.; Sarroca, S.; Ivanova, A.; Puigoriol-Illamola, D.; Aguado, F.; Camins, A.; Sanfeliu, C.; Pallàs, M. Epigenetic mechanisms underlying cognitive impairment and Alzheimer disease hallmarks in 5XFAD mice. *Aging* **2016**, *8*, 664–684. [CrossRef]
52. Ji, S.R.; Ma, L.; Bai, C.J.; Shi, J.M.; Li, H.Y.; Potempa, L.A.; Filep, J.G.; Zhao, J.; Wu, Y. Monomeric C-reactive protein activates endothelial cells via interaction with lipid raft microdomains. *FASEB J.* **2009**, *23*, 1806–1816. [CrossRef] [PubMed]
53. Malpas, C.B.; Sharmin, S.; Kalincik, T. The histopathological staging of tau, but not amyloid, corresponds to antemortem cognitive status, dementia stage, functional abilities and neuropsychiatric symptoms. *Int. J. Neurosci.* **2020**, *30*, 1–10. [CrossRef]
54. Park, J.H.; Hong, J.H.; Lee, S.W.; Ji, H.D.; Jung, J.A.; Yoon, K.W.; Lee, J.I.; Won, K.S.; Song, B.I.; Kim, H.W. The effect of chronic cerebral hypoperfusion on the pathology of Alzheimer's disease: A positron emission tomography study in rats. *Sci. Rep.* **2019**, *9*, 14102. [CrossRef]
55. Wen, Y.; Yang, S.; Liu, R.; Simpkins, J.W. Transient cerebral ischemia induces site-specific hyperphosphorylation of tau protein. *Brain Res.* **2004**, *1022*, 30–38. [CrossRef]
56. Khreiss, T.; József, L.; Potempa, L.A.; Filep, J.G. Conformational rearrangement in C-reactive protein is required for proinflammatory actions on human endothelial cells. *Circulation* **2004**, *109*, 2016–2022. [CrossRef]
57. Li, H.Y.; Wang, J.; Wu, Y.X.; Zhang, L.; Liu, Z.P.; Filep, J.G.; Potempa, L.A.; Wu, Y.; Ji, S.R. Topological localization of monomeric C-reactive protein determines proinflammatory endothelial cell responses. *J. Biol. Chem.* **2014**, *289*, 14283–14290. [CrossRef] [PubMed]
58. Zhang, Y.; Cao, H. Monomeric C-reactive protein affects cell injury and apoptosis through activation of p38 MAPK in human coronary artery endothelial cells. *Bosn. J. Basic Med. Sci.* **2020**. [CrossRef]
59. Colié, S.; Sarroca, S.; Palenzuela, R.; Garcia, I.; Matheu, A.; Corpas, R.; Dotti, C.G.; Esteban, J.A.; Sanfeliu, C.; Nebreda, A.R. Neuronal p38$\alpha$ mediates synaptic and cognitive dysfunction in an Alzheimer's mouse model by controlling $\beta$-amyloid production. *Sci. Rep.* **2017**, *7*, 45306. [CrossRef]
60. Sproston, N.R.; El Mohtadi, M.; Slevin, M.; Gilmore, W.; Ashworth, J.J. The effect of C-reactive protein isoforms on nitric oxide production by U937 monocytes/macrophages. *Front. Immunol.* **2018**, *9*, 1500. [CrossRef] [PubMed]
61. Cinelli, M.A.; Do, H.T.; Miley, G.P.; Silverman, R.B. Inducible nitric oxide synthase: Regulation, structure, and inhibition. *Med. Res. Rev.* **2020**, *40*, 158–189. [CrossRef] [PubMed]
62. Aldana, B.I. Microglia-specific metabolic changes in neurodegeneration. *J. Mol. Biol.* **2019**, *431*, 1830–1842. [CrossRef] [PubMed]
63. Wake, H.; Fields, R.D. Physiological function of microglia. *Neuron Glia Biol.* **2011**, *7*, 1–3. [CrossRef]
64. Chen, Y.; Tian, H.; Yao, E.; Tian, Y.; Zhang, H.; Xu, L.; Yu, Z.; Fang, Y.; Wang, W.; Du, P.; et al. Soluble epoxide hydrolase inhibition promotes white matter integrity and long-term functional recovery after chronic hypoperfusion in mice. *Sci. Rep.* **2017**, *7*, 7758. [CrossRef]
65. Tu, R.; Armstrong, J.; Lee, K.S.S.; Hammock, B.D.; Sapirstein, A.; Koehler, R.C. Soluble epoxide hydrolase inhibition decreases reperfusion injury after focal cerebral ischemia. *Sci. Rep.* **2018**, *8*, 5279. [CrossRef]
66. Hung, T.H.; Shyue, S.K.; Wu, C.H.; Chen, C.C.; Lin, C.C.; Chang, C.F.; Chen, S.F. Deletion or inhibition of soluble epoxide hydrolase protects against brain damage and reduces microglia-mediated neuroinflammation in traumatic brain injury. *Oncotarget* **2017**, *8*, 103236–103260. [CrossRef]
67. Slastnikova, T.A.; Ulasov, A.V.; Rosenkranz, A.A.; Sobolev, A.S. Targeted Intracellular Delivery of Antibodies: The State of the Art. *Front. Pharmacol.* **2018**, *9*, 1208. [CrossRef]

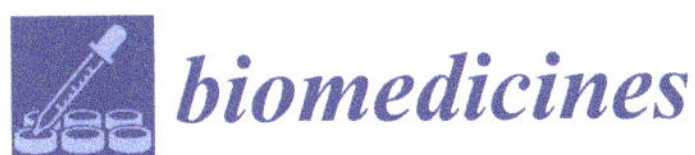

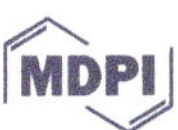

Article

# Transthyretin as a Biomarker to Predict and Monitor Major Depressive Disorder Identified by Whole-Genome Transcriptomic Analysis in Mouse Models

**Sung-Liang Yu [1,2,3,4], Selina Shih-Ting Chu [1], Min-Hui Chien [1], Po-Hsiu Kuo [5], Pan-Chyr Yang [6] and Kang-Yi Su [1,2,7,*]**

1 Department of Clinical Laboratory Sciences and Medical Biotechnology, College of Medicine, National Taiwan University, Taipei 10051, Taiwan; slyu@ntu.edu.tw (S.-L.Y.); r98424014@ntu.edu.tw (S.S.-T.C.); julia861009@hotmail.com (M.-H.C.)
2 Department of Laboratory Medicine, National Taiwan University Hospital, Taipei 10051, Taiwan
3 Graduate Institute of Pathology, College of Medicine, National Taiwan University, Taipei 10051, Taiwan
4 Center for Optoelectronic Biomedicine, College of Medicine, National Taiwan University, Taipei 10051, Taiwan
5 Department of Public Health, Institute of Epidemiology and Preventive Medicine, College of Public Health, National Taiwan University, Taipei 100, Taiwan; phkuo@ntu.edu.tw
6 Department of Internal Medicine, College of Medicine, National Taiwan University, Taipei 10051, Taiwan; pcyang@ntu.edu.tw
7 Genome and Systems Biology Degree Program, College of Life Science, National Taiwan University, Taipei 10617, Taiwan
* Correspondence: suky@ntu.edu.tw; Tel.: +886-223123456 (ext. 66910)

**Citation:** Yu, S.-L.; Chu, S.S.-T.; Chien, M.-H.; Kuo, P.-H.; Yang, P.-C.; Su, K.-Y. Transthyretin as a Biomarker to Predict and Monitor Major Depressive Disorder Identified by Whole-Genome Transcriptomic Analysis in Mouse Models. *Biomedicines* **2021**, *9*, 1124. https://doi.org/10.3390/biomedicines9091124

Academic Editor: Arnab Ghosh

Received: 11 August 2021
Accepted: 30 August 2021
Published: 31 August 2021



**Abstract:** Background: Accumulations of stressful life events result in the onset of major depressive disorder (MDD). Comprehensive genomic analysis is required to elucidate pathophysiological changes and identify applicable biomarkers. Methods: Transcriptomic analysis was performed on different brain parts of a chronic mild stress (CMS)-induced MDD mouse model followed by systemic analysis. QPCR and ELISA were utilized for validation in mice and patients. Results: The highest numbers of genes with significant changes induced by CMS were 505 in the amygdala followed by 272 in the hippocampus (twofold changes; FDR, $p < 0.05$). Enrichment analysis indicated that the core-enriched genes in CMS-treated mice were positively enriched for IFN-$\gamma$ response genes in the amygdala, and hedgehog signaling in the hippocampus. Transthyretin (TTR) was severely reduced in CMS-treated mice. In patients with diagnosed MDD, serum concentrations of TTR were reduced by 48.7% compared to controls ($p = 0.0102$). Paired samples from patients with MDD demonstrated a further 66.3% increase in TTR at remission compared to the acute phase ($p = 0.0339$). Conclusions: This study provides comprehensive information on molecular networks related to MDD as a basis for further investigation and identifies TTR for MDD monitoring and management. A clinical trial with bigger patient cohort should be conducted to validate this translational study.

**Keywords:** major depressive disorder; transthyretin; chronic mild stress; transcriptome; amygdala

## 1. Introduction

Major depressive disorder (MDD) is a potentially life-threatening disorder with a complicated etiology that imposes a major public health and economic problem worldwide. According to a World Health Organization (WHO) report, it may become a leading cause of disability by the end of 2030 [1]. Patients with MDD exhibit a diverse range of symptoms, including psychomotor retardation, agitation, reduced motivation, depressed mood, and suicidality [2,3]. An epidemiological survey conducted on the working population highlighted the correlations between both chronic psychosocial stress and depression with heart disease, high blood pressure, and high blood glucose [4]. Stress and depression both cause neural atrophy and apoptosis in different areas of the brain, including reduction in the numbers and size of neurons and glial cells, and decreased neurogenesis in the prefrontal cortex (PFC) or hippocampus of patients with depressive disorders [5]. Stress can also affect brain function and inflammatory activity by enhancing the expression of cytokines or suppressing the immune system [6–8]. In addition, it can increase activation of the hypothalamus–pituitary axis (HPA) and promote depressive-like behavior [9]. Therefore, several components of the HPA axis are involved in the development of MDD-related changes in the hippocampus, amygdala, and PFC [10]. However, the detailed molecular mechanism underlying these changes, as well as the pathogenesis of MDD, including onset and progression, have not yet been fully clarified due to the wide spectrum of symptoms and complicated etiology.

The prediction, diagnosis, and treatment of MDD has become an emerging issue, where current antidepressants are only effective in approximately 40–50% of patients [11]. In addition to subjective criteria, objective biomarkers that reveal the pathophysiological changes specific to MDD are required to ensure that effective treatments are developed. Therefore, an animal model of MDD may facilitate the development of applicable biomarkers, novel drug discovery, and pre-clinical trials. Until now, the validated mouse model of human MDD induced by the unpredictable chronic mild stress (CMS) had been widely utilized. However, it is also subject to variability related to animal strain, environmental factors, the strength and frequency of treatment, stressor variety, and technical diversity, all of which are still unable to be avoided [12]. Several previous reports have highlighted that CMS reduces aggressiveness and male sexual behavior, and generates both behavioral and physiological abnormalities characteristic of human depression. One previous study suggested that CMS is associated with behavioral changes, body weight loss, and learning and memory impairments [13]. Another study using microarray analysis showed that CMS affects several genes in the cerebral cortex and hippocampus, and that these genes are involved in multiple functions, such as the regulation of neurotransmitters and growth factors [14]. Further to this, using microarray analysis, Yamanishi et al. reported that Hnf4a directly affects various genes associated with several metabolic processes in the prefrontal cortex [15]. Therefore, a comprehensive, systemic, and comparative analysis of different brain areas involved in emotion and the stress response should be conducted. In addition, developing a potential biomarker to predict MDD and monitor outcomes from genomic studies would be extremely beneficial; however, this remains to be identified. In this study, we provided comprehensive genomic information related to MDD, and identified transthyretin (TTR) as a gene significantly downregulated in most brain areas as well as in the peripheral blood of CMS-treated mice. Importantly, we found TTR to be significantly elevated in the serum of MDD patients during the remission phase compared to paired serum samples from the acute phase. Thus, this study identified TTR as a possible biomarker for MDD monitoring.

## 2. Materials and Methods

### 2.1. Animals

Six- to eight-week-old adult male C57BL/6 mice were purchased from the National Taiwan University Laboratory Animal Center. To minimize variation, the mice were allowed to remain in the transport cage for seven days prior to stress induction. Mice had free access to food and water, and were housed at 22 $\pm$ 1 °C with 50 $\pm$ 2% humidity and a 12 h light/12 h dark schedule, except for when the CMS procedure required continuous overnight illumination. All experiments were carried out with the agreement and approval of the Institutional Animal Care and Use Committee (IACUC) of National Taiwan University Medical College (approval number 20120060).

### 2.2. Chronic Mild Stress Procedures

Mice were randomly divided into two groups ($n$ = 6 each), the CMS group and the control group. The CMS experimental group underwent unpredicted unique or combined stressors exposure 6 days a week for 4 weeks. All CMS treated mice experienced the same sequence of stressors. The stressors consisted of the followings.

2.2.1. Fear Stress

Mice were housed together with a rat. They were introduced in a customized metallic mesh cage (21 cm × 18 cm × 14 cm), which were place in the central of a rat home space (60 cm × 45 cm × 30 cm). The exposed time was about 8 to 12 h; food and water were freely available.

2.2.2. Cage Tilting

Mice were placed in a 45° tilted cage for 2 or 8 h according to CMS schedule.

2.2.3. Cage Shaking

Mice were placed in the cage on the shaking machine with 80 to 100 rpm horizontal shaking for 10 min and rest for next 10 min. The procedure was repeated 6 times within 2 h period.

2.2.4. Wet Sawdust Bedding

Three hundred ml water was added to wet the bedding and mice were placed in this cage for 2 or 8 h according to the CMS schedule.

2.2.5. Physical Restraint and Social Stress

Mice were separated individually in a restraint space for physical restraint stress and ten mice were placed together in one cage for social stress. The duration was according to the CMS schedule. During treatment, mice had free access to food and water.

2.2.6. Water Emergency

The mice were placed in another cage without sawdust bedding and filled with tepid water (about 2 cm in depth) for 10 min and rest for next 10 min. The procedure was repeated 6 times within 2 h period.

2.2.7. Tail Pinching

A 3 cm long artery clip with the branches of 1 cm long, 1.5 mm in diameter is used to press the base of mice's tail for ten minutes. This was repeated 6 times at 10 min intervals.

2.2.8. Continuous Overnight Illumination

Mice mere housed in a separated cage with converted dark to light cycle for 12 h.

*2.3. Behavioral Testing Assessments*

2.3.1. Running Wheel Test

Mice were placed into a customized running wheel (5 cm wide, 15 cm diameter) and allowed to run freely for five minutes. Running cycles were counted manually.

2.3.2. Forced Swimming Test (FST)

The FST was performed according to the protocol of a previous study [16]. Briefly, mice were placed in a glass cylinder (45 cm high, 15 cm diameter) filled with water to a depth of 30 cm (23–25 °C). Water was changed between each mouse test. Immobility time was recorded over a 6 min period with a digital camera and analyzed using DepressionScan Suite software (CLEVER Sys. Inc., Reston, VA, USA).

2.3.3. Tail Suspension Test (TST)

The TST was carried out according to the protocol of a previous study [17]. Briefly, mice were securely fastened by the 1.0–1.5 cm tip of their tail to a flat metallic surface using medical adhesive tape and suspended ~30 cm above the ground in a 40 $cm^3$ box, thus isolating the mice from visual distractions while permitting observation of their behavior from above. Immobility time was defined as the absence of limb or body movement within the 6 min testing period. Criteria were defined and data analyses were performed using DepressionScan Suite.

### 2.4. Expression Microarray Experiments and Data Analysis

The GeneChip Mouse Genome 430 2.0 Array (Affymetrix, Santa Clare, CA, USA) was used to perform whole genome expression profiling. The procedures were performed according to the manufacturer's manual. Briefly, 100 ng of pooled RNA was used for the Two-Cycle cDNA Synthesis Kit. Biotin-labelled cRNA was produced through in vitro cDNA transcription (IVT Labeling Kit, Affymetrix). Fragmented cRNA (20 μg) was hybridized to the chip by using the Affymetrix Fluidics Station 450 (Affymetrix). The arrays were washed and stained according to the supplied protocols followed by GeneChip Scanner 3000 (Affymetrix) scanning. The raw data contained in the CEL file were further analyzed using GeneSpring GX software (Agilent Technologies, Santa Clare, CA, USA) with the GCRMA summarization algorithm and baseline to mean normalization. The original CEL files, normalized data, and experimental information were deposited in the Gene Expression Omnibus (accession number GSE151807). Significant genes were selected by statistical analysis performed with false discovery rate (FDR) correlated $p$ value < 0.05 and fold change greater than 2 in CMS treated mice compared with control mice for Metacore software (Thomson Reuters) pathway analysis. The gene expression data generated by cDNA expression microarray were analyzed using GSEA 4.1.0linebreak (http://software.broadinstitute.org/gsea/index.jsp, accessed on 30 July 2020) to extract biological knowledge. Highly significant enriched gene sets are shown. The false discovery rate (FDR) is calculated by comparing the actual data with 1000 Monte Carlo simulations. The normalized enrichment score (NES) computes the density of modified genes in the data set with the random expectancies, normalized by the number of genes found in a given gene cluster, to consider the size of the cluster.

### 2.5. QPCR Validation

Quantitative PCR (QPCR) was performed in a 96-well format. The SYBR green primers of the genes were designed by Primer Express 3.0. The cDNA amplification was carried out using an ABI 7700 Sequence Detection System (Applied Biosystems), and the detection was carried out by measuring the binding of the fluorescence dye SYBR Green I to double-stranded DNA. The relative expression level of the target gene compared with that of the mouse TBP (TATA box binding protein) was defined as $-\Delta CT = (CTgene - CTmTBP)$. The gene mRNA/mTBP mRNA ratio was calculated as $2^{-\Delta CT}$. The primers used for qPCR are listed in Supplementary Table S1.

### 2.6. Immunohistochemical (IHC) Staining

Mice brains at the end of experiments were isolated for post fixation overnight in the 4% paraformaldehyde at 4 °C and embedded in paraffin. Five-micrometer-thick coronal sections were deparaffinized followed by epitope retrieval with citrate buffer. After treating with 3% $H_2O_2$, primary antibodies were incubated for overnight at 4 °C. Immunostaining was performed by liquid DAB-substrate-chromogen system (DAKO,Cat. K3467, Santa Clare, CA, USA) for 10 min and counterstain with hematoxylin (Sigma-Aldrich, Cat. GHS316, Burlington, MA, USA) for 10 s. Slides were stained with anti-Tau1 (Sigma-Aldrich, Cat. MAB3420, Burlington, MA, USA), anti-MAP2 (Abcam, Cat. ab5392), anti-synapsin (Abcam, Cat. ab64581, Cambridge, UK), and anti-ki-67 (Abcam, Cat. ab15580, Cambridge, UK) antibodies.

### 2.7. TTR ELISA

TTR ELISA was performed by Enzyme-linked Immunosorbent Assay Kit for Transthyretin (TTR) (Cat. E90726Mu) (Uscn Life Science, Wuhan, China) according to the user manual.

### 2.8. Patient Samples

Twelve patients who were diagnosed with MDD according to the criteria of the Diagnostic and Statistical Manual of Mental Disorders, 5th version (DSM-5) and had sufficient specimens for testing were consecutively referred to the study by psychiatrists from central and regional hospitals in Taipei. Twelve case-control participants were obtained from the community in matched catchment areas. Case-controls had no past diagnosis of major psychiatric disorders, including anxiety disorder, mood disorder, schizophrenia, mental retardation, or substance use disorder. Acute manic patients were followed until they achieved full remission or for at least 2 months. In total, six patients with paired and sufficient serum samples were collected for testing. All participants signed informed consent forms after the study procedures were fully explained. The tests used in this study were approved by the institutional review board of all participating hospitals.

### 2.9. Statistical Analysis

All results are shown as the mean ± standard deviation (SD) of $n$ observations. The sample size was determined based on the results from pilot studies and previous experience regarding the variability of each data set within experimental and control groups. Each experiment was repeated at least three times, resulting in the same conclusion. Data analysis was performed using GraphPad Prism 8. Statistical analysis for behavioral tests was performed using two-way ANOVA and mixed-effects model. Statistical analysis for expression data was performed using an unpaired, two-tailed Student's $t$-test. TTR concentrations in paired patient serum samples were analyzed using a paired, two-tailed Student's $t$-test. Differences between the means of two compared groups considered to be statistically significant were denoted as * $p < 0.05$, ** $p < 0.01$, and *** $p < 0.001$.

## 3. Results

### 3.1. Mice That Underwent CMS Gained Less Body Weight and Exhibited Reduced Mobility

The CMS procedure involved the combination of ten various, unpredictable, mild stressors (Figure 1). To evaluate the induction efficacy of CMS, body weight monitoring and behavioral tests, including the running wheel test (RWT), forced swimming test (FST), and tail suspension test (TST), were performed before and each week after CMS treatments according to the schedule (Figure 2). Mice that underwent CMS ($n = 6$) gained significantly less weight over the 4-week treatment period compared to controls ($n = 6$; Figure 2a). Using ANOVA, time [F (4, 40) = 23.00, $p < 0.001$] and CMS treatment [F (1, 10) = 20.42, $p < 0.01$] were identified as significant main effects. In addition, a significant interaction was identified between time and CMS treatment [F (4, 40) = 10.31, $p < 0.001$]. CMS was also found to significantly reduce motor activities according to a RWT performed in CMS mice ($n = 6$) compared to control mice ($n = 6$; Figure 2b). Again, ANOVA revealed time [F(4, 40) = 7.86, $p < 0.001$] and CMS treatment [F (1, 10) = 27.88, $p < 0.001$] to be significant main effects. In addition, a significant interaction was found between time and CMS treatment [F (4, 40) = 15.88, $p < 0.001$]. Significant increases in immobility during the FST and TST were also observed in CMS mice ($n = 6$) compared to control mice ($n = 6$; Figure 2c,d). ANOVA revealed time [F (4, 40) = 20.82, $p < 0.001$] and CMS treatment [F (1, 10) = 61.47, $p < 0.001$] to be significant main effects, and an interaction between time and CMS treatment [F (4, 40) = 14.05, $p < 0.001$] in FST was also found. Meanwhile, a significant main effect of time [F (4, 40) = 7.739, $p < 0.001$] and an interaction between time and CMS treatment [F (4, 40) = 3.164, $p = 0.0238$] were observed for TST, but no significant effect was found for CMS treatment [F (1, 10) = 1.209, $p = 0.2972$].

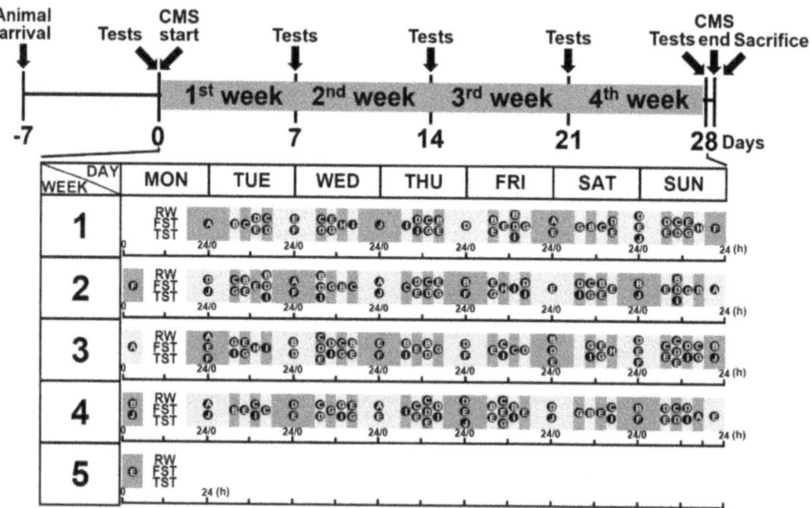


**Figure 1.** The induction schedule of chronic mild stress (CMS) treatment. Mice were allowed to remain in cages for a week before stress induction to eliminate the environment as a potential confounding factor. According to the protocol, CMS-treated mice underwent unpredicted unique or combined stressor exposure at a frequency of 6 days per week for 4 weeks. All CMS-treated mice experienced the same sequence of stressors; meanwhile, control mice were housed in standard conditions. At the end of the experiments, mice were sacrificed, and brain areas including the amygdala, hippocampus, prefrontal cortex, and cerebral cortex were isolated and collected. A, housing of rats; B, 45° cage tilt; C, cage shaking every 10 min; D, wet sawdust bedding; E, physical restraint; F, flash lighting; G, water emergency every 10 min; H, physical and social stress; I, tail pinching every 10 min; J, continuous overnight illumination; RW, running wheel; FST, forced swimming test; TST, tail suspension test.

### 3.2. Histopathological Analysis of CMS-Treated Mouse Brains

To test the impact of CMS on histopathological and anatomical brain changes, immunohistochemical staining was performed on axons and dendrites using antibodies against Tau-1 and MAP2, respectively (Supplementary Figures S1 and S2). No obvious significant abnormality in neurite structures was found. However, the MAP-2-positive neurites in the hippocampus CA1 region of CMS-treated mice seemed to be mildly shrunken and disorganized in appearance. There were no obvious differences between CMS and control mice.

### 3.3. Identification of MDD-Related Gene Signatures Using Whole-Genome Transcriptomic Analysis

Whole-genome transcriptomic analysis was performed using expression cDNA microarrays to identify genetic biomarkers associated with MDD-like behavior in the CMS-induced mouse model. Brain areas, including the amygdala (Amy), hippocampus (Hippo), prefrontal cortex (PFC), and cerebral cortex (CC), were separated into independent analyses comparing CMS and control mice. Each brain area from three independent mice in both the CMS and control groups was assessed in the described assays, and data were analyzed (Figure 3). Principal component analysis (PCA) was used to illustrate the global gene expression changes among the different areas and treatments (Figure 3a). A Pearson correlation cluster heatmap showed that the gene expression profiles were more similar between CMS treatments than between brain areas (Figure 3b). Interestingly, the hippocampus exhibited relatively unique patterns in comparison with other areas. Volcano plot analysis demonstrated that probes of genes were significantly correlated in each of the four brain areas (FDR $p < 0.05$ and over twofold change [blue dots]; Figure 3c). Among these brain areas, the amygdala exhibited the greatest number of probes with significant changes in abundance. Probes of genes with significant changes included the following: 182 upregulated and 323 downregulated in Amy; 266 upregulated and 65 downregulated in CC; 229 upregulated and 43 downregulated in Hippo; and 23 upregulated and 28 downregulated in PFC (Figure 3d). The expression levels of the top ten CMS-affected genes in all brain areas ranged from 39.30 to 3.94 among upregulated genes and 100.00 to 2.33 among downregulated genes (Supplementary Table S2). A Venn diagram was generated to visualize the intersecting and unique genes that were significantly affected among the four brain areas (Figure 3d). Furthermore, 16 genes with significant changes were present in at least three brain areas, where S100a8 commonly affected by CMS in all four brain areas. A heat map was created with unsupervised clustering using a total of 1006 probes with significant changes in the four brain areas, and demonstrated that all conditions were well differentiated according to treatment groups and brain areas (Figure 3e).

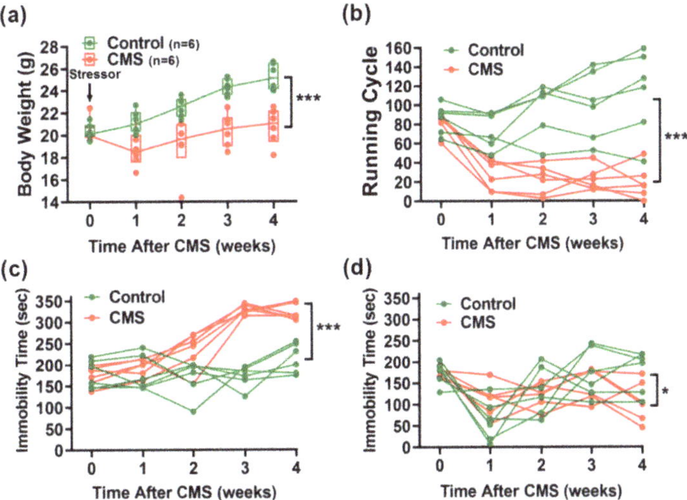


**Figure 2.** Behavioral tests of mice after CMS stimulation. (**a**) Body weight recording during 4-week CMS treatments. (**b**) Running wheel test results. Mice were placed on the running wheel for 5 min. Running cycles were recorded using a video camera then counted manually. (**c**) Forced swimming test results. Mice were placed in a glass cylinder filled with water for 6 min. Their time spent immobile was recorded, followed by analysis with DepressionScan Suite software. (**d**) Tail suspension test results. Mice were placed in a box to isolate them from visual distractions, and securely fastened and suspended for 6 min. Their time spent immobile was recorded, followed by analysis with DepressionScan Suite software. Statistical analyses were performed using two-way ANOVA and mixed-effects model ($n$ = 6 for CMS and control groups). The significant interaction between time and CMS treatment was analyzed. *, $p < 0,05$; ***, $p < 0.001$.

### 3.4. GSEA Predicts Potential Biological Function Related to CMS Induction

To clarify the potential underlying pathways involved in CMS stimulation, GSEA was further utilized as a means to identify hallmark gene signatures differentially regulated by stimuli (Figure 4 and Supplementary Table S3). According to combined four parts analysis, we identified several core gene clusters which were enriched in CMS-treated or control mice and were involved in several hallmarks among the four brain areas (Figure 4a). Among these hallmarks, specifically, the most enriched hallmark in Amy (Figure 4b), CC (Figure 4d), and PFC (Figure 4e) of CMS-treated mice were IFN-γ response, oxidative phosphorylation, and oxidative phosphorylation, respectively. Interestingly, Hippo was a unique part with only a hallmark enriched in hedgehog signaling (Figure 4c).

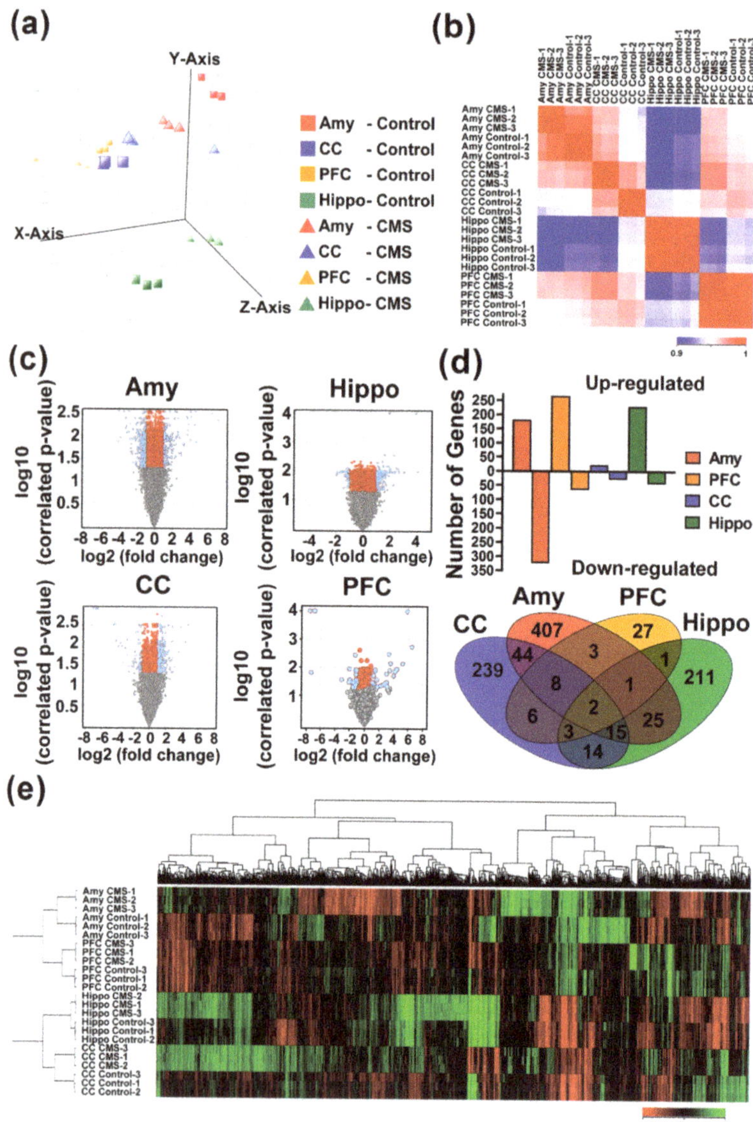


**Figure 3.** Whole-genome transcriptomic analysis for genes with significant alterations in brain areas due to chronic mild stress (CMS) stimuli. Brain areas from CMS and control mice ($n = 3$ for each group, biological repeats) were assessed for expression microarray experiments followed by Genespring (Agilent Technologies, Santa Clara, CA, USA) software analysis. (**a**) PCA correlation of individual samples. (**b**) Pearson correlation coefficient-based heat map of individual experiments. (**c**) Volcano plot of log2 fold change versus log10 false discovery rate (FDR)-correlated $p$ value for all genes among four brain areas. Blue dots represent significant correlated genes with FDR $p < 0.05$ and fold-change >2. (**d**) Comparison of genes with significant changes and Venn diagram illustration of the four brain areas. (**e**) Heat map diagram with two-way unsupervised hierarchical clustering of significant union genes and samples. Each column represents a gene and each row represents a sample. The gene clustering tree is shown on the top, and the sample clustering tree is shown on the left. The color scale shown in the map illustrates the relative expression level of a gene across all samples: red represents an expression level above the mean and green represents expression lower than the mean. Amy, amygdala; hippo, hippocampus; PFC, prefrontal cortex; CC, cerebral cortex.

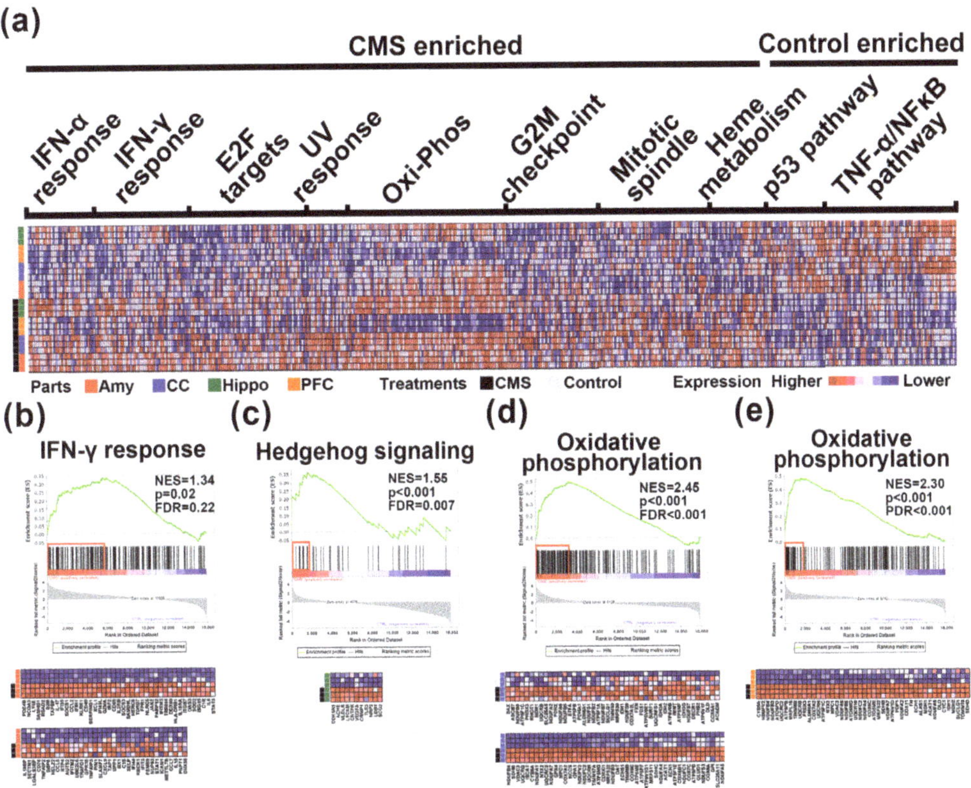


**Figure 4.** Gene set enrichment analysis (GSEA) of expression results in brain areas induced by chronic mild stress (CMS) stimuli. (**a**) Heat map showing core enriched gene clusters involved in several significant differences in hallmark signatures among the four brain areas, including IFN-α response, IFN-γ response, E2F targets, UV response, oxidative phosphorylation, G2M checkpoint, mitotic spindle, heme metabolism, p53 pathway, and TNF-α signaling. (**b**) Graphical representation of core-enriched genes in the CMS-treated amygdala showed positive enrichment for the IFN-γ response. (**c**) Graphical representation of core-enriched genes in the CMS-treated hippocampus showed positive enrichment for Hedgehog signaling. (**d**) Graphical representation of core-enriched genes in the CMS-treated CC showed positive enrichment for oxidative phosphorylation. (**e**) Graphical representation of core-enriched genes in the CMS-treated PFC showed positive enrichment for oxidative phosphorylation. Amy, amygdala; hippo, hippocampus; PFC, prefrontal cortex; CC, cerebral cortex; NES, normalized enrichment score; FDR, false discovery rate.

### *3.5. Pathway Prediction and Regulatory Network Construction in CMS-Treated Mice*

Metacore software was utilized to analyze regulatory signaling affected by CMS in all four brain areas. The differentially expressed genes were then categorized according to process networks, disease, and GO processes (Supplementary Table S4). The top ten significantly enriched terms were listed for each brain area after analysis using a threshold of FDR $p < 0.01$. The results indicated that CMS may affect several developmental processes in neurons and in the immune system. The most abundant gene alterations were found in the amygdala; therefore, we focused on this area for further analysis and regulatory network construction. Firstly, we validated transcriptomic results in Amy using qPCR (Figure 5a). The top three upregulated and downregulated genes in Amy also demonstrated significant changes, consistent with the transcriptomic results. The underlying regulatory network was constructed based on the transcriptional regulation module. We determined that two core transcription factors, NRSF and E2F1, which are downstream of BRM/SWI2-related gene 1 (BRG1) and GSK3β, respectively, had direct interactions with many genes related to neuronal functions (Figure 5b). Specifically, CMS may affect processes including cell–cell signaling, brain development, intracellular transport, neurogenesis, forebrain development, and nervous system development via modulation of NRSF and E2F1. Moreover, two important genes in this network, neuropillin-1 and cerebellin-1, related to neurite outgrowth were significantly downregulated in CMS-treated mice (Figure 5c), which further validates the impact of CMS on neurite trajectory observed through IHC staining (Supplementary Figures S1 and S2).

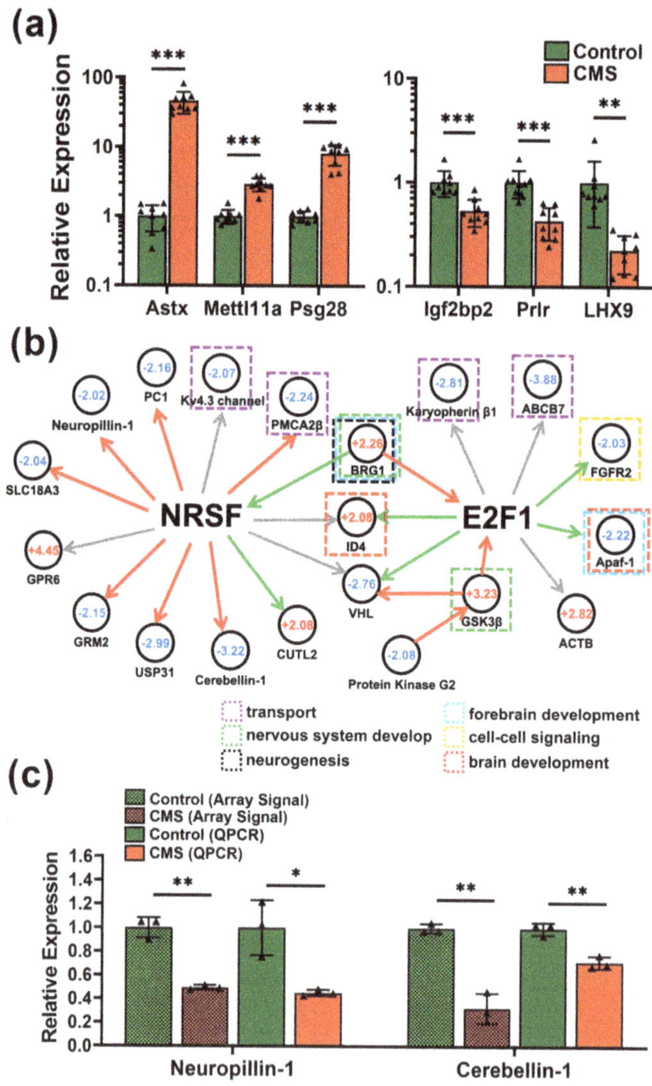


**Figure 5.** qPCR validation and network construction for underlying chronic mild stress (CMS)-induced molecular regulation. (**a**) qPCR validation for CMS-induced genes with significant alterations. Top three upregulated genes (**left** panel) and top three downregulated genes (**right** panel) in the CMS-treated

amygdala. (**b**) Regulatory network construction based on transcriptional regulation. Genes displaying significant changes in the CMS-treated amygdala were subjected to further pathway analysis using Metacore software. NRSF and E2F functioned as two core transcription factors under BRG1 and GSK3β stimulation, respectively. Fold changes in gene expression are indicated with numbers, and genes with functions related to neurodevelopment and neurogenesis are highlighted. Green arrows indicate positive regulation/activation, red arrows indicate negative regulation/inhibition, and gray arrows indicate inconclusive regulation. (**c**) qPCR validation for neurite growth-related genes, neuropillin-1 and cerebellin-1. The results from both the expression array and qPCR were compared in parallel. GPR6, G protein-coupled receptor 6; GRM2, glutamate receptor metabotropic 2; USP31, ubiquitin specific peptidase 31; KCNQ5, potassium voltage-gated channel KQT-like subfamily 5; CUTL2, cut-like homeobox 2; PMCA2b, plasma membrane calcium ATPase 2; SLC18A3, solute carrier family 18; PC1, proprotein convertase subtilisin/kexin type 1; BRG1, BRM/SWI2-related gene 1; ID4, inhibitor of DNA binding 4; VHL, von Hippel-Lindau tumor suppressor; ACTB, beta-actin; Apaf-1, apoptotic peptidase activating factor 1; FGFR2, fibroblast growth factor receptor 2; ABCB7, ATP-binding cassette B7. Statistical analysis was performed using unpaired, two-tailed Student's $t$ tests. * $p < 0.05$, ** $p < 0.01$, and *** $p < 0.001$.

### 3.6. Transthyretin (TTR) Is a Biomarker for MDD Monitoring

The identification of an applicable biomarker for MDD is necessary to improve diagnosis and monitoring in clinical settings. We filtered the results of the transcriptomic analysis to identify genes with a greater than twofold change in at least three of the four brain areas based on the previous analysis (Figure 3d). A total of 17 genes were selected for further analysis (Figure 6a). Notably, TTR was dramatically reduced in Amy, CC, and PFC after CMS treatment. We further confirmed this by three independent qPCR primer sets in Amy highly related to emotion regulation (Figure 6b). ELISA also validated the finding of reduced serum TTR concentrations in CMS-treated mice (Figure 6c). Finally, we assessed whether the TTR concentration in the serum could distinguish patients with MDD (Supplementary Table S5; Figure 6d). Patients with diagnosed MDD were found to exhibit significantly reduced serum TTR compared with health controls. Furthermore, paired serum samples from MDD patients in acute and remission stages showed that TTR levels were significantly enhanced in the remission stage compared with the acute stage (Figure 6e).

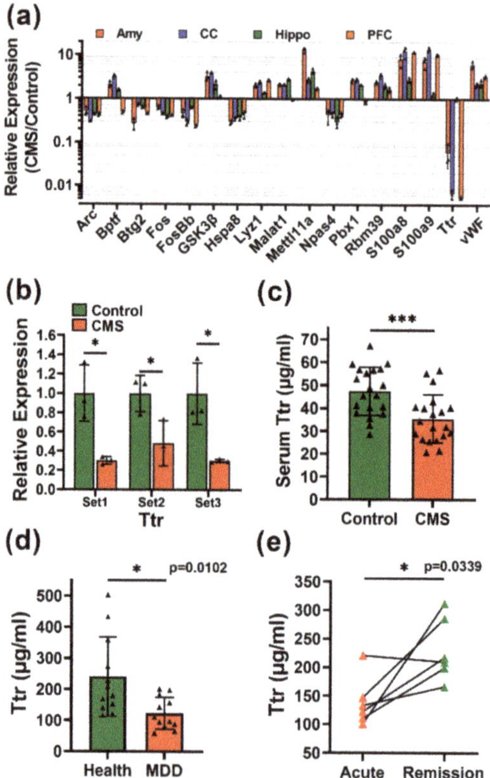


**Figure 6.** Transthyretin (TTR) is a serum biomarker for major depressive disorder (MDD). (**a**) Expression profiling of genes with significant changes and consistent trends in response to CMS treatment in at least three of the four brain areas. TTR exhibited significant downregulation in the amygdala, prefrontal cortex, and cerebral cortex after CMS treatments. (**b**) qPCR validation of TTR expression in the amygdala using three independent sets of primers. (**c**) Serum TTR concentrations in CMS-treated and control mice according to ELISA ($n$ = 20 independent mouse serum samples from three independent CMS treatments per group). (**d**) Serum TTR concentrations in patients with diagnosed MDD and case-controls. (**e**) TTR concentrations in paired serum samples from patients at acute and remission phases of MDD. Statistical analysis was performed using an unpaired, two-tailed Student's $t$-test (**d**) and a paired, two-tailed Student's $t$-test (**e**). Amy, amygdala; hippo, hippocampus; PFC, prefrontal cortex; CC, cerebral cortex. * $p < 0.05$, and *** $p < 0.001$.

## 4. Discussion

Although novel antidepressant therapies are currently emerging, challenges remain due to very limited knowledge of the molecular etiology and clinical complexity of MDD. CMS animal models are valuable tools to help improve understanding of the pathological processes underlying MDD. They can be used to identify specific biomarkers for disease monitoring and support the development of novel antidepressant treatment strategies [18]. In the present study, we found that the amygdala of CMS-treated mice displayed the greatest number of altered genes compared with other areas, which suggests that it was highly affected by CMS. It is not surprising that the amygdala exhibited the greatest number of gene expression changes following CMS treatment, since it plays a crucial role in regulation of the stress response and mediates the influence of stress on memory consolidation and recall [19]. Patients with depression and anxiety have been found to exhibit specific amygdala reactivity [20]. Furthermore, the amygdala represents the node of an extended corticolimbic circuit that supports emotion processing and stress responsiveness [21]. It interacts with other areas in the brain, including the hippocampus and prefrontal cortex, to promote enhancement of several forms of perceptual processing as well as attention, which serve to create memory of emotional material [22]. Accumulating evidence has shown that in the hippocampus, chronic stress may alter cellular functions and plasticity of neurons, and result in dendritic atrophy as well as inhibition of neurogenesis [23]. In particular, chronic stress can also induce dendritic atrophy and reduce the length of apical dendrites of pyramidal neurons in the CA1 and CA3 regions, which may reduce neuroplasticity [24–26]. Furthermore, since GABAergic interneurons of the hippocampus are important in the regulation of cellular and neural circuit function, their roles in the pathogenesis of MDD have been well documented [27]. Our results indicate that neurite outgrowth may also be affected by CMS.

In CMS-induced physiological and functional alterations, firstly, based on GSEA results, gene changes related to CMS in the amygdala are highly enriched in IFN-$\gamma$ responses (Figure 4b). This indicates that the immune system and inflammatory response of mice may be induced by CMS. It has been reported that subjects with depression exhibit elevated levels of inflammatory immune activation [28]. Increases in pro-inflammatory cytokines, especially IL-1, IL-6, TNF-$\alpha$, and IFN-$\gamma$, may exert neurotoxic effects on specific brain areas implicated in emotional regulation, including the amygdala, hippocampus, and cerebral cortex [29]. Secondly, sonic hedgehog signaling (Shh) was found to be significantly enriched in the hippocampus (Figure 4c). This is supported by a previous study, which found that impaired Shh signaling contributes the pathogenesis of several neurological disorders, including MDD [30]. Thirdly, both PFC and CC exhibited enrichment in the oxidative phosphorylation family of genes, suggesting that metabolic alterations may reflect the consequence of CMS stimulation. Accumulated evidence has revealed the link between CMS and alteration of metabolism. For example, stressed animals demonstrate decreased food intake and preference, as well as decreased appetite hormone homeostasis and systematic metabolome changes [31,32]. Upon deeper examination, we found significant changes in gene families related to electron transfer in the mitochondria complexes of stressed mice, suggesting that energy consumption may be affected by CMS (Figure 4d,e).

According to enrichment analysis, significant changed genes were highly correlated with pathways and signaling involved in the neural system (Supplementary Table S4). Specifically, we found alteration in NRSF and E2F1 transcriptional networks under BRG1 gene regulation in the amygdala (Figure 5b). In particular, NRSF exerted direct effects on various genes related to neurogenesis, metabolic processes, axonal guidance, and immunological regulation in the amygdala. The genes downstream of NRSF were also significantly altered in CMS-induced mice. Although NRSF is a well-known transcriptional regulator involved in neurogenesis and differentiation, its role in neurological disorders and diseases such as schizophrenia [33], Alzheimer's disease [34], mood disorders [35], and other physiological functions remains controversial [36]. From a clinical perspective, NRSF may be a specific molecular target able to be suppressed by lithium, a mood-stabilizing drug [37]. Other previous studies have found, using transcriptional analysis, that the GSK3$\beta$-E2F1 axis may be involved in neuronal apoptosis and differentiation [38], as well as tumor growth [39], and has several direct effects on its downstream effectors. This implies that targeting of GSK3$\beta$-E2F1 or NRSF signaling may be able to reduce the effects of CMS-induced bipolar disorder.

In terms of the regulatory network, our results show that two important genes, GSK3$\beta$ and BRG1, were significantly upregulated after CMS administration (Figure 5). This upregulation consequently resulted in downstream gene expression changes related to several neurophysiological functions, predominantly through two core transcription factors, E2F1 and NRSF. Although GSK3$\beta$ and BRG1 have been suggested to have an integral role in neurophysiological function, the molecular basis remains difficult to characterize in MDD [40,41]. This may support the development of therapeutic targets by identifying potential drugs that can reverse or regulate genes involved in MDD pathogenesis.

It has been demonstrated that stress can induce not only depressive-like behaviors, but also alterations in oxidative stress, inflammation, neurogenesis, DNA damage, and apoptosis, where the reduction of these changes can efficiently reverse psychopathological and behavioral abnormalities [42,43]. Our enrichment analysis results are also consistent with these studies, and indicate that greater numbers of physiological processes are enriched after CMS treatment (Supplementary Table S2). For example, accumulating evidence has shown that MDD is accompanied by the activation of immune/inflammatory-related cytokines and acute-phase proteins [44,45]. Two meta-analyses have demonstrated a correlation between the expression of several inflammatory cytokines and clinical bipolar disorder using a case-control study [46,47].

This study identified TTR as an applicable biomarker not only for MDD evaluation, but also for disease monitoring (Figure 6). TTR is a protein synthesized and secreted into peripheral blood and CSF, responsible for retinol and thyroxin transportation, and known as prealbumin [13]. It had been reported to associate with several diseases as well as neurological disease. It may aggregate into fibrils and be deposited into the nervous system and result in neuropathy called transthyretin amyloidosis. Some foster the dissociation of TTR tetramer and some facilitate misfolding and denaturation of monomers to cause the irreversible formation of amyloid fibrils. Furthermore, in addition to deposited amyloid fibrils, non-fibrillar circulating formations confer to neurotoxicity and organ disfunction [48]. This can support that lower TTR in peripheral blood may indicate neuropathogenesis. On the other hand, increasing of serum TTR levels by administrating TTR stabilizers may indicate a positive prognostic response to therapy [49]. Patients treated with TTR stabilizers by binding TTR to reduce dissociation of TTR showed reduced morbidity and mortality in a large clinical trial [50]. On the other hand, lower levels of TTR were observed during malnutrition or inflammation as a negative acute-phase reactant [51,52]. This evidence supports our transcriptomic findings that CMS may cause alterations in immune responses, inflammation, and metabolism (Figure 4; Supplementary Table S4) that may be correlated with TTR reduction. Although low TTR may be highly correlated with MDD, and suicidal ideation and low serotonin function in patients have been documented [53,54], the mechanism involved in CMS induced TTR reduction is still enigmatic. It is possible that CMS-induced GSK3β (Figure 5) reduces TTR expression via repressing heat shock factor 1 (HSF1) activation [55–57]. Manipulation including exogenous overexpression or endogenous knockdown as well as inhibition by drugs of GSK3β followed by TTR characterization should be considered to reveal the relationship between TTR and GSK3β pathways in the future. This may provide a potential actionable strategy for MDD treatments.

The current study was limited by several factors. Firstly, choosing the most ideal MDD animal model remains a controversial question. Therefore, it cannot be excluded that several confounding factors, such as environments, stressors, animal strains, and treatment strategies, may influence gene expression patterns. We used a CMS strategy with various unpredictable stressors to model MDD. It should be noted that MDD is not a homogenous disorder; it is diagnosed when a certain minimal number of symptoms are displayed in humans. Thus, a limitation of this study was that it may not have allowed clear differentiation of MDD depression subtypes, such as melancholic or atypical depression. Secondly, it should be noticed that MDD is a sex-biased (high occurrence in females) disease. Although only male mice were included for the CMS-induced MDD model, based on the consideration of estrogen interference, it cannot be excluded that some biases may exist. However, the validation in patients (75% females), which indicated that TTR was still highly correlated to MDD, suggested that it may be independent from sex. Thirdly, the sample size of patients with MDD was few and several confounding factors that may affect the power of TTR were difficult to analyze.

In order to validate the clinical utilities of TTR, it is necessary to conduct a clinical trial with a large and comprehensive cohort in the future.

## 5. Conclusions

The current study utilized an MDD animal model to comprehensively dissect the underlying molecular mechanisms of MDD. CMS may induce MDD-like pathogenesis accompanied by physiological changes such as IFN-$\gamma$ response, hedgehog signaling, and oxidative phosphorylation in different brain parts. This provided rationales for further MDD-related investigations. Furthermore, current results also identified TTR as a potential diagnostic and monitoring marker for clinical applications in the future.

**Supplementary Materials:** The following are available online at https://www.mdpi.com/article/10.3390/biomedicines9091124/s1. Figure S1: Immunohistochemical staining of Tau-1. Figure S2: Immunohistochemical staining of MAP2. Table S1: Primer List for SYBR Green Quantitative PCR. Table S2: Genes differentially expression in prefrontal cortex, cerebral cortex, amygdala and hippocampus with CMS. Table S3: Gene Enrichment Analysis for CMS vs. Control Mouse Model in Amygdala, Hippocampus, Cerebral Cortex and Prefrontal Cortex. Table S4: Characteristics of patients with MDD and control individuals in the TTR testing cohort.

**Author Contributions:** Conceptualization, S.-L.Y., P.-C.Y., K.-Y.S.; methodology, S.S.-T.C., M.-H.C., K.-Y.S.; software, S.S.-T.C., K.-Y.S.; validation, S.S.-T.C., M.-H.C., K.-Y.S.; formal analysis, S.-L.Y., S.S.-T.C., K.-Y.S.; resources, S.-L.Y., P.-H.K., P.-C.Y., K.-Y.S.; data curation, S.-L.Y., K.-Y.S.; writing—original draft preparation, S.S.-T.C., K.-Y.S.; writing—review and editing, S.-L.Y., S.S.-T.C., M.-H.C., P.-H.K., P.-C.Y., K.-Y.S.; supervision, P.-C.Y., K.-Y.S.; project administration, S.-L.Y., K.-Y.S.; funding acquisition, S.-L.Y., P.-C.Y., K.-Y.S. All authors have read and agreed to the published version of the manuscript.

**Funding:** This work was funded by grants from the Ministry of Science and Technology, Taiwan. (MOST103-2320-B-002-052, MOST104-2320-B-002-030, MOST109-2314-B-002-186, MOST110-2314-B-002-269 to Kang-Yi Su).

**Institutional Review Board Statement:** All animal experiments were carried out with the agreement and approval of the Institutional Animal Care and Use Committee (IACUC) of National Taiwan University Medical College (approval number 20120060).

**Informed Consent Statement:** Informed consent was obtained from all subjects involved in the study. All participants signed informed consent forms after the study procedures were fully explained.

**Data Availability Statement:** All data generated or analyzed during this study are included in this published article.

**Acknowledgments:** We would like to thank the technical support from the Center of Genomic and Precision Medicine and Pharmacogenomics Labs (TR6), National Taiwan University.

**Conflicts of Interest:** All authors of this work declare no conflict of interest.

## References

1. World Health Assembly. Global Burden of Mental Disorders and the Need for a Comprehensive, Coordinated Response from Health and Social Sectors at the Country Level: Report by the Secretariat. 2012. Available online: https://apps.who.int/gb/ebwha/pdf_files/eb130/b130_9-en.pdf (accessed on 1 December 2011).
2. Kessler, R.C.; Chiu, W.T.; Demler, O.; Merikangas, K.R.; Walters, E.E. Prevalence, severity, and comorbidity of 12-month DSM-IV disorders in the National Comorbidity Survey Replication. *Arch. Gen. Psychiatry* **2005**, *62*, 617–627. [CrossRef]
3. Tye, K.M.; Mirzabekov, J.J.; Warden, M.R.; Ferenczi, E.A.; Tsai, H.C.; Finkelstein, J.; Kim, S.Y.; Adhikari, A.; Thompson, K.R.; Andalman, A.S.; et al. Dopamine neurons modulate neural encoding and expression of depression-related behaviour. *Nature* **2013**, *493*, 537–541. [CrossRef]
4. Goetzel, R.Z.; Pei, X.; Tabrizi, M.J.; Henke, R.M.; Kowlessar, N.; Nelson, C.F.; Metz, R.D. Ten modifiable health risk factors are linked to more than one-fifth of employer-employee health care spending. *Health Aff.* **2012**, *31*, 2474–2484. [CrossRef] [PubMed]
5. Duman, R.S.; Malberg, J.; Nakagawa, S.; D'Sa, C. Neuronal plasticity and survival in mood disorders. *Biol. Psychiatry* **2000**, *48*, 732–739. [CrossRef]

6. Hannestad, J.; DellaGioia, N.; Bloch, M. The effect of antidepressant medication treatment on serum levels of inflammatory cytokines: A meta-analysis. *Neuropsychopharmacology* **2011**, *36*, 2452–2459. [CrossRef] [PubMed]
7. Pan, Y.; Lin, W.; Wang, W.; Qi, X.; Wang, D.; Tang, M. The effects of central pro-and anti-inflammatory immune challenges on depressive-like behavior induced by chronic forced swim stress in rats. *Behav. Brain Res.* **2013**, *247*, 232–240. [CrossRef] [PubMed]
8. Schiepers, O.J.; Wichers, M.C.; Maes, M. Cytokines and major depression. *Prog. Neuropsychopharmacol. Biol Psychiatry* **2005**, *29*, 201–217. [CrossRef] [PubMed]
9. Duman, R.S.; Monteggia, L.M. A neurotrophic model for stress-related mood disorders. *Biol. Psychiatry* **2006**, *59*, 1116–1127. [CrossRef]
10. Ulrich-Lai, Y.M.; Herman, J.P. Neural regulation of endocrine and autonomic stress responses. *Nat. Rev. Neurosci.* **2009**, *10*, 397–409. [CrossRef]
11. Trivedi, M.H.; Rush, A.J.; Wisniewski, S.R.; Nierenberg, A.A.; Warden, D.; Ritz, L.; Norquist, G.; Howland, R.H.; Lebowitz, B.; McGrath, P.J.; et al. Evaluation of outcomes with citalopram for depression using measurement-based care in STAR*D: Implications for clinical practice. *Am. J. Psychiatry* **2006**, *163*, 28–40. [CrossRef]
12. Hill, M.N.; Hellemans, K.G.; Verma, P.; Gorzalka, B.B.; Weinberg, J. Neurobiology of chronic mild stress: Parallels to major depression. *Neurosci. Biobehav. Rev.* **2012**, *36*, 2085–2117. [CrossRef]
13. Alfarez, D.N.; Joels, M.; Krugers, H.J. Chronic unpredictable stress impairs long-term potentiation in rat hippocampal CA1 area and dentate gyrus in vitro. *Eur. J. Neurosci.* **2003**, *17*, 1928–1934. [CrossRef] [PubMed]
14. Liu, Y.; Yang, N.; Zuo, P. cDNA microarray analysis of gene expression in the cerebral cortex and hippocampus of BALB/c mice subjected to chronic mild stress. *Cell. Mol. Neurobiol.* **2010**, *30*, 1035–1047. [CrossRef]
15. Yamanishi, K.; Doe, N.; Sumida, M.; Watanabe, Y.; Yoshida, M.; Yamamoto, H.; Xu, Y.; Li, W.; Yamanishi, H.; Okamura, H.; et al. Hepatocyte nuclear factor 4 alpha is a key factor related to depression and physiological homeostasis in the mouse brain. *PLoS ONE* **2015**, *10*, e0119021. [CrossRef] [PubMed]
16. Hines, L.M.; Hoffman, P.L.; Bhave, S.; Saba, L.; Kaiser, A.; Snell, L.; Goncharov, I.; LeGault, L.; Dongier, M.; Grant, B.; et al. A sex-specific role of type VII adenylyl cyclase in depression. *J. Neurosci.* **2006**, *26*, 12609–12619. [CrossRef] [PubMed]
17. Holmes, A.; Li, Q.; Koenig, E.A.; Gold, E.; Stephenson, D.; Yang, R.J.; Dreiling, J.; Sullivan, T.; Crawley, J.N. Phenotypic assessment of galanin overexpressing and galanin receptor R1 knockout mice in the tail suspension test for depression-related behavior. *Psychopharmacology* **2005**, *178*, 276–285. [CrossRef]
18. Czeh, B.; Fuchs, E.; Wiborg, O.; Simon, M. Animal models of major depression and their clinical implications. *Prog. Neuropsychopharmacol. Biol. Psychiatry* **2016**, *64*, 293–310. [CrossRef]
19. Roozendaal, B.; McEwen, B.S.; Chattarji, S. Stress, memory and the amygdala. *Nat. Rev. Neurosci.* **2009**, *10*, 423–433. [CrossRef]
20. Groenewold, N.A.; Opmeer, E.M.; de Jonge, P.; Aleman, A.; Costafreda, S.G. Emotional valence modulates brain functional abnormalities in depression: Evidence from a meta-analysis of fMRI studies. *Neurosci. Biobehav. Rev.* **2013**, *37*, 152–163. [CrossRef]
21. Swartz, J.R.; Knodt, A.R.; Radtke, S.R.; Hariri, A.R. A neural biomarker of psychological vulnerability to future life stress. *Neuron* **2015**, *85*, 505–511. [CrossRef]
22. Murty, V.P.; Ritchey, M.; Adcock, R.A.; LaBar, K.S. fMRI studies of successful emotional memory encoding: A quantitative meta-analysis. *Neuropsychologia* **2010**, *48*, 3459–3469. [CrossRef]
23. McEwen, B.S.; Akil, H. Revisiting the Stress Concept: Implications for Affective Disorders. *J. Neurosci.* **2020**, *40*, 12–21. [CrossRef]
24. Qiao, H.; An, S.C.; Xu, C.; Ma, X.M. Role of proBDNF and BDNF in dendritic spine plasticity and depressive-like behaviors induced by an animal model of depression. *Brain Res.* **2017**, *1663*, 29–37. [CrossRef]
25. Sousa, N.; Lukoyanov, N.V.; Madeira, M.D.; Almeida, O.F.; Paula-Barbosa, M.M. Erratum to "Reorganization of the morphology of hippocampal neurites and synapses after stress-induced damage correlates with behavioral improvement". *Neuroscience* **2000**, *101*, 483. [CrossRef]
26. Zhuang, P.C.; Tan, Z.N.; Jia, Z.Y.; Wang, B.; Grady, J.J.; Ma, X.M. Treadmill Exercise Reverses Depression Model-Induced Alteration of Dendritic Spines in the Brain Areas of Mood Circuit. *Front. Behav. Neurosci.* **2019**, *13*, 93. [CrossRef]
27. Duman, R.S.; Sanacora, G.; Krystal, J.H. Altered Connectivity in Depression: GABA and Glutamate Neurotransmitter Deficits and Reversal by Novel Treatments. *Neuron* **2019**, *102*, 75–90. [CrossRef]
28. Kohler, C.A.; Freitas, T.H.; Maes, M.; de Andrade, N.Q.; Liu, C.S.; Fernandes, B.S.; Stubbs, B.; Solmi, M.; Veronese, N.; Herrmann, N.; et al. Peripheral cytokine and chemokine alterations in depression: A meta-analysis of 82 studies. *Acta Psychiatr. Scand.* **2017**, *135*, 373–387. [CrossRef] [PubMed]
29. Shim, H.S.; Park, H.J.; Woo, J.; Lee, C.J.; Shim, I. Role of astrocytic GABAergic system on inflammatory cytokine-induced anxiety-like behavior. *Neuropharmacology* **2019**, *160*, 107776. [CrossRef] [PubMed]
30. Yao, P.J.; Petralia, R.S.; Mattson, M.P. Sonic Hedgehog Signaling and Hippocampal Neuroplasticity. *Trends Neurosci.* **2016**, *39*, 840–850. [CrossRef] [PubMed]
31. Geng, C.; Guo, Y.; Wang, C.; Liao, D.; Han, W.; Zhang, J.; Jiang, P. Systematic impacts of chronic unpredictable mild stress on metabolomics in rats. *Sci. Rep.* **2020**, *10*, 700. [CrossRef] [PubMed]
32. Lopez Lopez, A.L.; Escobar Villanueva, M.C.; Brianza Padilla, M.; Bonilla Jaime, H.; Alarcon Aguilar, F.J. Chronic Unpredictable Mild Stress Progressively Disturbs Glucose Metabolism and Appetite Hormones in Rats. *Acta Endocrinol.* **2018**, *14*, 16–23. [CrossRef]

33. Warburton, A.; Breen, G.; Rujescu, D.; Bubb, V.J.; Quinn, J.P. Characterization of a REST-Regulated Internal Promoter in the Schizophrenia Genome-Wide Associated Gene MIR137. *Schizophr. Bull.* **2015**, *41*, 698–707. [CrossRef]
34. Lu, T.; Aron, L.; Zullo, J.; Pan, Y.; Kim, H.; Chen, Y.; Yang, T.H.; Kim, H.M.; Drake, D.; Liu, X.S.; et al. REST and stress resistance in ageing and Alzheimer's disease. *Nature* **2014**, *507*, 448–454. [CrossRef]
35. Warburton, A.; Savage, A.L.; Myers, P.; Peeney, D.; Bubb, V.J.; Quinn, J.P. Molecular signatures of mood stabilisers highlight the role of the transcription factor REST/NRSF. *J. Affect. Disord.* **2014**, *172*, 63–73. [CrossRef]
36. Song, Z.; Zhao, D.; Zhao, H.; Yang, L. NRSF: An Angel or a Devil in Neurogenesis and Neurological Diseases. *J. Mol. Neurosci.* **2015**, *56*, 131–144. [CrossRef] [PubMed]
37. Ishii, T.; Hashimoto, E.; Ukai, W.; Tateno, M.; Yoshinaga, T.; Saito, S.; Sohma, H.; Saito, T. Lithium-induced suppression of transcription repressor NRSF/REST: Effects on the dysfunction of neuronal differentiation by ethanol. *Eur. J. Pharmacol.* **2008**, *593*, 36–43. [CrossRef] [PubMed]
38. Espada, L.; Udapudi, B.; Podlesniy, P.; Fabregat, I.; Espinet, C.; Tauler, A. Apoptotic action of E2F1 requires glycogen synthase kinase 3-beta activity in PC12 cells. *J. Neurochem.* **2007**, *102*, 2020–2028. [CrossRef]
39. Zhu, Q.; Yang, J.; Han, S.; Liu, J.; Holzbeierlein, J.; Thrasher, J.B.; Li, B. Suppression of glycogen synthase kinase 3 activity reduces tumor growth of prostate cancer in vivo. *Prostate* **2011**, *71*, 835–845. [CrossRef] [PubMed]
40. Lessard, J.; Wu, J.I.; Ranish, J.A.; Wan, M.; Winslow, M.M.; Staahl, B.T.; Wu, H.; Aebersold, R.; Graef, I.A.; Crabtree, G.R. An essential switch in subunit composition of a chromatin remodeling complex during neural development. *Neuron* **2007**, *55*, 201–215. [CrossRef] [PubMed]
41. Manduca, J.D.; Theriault, R.K.; Perreault, M.L. Glycogen synthase kinase-3: The missing link to aberrant circuit function in disorders of cognitive dysfunction? *Pharmacol. Res.* **2020**, *157*, 104819. [CrossRef] [PubMed]
42. Banagozar Mohammadi, A.; Torbati, M.; Farajdokht, F.; Sadigh-Eteghad, S.; Fazljou, S.M.B.; Vatandoust, S.M.; Golzari, S.E.J.; Mahmoudi, J. Sericin alleviates restraint stress induced depressive- and anxiety-like behaviors via modulation of oxidative stress, neuroinflammation and apoptosis in the prefrontal cortex and hippocampus. *Brain Res.* **2019**, *1715*, 47–56. [CrossRef] [PubMed]
43. Fatima, M.; Srivastav, S.; Ahmad, M.H.; Mondal, A.C. Effects of chronic unpredictable mild stress induced prenatal stress on neurodevelopment of neonates: Role of GSK-3beta. *Sci. Rep.* **2019**, *9*, 1305. [CrossRef]
44. Maes, M.; Meltzer, H.Y.; Bosmans, E.; Bergmans, R.; Vandoolaeghe, E.; Ranjan, R.; Desnyder, R. Increased plasma concentrations of interleukin-6, soluble interleukin-6, soluble interleukin-2 and transferrin receptor in major depression. *J. Affect. Disord.* **1995**, *34*, 301–309. [CrossRef]
45. Maes, M.; Delange, J.; Ranjan, R.; Meltzer, H.Y.; Desnyder, R.; Cooremans, W.; Scharpe, S. Acute phase proteins in schizophrenia, mania and major depression: Modulation by psychotropic drugs. *Psychiatry Res.* **1997**, *66*, 1–11. [CrossRef]
46. Munkholm, K.; Brauner, J.V.; Kessing, L.V.; Vinberg, M. Cytokines in bipolar disorder vs. healthy control subjects: A systematic review and meta-analysis. *J. Psychiatr. Res.* **2013**, *47*, 1119–1133. [CrossRef]
47. Modabbernia, A.; Taslimi, S.; Brietzke, E.; Ashrafi, M. Cytokine alterations in bipolar disorder: A meta-analysis of 30 studies. *Biol. Psychiatry* **2013**, *74*, 15–25. [CrossRef] [PubMed]
48. Sousa, M.M.; Cardoso, I.; Fernandes, R.; Guimaraes, A.; Saraiva, M.J. Deposition of transthyretin in early stages of familial amyloidotic polyneuropathy: Evidence for toxicity of nonfibrillar aggregates. *Am. J. Pathol.* **2001**, *159*, 1993–2000. [CrossRef]
49. Judge, D.P.; Heitner, S.B.; Falk, R.H.; Maurer, M.S.; Shah, S.J.; Witteles, R.M.; Grogan, M.; Selby, V.N.; Jacoby, D.; Hanna, M.; et al. Transthyretin Stabilization by AG10 in Symptomatic Transthyretin Amyloid Cardiomyopathy. *J. Am. Coll. Cardiol.* **2019**, *74*, 285–295. [CrossRef]
50. Maurer, M.S.; Schwartz, J.H.; Gundapaneni, B.; Elliott, P.M.; Merlini, G.; Waddington-Cruz, M.; Kristen, A.V.; Grogan, M.; Witteles, R.; Damy, T.; et al. Tafamidis Treatment for Patients with Transthyretin Amyloid Cardiomyopathy. *N. Engl. J. Med.* **2018**, *379*, 1007–1016. [CrossRef]
51. Dickson, P.W.; Howlett, G.J.; Schreiber, G. Metabolism of prealbumin in rats and changes induced by acute inflammation. *Eur. J. Biochem.* **1982**, *129*, 289–293. [CrossRef]
52. Ingenbleek, Y.; Young, V. Transthyretin (prealbumin) in health and disease: Nutritional implications. *Annu. Rev. Nutr.* **1994**, *14*, 495–533. [CrossRef]
53. Fava, M.; Labbate, L.A.; Abraham, M.E.; Rosenbaum, J.F. Hypothyroidism and hyperthyroidism in major depression revisited. *J. Clin. Psychiatry* **1995**, *56*, 186–192.
54. Sullivan, G.M.; Mann, J.J.; Oquendo, M.A.; Lo, E.S.; Cooper, T.B.; Gorman, J.M. Low cerebrospinal fluid transthyretin levels in depression: Correlations with suicidal ideation and low serotonin function. *Biol. Psychiatry* **2006**, *60*, 500–506. [CrossRef]
55. Bijur, G.N.; Jope, R.S. Opposing actions of phosphatidylinositol 3-kinase and glycogen synthase kinase-3beta in the regulation of HSF-1 activity. *J. Neurochem.* **2000**, *75*, 2401–2408. [CrossRef]
56. Chu, B.; Zhong, R.; Soncin, F.; Stevenson, M.A.; Calderwood, S.K. Transcriptional activity of heat shock factor 1 at 37 degrees C is repressed through phosphorylation on two distinct serine residues by glycogen synthase kinase 3 and protein kinases Calpha and Czeta. *J. Biol. Chem.* **1998**, *273*, 18640–18646. [CrossRef]
57. Wang, X.; Cattaneo, F.; Ryno, L.; Hulleman, J.; Reixach, N.; Buxbaum, J.N. The systemic amyloid precursor transthyretin (TTR) behaves as a neuronal stress protein regulated by HSF1 in SH-SY5Y human neuroblastoma cells and APP23 Alzheimer's disease model mice. *J. Neurosci.* **2014**, *34*, 7253–7265. [CrossRef] [PubMed]

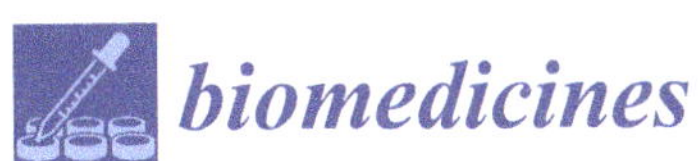

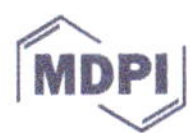

*Article*

# Low-Dose Niacin Supplementation Improves Motor Function in US Veterans with Parkinson's Disease: A Single-Center, Randomized, Placebo-Controlled Trial

**Chandramohan Wakade [1,2,3,4,5,*], Raymond Chong [1,6], Marissa Seamon [1,4], Sharad Purohit [1,2,7], Banabihari Giri [1,2] and John C. Morgan [1,5]**

1 Charlie Norwood VA Medical Center, Augusta, GA 30904, USA; rchong@augusta.edu (R.C.); mseamon@augusta.edu (M.S.); spurohit@augusta.edu (S.P.); bgiri@augusta.edu (B.G.); jmorgan@augusta.edu (J.C.M.)
2 Center for Biotechnology and Genomic Medicine, Medical College of Georgia, Augusta University, Augusta, GA 30912, USA
3 Department of Physical Therapy, College of Allied Health Sciences, Augusta University, Augusta, GA 30912, USA
4 Department of Neuroscience and Regenerative Medicine, Medical College of Georgia, Augusta University, Augusta, GA 30912, USA
5 Department of Neurology, Medical College of Georgia, Augusta University, Augusta, GA 30912, USA
6 Department of Interdisciplinary Health Sciences, College of Allied Health Sciences, Augusta University, Augusta, GA 30912, USA
7 Department of Undergraduate Health Professions, College of Allied Health Sciences, Augusta University, Augusta, GA 30912, USA
* Correspondence: cwakade@augusta.edu

**Citation:** Wakade, C.; Chong, R.; Seamon, M.; Purohit, S.; Giri, B.; Morgan, J.C. Low-Dose Niacin Supplementation Improves Motor Function in US Veterans with Parkinson's Disease: A Single-Center, Randomized, Placebo-Controlled Trial. *Biomedicines* **2021**, *9*, 1881. https://doi.org/10.3390/biomedicines9121881

Academic Editor: Arnab Ghosh

Received: 25 October 2021
Accepted: 7 December 2021
Published: 10 December 2021



**Abstract:** A six-month double-blind, placebo-controlled randomized study was conducted to ascertain whether low-dose daily niacin supplementation would improve motor symptoms in Parkinson's disease (PD) patients. A total of 47 PD patients were assigned to receive low-dose niacin or a placebo. At the end of the double-blind phase, all participants received open-label niacin for the next six months. All patients were evaluated at baseline, after six months, and after one year of treatment. The primary outcome measure was the Unified Parkinson's Disease Rating Scale III (UPDRS III) scores. Secondary outcome measures were depression, sleep quality, mental flexibility and cognition, and physical fatigue. Niacin treatment was well-tolerated by forty-five subjects. The mean [95% CI] change in UPDRS III scores at six months of placebo was −0.05 [95% CI, −2.4 to 2.32], and niacin was −1.06 [95% CI, −3.68 to 1.57]. From six to twelve months when both groups received open-label niacin supplementation, the average UPDRS III scores significantly decreased for the placebo group by 4.58 [95% CI, −0.85 to 8.30] and the niacin group by 4.63 [95% CI, 1.42 to 7.83] points. Low-dose niacin supplementation is a well-tolerated adjunct therapy and may improve motor function in PD when taken over a longer period.

**Keywords:** Parkinson's disease; movement disorder; niacin; UPDRS III; fatigue

## 1. Introduction

Parkinson's disease (PD) is one of the most common movement disorders afflicting approximately 1% of the population above the age of 60 and 4% by age 80. A definitive diagnosis for PD requires an autopsy, and there is no cure or definitive disease-slowing therapy despite extensive investigation [1]. Sinemet (carbidopa/levodopa) remains the cornerstone of PD therapy but can lead to significant motor complications (wearing off and dyskinesia) over time [2].

Numerous pathophysiological processes interplay in PD, but neuroinflammation and mitochondrial dysfunction remain at the core of PD pathology [3–6]. Niacin is, therefore, a promising choice as an adjunct therapy in PD since it is anti-inflammatory and boosts mitochondrial function by providing NAD [5,6]. Parkinson's disease is accompanied by non-motor symptoms such as lack of sleep, depression, and fatigue, resulting in poor quality of life [7–9]. Medications that reduce motor symptoms further aggravate non-motor symptoms in PD patients [10]. Moreover, carbidopa in Sinemet is known to deplete niacin levels in treated PD patients [11]. Chong et al. recently investigated niacin in a three-month effectiveness trial, showing improvements in quality of life and motor symptoms in PD patients [12]. Our group and others have indicated that niacin supplementation may influence outcomes in PD patients [5,12,13].

The present study investigates the effects of low-dose niacin treatment and improvement in tremor, rigidity, and overall Unified Parkinson's Disease Rating Scale III (UPDRS III) scores in US veterans with PD. Compared to the study by Chong et al. [12], this trial has a longer randomized, double-blind, placebo-controlled phase, followed by an additional six months of open-label niacin.

## 2. Materials and Methods

### 2.1. Participants

The study was a single-center prospective trial conducted at Charlie Norwood Veterans Affairs Medical Center (CNVAMC, GA, USA) neurology clinic and Augusta University Medical Center (AUMC, GA, USA) Tertiary Movement Disorders Center (clinicaltrials.gov identifier: NCT03462680). The patients were enrolled from October 5th, 2016 to September 18th, 2019, and tested every six months. The inclusion criteria were: (1) mild to moderately severe PD patients according to the United Kingdom Parkinson's Disease Society Brain Bank Diagnostic Criteria [14], (2) Hoehn and Yahr (H&Y) scores between 0.5–4, (3) stabilized on all PD medications prior to enrollment with expected medication stability for at least six months, and (4) mini-mental state exam (MMSE) scores above 24. The exclusion criteria were: (1) other severe neurological problems, previous brain surgery, functional blindness, inability to participate in visuomotor or gait assessments, (2) an allergy to niacin, (3) other severe illnesses, (4) previously undergone deep brain stimulation, or (5) dementia. An attending expert neurologist used his clinical judgment to determine if a patient was suitable for the study, including an optional spinal tap. The study was conducted according to the Declaration of Helsinki (1997) and approved by The Institutional Review Board at AUMC (750415). Demographic, clinical, and medication data were captured from the patient database. All subjects signed a written informed consent to participate in the study.

### 2.2. Intervention

A total of 47 patients, stabilized on medications three months prior, were enrolled in the study. The subjects were kept on the same dose of medications for the first six months of the study. Patients were randomized and blinded to receive either 250 mg of niacin once daily or placebo in accordance with the sequestered fixed randomization schedule (Figure 1), using balanced blocks to ensure an approximate 1:1 ratio of the two treatment arms for early-stage (H&Y 0.5–2) or late-stage patients (H&Y 2.5–4). The VAMC pharmacy generated the randomized sequence for the group assignment. Study subjects and the researchers were blinded to the allocation. Grouping was also concealed by dispensing the supplements (placebo and niacin) in an opaque pouch. The randomization code was not revealed to the investigators until the study was completed in April 2020. The facility for performing outcome measures was provided by the CNVAMC.

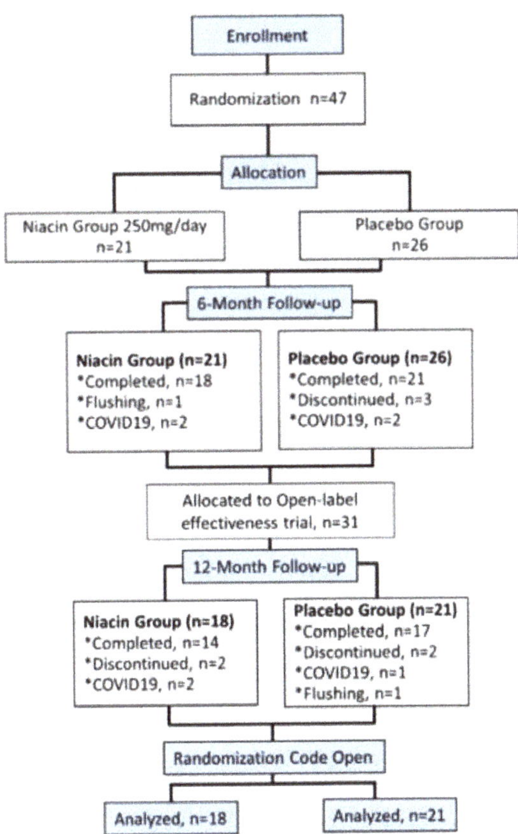


**Figure 1.** Flowchart showing participant flow in the Niacin for Parkinson's disease trial. A total of 47 participants enrolled in the study were randomly placed into the placebo or niacin-treated group. The randomized, double-blind portion lasted six months; then, a subsequent open-label niacin phase was implemented from six to twelve months.

## 2.3. Outcomes of the Study

The study's primary outcome was a change in the UPDRS III scores from baseline to six months and one year. Based on pilot data, the margin of superiority representing the minimal clinically meaningful change in score, δ, is 5. This value is the expected median annual rate of decline in the UPDRS III score of +5.5 points [15,16]. Secondary outcomes included depression rating by the Geriatric Depression Scale (GDS), fatigue rating by the Fatigue Severity Scale (FSS) and Visual Analogue Fatigue Scale (VAFS), mental resilience measured by Trail Making Test (TMT) A and B (the difference between TMT-B and TMT-A was considered as a measurement of cognitive flexibility) [17], cognitive ability and mental fatigue through the Stroop Test, overall cognitive function by MMSE, amino acid and serotonin levels, and physical strength and fatigue through a grip strength test. A single assessor took all measurements to eliminate interrater differences. Patients were tested at baseline, after six months of daily 250 mg niacin or placebo, and then again after six months of open-label 250 mg daily niacin. There were no treatment changes (regarding medications and dosages) made during the double-blind trial period.

### 2.4. Statistical Analysis

The trial data was analyzed according to the intent to treat and per-protocol methods. Means, standard deviations or standard errors, and ranges were calculated for continuous and numerical data. Categorical data were presented as counts and percentages, analyzed by chi-sq test. Statistical differences were tested between the treatment groups and time points by ANOVA with Tukey's post hoc corrections for primary outcomes. All $p$-values were adjusted for multiple comparisons according to Bonferroni's correction. A $p \leq 0.05$ was considered statistically significant; all $p$ values were two-sided.

The sample size of thirty-nine analyzed patients was determined to give 80% power ($\alpha$ = 0.05) to detect a reduction of 2.5 points in UPDRS III scores after six months of treatment [15,16]. For a significance level ($\alpha$) of 5% and a power (1-$\beta$) of 80%, an expected standard deviation of the difference between data pairs was 3.9, and the minimum sample size was 13 participants per group. Our study sample was substantially increased to take into account potential dropouts or unexpected increases in variability.

Data for age, sex, race, and PD medications and dose were documented from the patient records system. Laboratory data on serum levels of serotonin was also obtained. Data for all participants was entered into an Excel sheet (Microsoft Excel v2016) for subsequent analysis. Outcomes of all 39 participants who completed the six-month trial were analyzed according to their randomization groups, comparing differences between treatments and differences between time points of baseline, six months, and one year.

One outlier was removed from UPDRS III scores based on the ordinary least-squares regression test (Q = 10%). All other outcome data had no outliers removed by the robust regression and outlier removal test. All analyses were performed using Prism (v8.0, Graphpad, San Deigo, CA, USA).

## 3. Results

### 3.1. Subjects

Between 2016–2019, 47 participants were enrolled at the CNVAMC; 39 returned for the six-month evaluation. Participants were randomly assigned to the placebo (n = 21) or 250 mg daily niacin (n = 18) group (Figure 1). The mean age was 68.4, with a mean duration of PD being 5.8 years (Table 1). A total of 36 participants were Caucasian, and three were African American; four participants were women. Based on H&Y scores, the subjects were divided into early (n = 28) and late-stage (n = 11) groups. Veterans (n = 25) constituted 64 % of the total study subjects (n = 39), while remaining patients were non-veterans (n = 14) (Table 1).

A total of 35 subjects were on Sinemet as their primary Parkinson's medication throughout the study. The neurologist changed the medication dose of five patients during the open-label phase of the study (Table 1). Other medications or supplements taken by subjects included Trihexyphenidyl (n = 2), Donepezil (n = 1), Simvastatin (n = 1), Diclofenac (n = 1), Temazepam (n = 1), Aspirin (n = 7), Ropinirole (n = 8), Rasagiline (n = 9), Pramipexole (n = 13), Amantadine (n = 1), Vitamin D3 (n = 2), multivitamin (n = 5), and Vitamin C (n = 1). None of the subjects in this study were on SSRIs.

The six-month follow-up was completed by 39 of the 47 enrolled patients. Of these, eight of the 39 patients did not complete the optional six-month open-label portion of the study (Figure 1). Participants discontinued due to the flushing effect of niacin (n = 2), voluntary discontinuation (n = 7), or the SARS-CoV-2 shut-down of clinical research (n = 7). Chi-squared and Fisher tests showed no significant differences in the dropout rate between the groups, $p$ = 0.65 and 0.72, respectively. Although both groups took niacin from six to twelve months, the group who took the placebo for the first six months will continue to be referred to as the placebo group for this study (Figure 1).

**Table 1.** Demographic and baseline characteristics of the participants (n = 39).

| Characteristics | Treatment Groups Placebo (n = 21) | Niacin (n = 18) | p-Value |
|---|---|---|---|
| Sex, N (%) | | | |
| Men | 19 (90.5) | 16 (88.9) | 1 [a] |
| Women | 2 (9.5) | 2 (11.1) | |
| Race/ethnicity, N (%) | | | |
| Non-Hispanic White | 18 (85.7) | 18 (100) | 0.29 [a] |
| Non-Hispanic Black | 3 (14.3) | 0 (0) | |
| Veteran status, N (%) | | | |
| Veterans | 15 (71.4) | 10 (55.6) | 0.5 [a] |
| Non-Veterans | 6 (28.6) | 8 (44.4) | |
| Age, mean (SD), y | 68.0 (10.7) | 68.2 (6.0) | |
| Duration of PD, mean (SD), y | 5.6 (4.2) | 6.0 (6.0) | |
| Age of Onset, mean (SD), y | 61.6 (10.9) | 63.3 (7.2) | |
| Disease Stage, N (%) | | | |
| Early (H&Y < 2.5) | 14 (66.7) | 14 (77.8) | 0.68 [a] |
| Late (H&Y ≥ 2.5) | 7 (33.3) | 4 (22.2) | |
| Medications, mg/day | | | |
| Sinemet intake, N (%) | 20 (95.2) | 15 (83.3) | 0.5 [a] |
| Levodopa dosage, mean (range) | 488.9 (300–1000) | 480.8 (200–800) | |
| H&Y staging, mean (range) | 2.2 (1.5–4) | 1.8 (0.5–4) | |
| UPDRS III Scores, mean (SD) | 22.4 (11.8) | 21.3 (15.8) | 0.99 [b] |
| Rigidity | 1.69 (2.23) | 1.5 (1.92) | 0.99 [b] |
| Resting Tremor | 4.52 (2.87) | 3.11 (2.82) | 0.34 [b] |
| Bradykinesia | 4.5 (4.6) | 4 (4.5) | 0.98 [b] |
| Cognitive flexibility | 73.38 (57.11) | 79.42 (62.46) | 0.99 [b] |
| Grip Strength, PSI | | | |
| First affected hand | 305.09 (105.26) | 297.04 (125.68) | 0.99 [b] |
| Non (or later) affected hand | 300.43 (80.49) | 284.1 (123.09) | 0.98 [b] |
| FSS | 36.65 (13.02) | 40.28 (11.99) | 0.76 [b] |
| VAFS | 5.4 (2.23) | 5.17 (2.23) | 0.96 [b] |
| REM sleep, % | 15.19 (12.1) | 22.5 (13.36) | 0.32 [b] |
| GDS | 6.2 (5.87) | 7.89 (7.31) | 0.66 [b] |
| Stroop 3 trial | 8.13 (6.64) | 6.18 (7.92) | 0.81 [b] |
| Walk and Turn, s | 11.47 (3.46) | 10.33 (3.16) | 0.66 [b] |
| Valine, mg/dL | 229.33 (51.78) | 245.64 (33.42) | 0.69 [b] |
| Tyrosine, mg/dL | 73.93 (14.77) | 64.93 (16.28) | 0.35 [b] |
| Tryptophan, mg/dL | 60.87 (11.39) | 53.5 (10.81) | 0.23 [b] |
| Serotonin, mg/dL | 89.56 (60.5) | 84.21 (68.17) | 0.99 [b] |
| Phenylalanine, mg/dL | 74.47 (12.59) | 73.07 (9.74) | 0.98 [b] |
| Leucine, mg/dL | 136.87 (38.75) | 143.07 (27.71) | 0.95 [b] |
| Isoleucine, mg/dL | 72.14 (24.2) | 73.36 (15) | 0.99 [b] |

Values presented are proportions and mean (SD). a—differences were tested by chi-squared test, b—differences in means was test by t-test. UPDRS III–Unified Parkinson's disease Rating Scale III, H&Y-Hoehn and Yahr Scale for Parkinson's Disease Staging. Levodopa dosage was determined as mg/day. * Medication information on two subjects in the niacin group was not available.

### 3.2. *Primary Outcome: UPDRS III*

#### 3.2.1. Six Months of 250 mg Niacin vs. Placebo

In intention-to-treat (ITT) analysis, there were no significant differences (Figure 2a,c,e,f). We then analyzed the data on a per-protocol (PP) basis (Figure 2b,d,f,h). The mean UPDRS III scores at baseline for placebo (22.4 ± 11.8) and niacin (21.3 ± 15.8) groups were comparable (Figure 2b and Supplementary Table S1). The mean changes in UPDRS III scores at six months for niacin (−1.06 [−3.68 to 1.57]) and placebo (−0.05 [−2.4 to 2.32]) groups were not significant (Table 2). No significant changes were noted in rigidity, bradykinesia, or resting tremor in either placebo or niacin-treated subjects. However, non-significant differences in the mean scores between baseline and six months were observed in both groups for these variables (Table 2). Average scores for rigidity non-significantly decreased in the placebo (0.14 [−0.14 to 0.42]) and niacin (0.03 [−0.26 to 0.31]) groups. The average score for resting tremor changed by 0.05 [−0.54 to 0.64] in the placebo group and −0.17 [−0.49 to 0.16] in the niacin-treated group. Mean scores for bradykinesia changed by 0.07 [−0.35 to 0.49] in the placebo group and by −0.39 [−1.42 to 0.65] in the niacin group (Table 2).

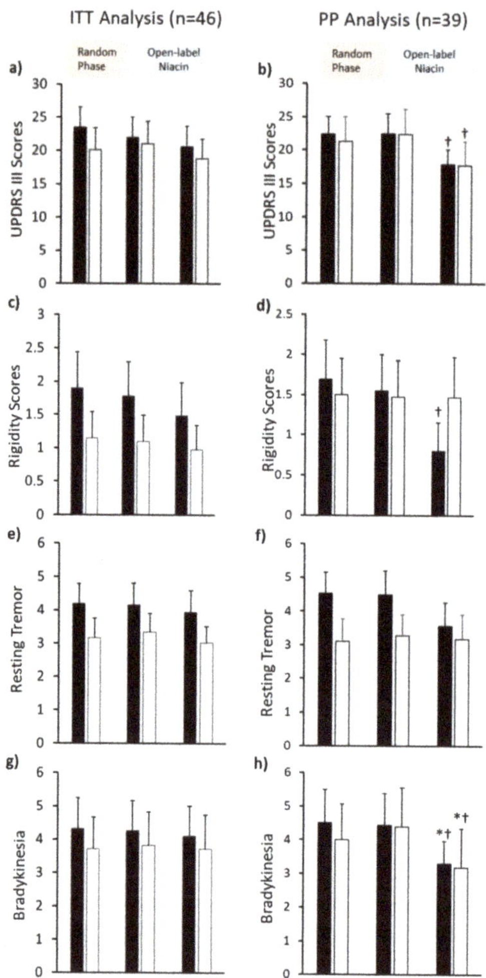


**Figure 2.** Mean Unified Parkinson's Disease Rating Scale III (UPDRS III) scores for two treatment groups analyzed per-protocol (right) and intention-to-treat with last observation carried forward (left). (**a**,**b**) Bar plot comparing changes in UPDRS III scores at baseline, after six months (6MO) of placebo (grey bars) or niacin (open bars), and after six months of niacin thereafter (12MO) (maximum points: 108). (**c**,**d**) Bar plot for rigidity scores (maximum points: 20), as a component of the UPDRS III scores, (**e**,**f**) Bar plot showing resting tremor scores (maximum points: 20), as a component of UPDRS III scores, and (**g**,**h**) Bar plot showing for bradykinesia scores (maximum points: 20), as a component of UPDRS III scores. * 12-month compared to baseline $p < 0.05$, † 12-month compared to 6-month $p < 0.05$. Values presented are mean ± SEM.

**Table 2.** Differences in motor and cognitive scores during the randomized trial period (baseline vs. 6MO).

| Clinical Variable, Units | Baseline Values, Mean ±SD | | 6-Month Change (Randomized, Placebo-Controlled Trial) | | |
|---|---|---|---|---|---|
| | Placebo Group | Niacin Group | Placebo Group Change | Niacin Group Change | Between Group Difference |
| UPDRS III Scores | 22.4 ± 11.8 | 21.3 ± 15.8 | −0.05 (−2.4–2.32) | −1.06 (−3.68–1.57) | 1.13 (−10.40–12.65) |
| Rigidity | 1.69 ± 2.23 | 1.5 ± 1.92 | 0.14 (−0.14–0.42) | 0.03 (−0.26–0.31) | 0.19 (−1.47–1.85) |
| Resting Tremor | 4.52 ± 2.87 | 3.11 ± 2.82 | 0.05 (−0.54–0.64) | −0.17 (−0.49–0.16) | 1.4 (−0.87–3.7) |
| Bradykinesia | 4.5 ± 4.6 | 4 ± 4.5 | 0.07 (−0.35–0.49) | −0.39 (−1.42–0.65) | 0.5 (−3.15–3.7) |
| Cognitive flexibility | 73.38 ± 57.11 | 79.42 ± 62.46 | −3.04 (−28.04–21.96) | 5.44 (−30.78–41.67) | −6.04 (−54.93–42.85) |
| Grip Strength, PSI | | | | | |
| First affected hand | 305.09 ± 105.26 | 297.04 ± 125.68 | 5.88 (−14.19–25.94) | −22.56 (−53.54–8.43) | 8.05 (−132.3–148.4) |
| Non (or later) affected hand | 300.43 ± 80.49 | 284.1 ± 123.09 | 3.73 (−35.11–42.56) | −31.67 (−63.74–0.39) | 16.33 (−110–142.7) |
| FSS | 36.65 ± 13.02 | 40.28 ± 11.99 | −0.06 (−2.5–2.37) | 1.78 (−5.5–9.05) | −3.63 (−13.79–6.53) |
| VAFS | 5.4 ± 2.23 | 5.17 ± 2.23 | −0.22 (−0.97–0.53) | −0.44 (−1.74–0.85) | 0.23 (−1.58–2.05) |
| REM sleep, % | 15.19 ± 12.1 | 22.5 ± 13.36 | −6.26 (−11.05–1.47) * | 1.39 (−5.42–8.2) | −7.31 (−17.62–3.0) |
| GDS | 6.2 ± 5.87 | 7.89 ± 7.31 | 0.25 (−0.53–1.03) | 1.17 (−1.75–4.08) | −1.69 (−7.14–3.76) |
| Stroop 3 trial | 8.13 ± 6.64 | 6.18 ± 7.92 | −0.59 (−3.17–1.99) | −2.19 (−5.93–1.54) | 1.96 (−4.16–8.08) |
| Walk and Turn, s | 11.47 ± 3.46 | 10.33 ± 3.16 | 0.44 (−1.08–1.96) | 0.18 (−0.61–0.96) | 1.14 (−1.61–3.88) |
| Valine, mg/dL | 229.33 ± 51.78 | 245.64 ± 33.42 | 1.83 (−27.05–30.72) | −0.71 (−35.17–33.74) | −16.31 (−57.55–24.93) |
| Tyrosine, mg/dL | 73.93 ± 14.77 | 64.93 ± 16.28 | 8.82 (−2.2–19.84) | −0.5 (−10.82–9.82) | 9.01 (−5.75–23.76) |
| Tryptophan, mg/dL | 60.87 ± 11.39 | 53.5 ± 10.81 | 7.48 (−0.39–15.34) | −0.07 (−6.1–5.96) | 7.37 (−3.13–17.86) |
| Serotonin, mg/dL | 89.56 ± 60.5 | 84.21 ± 68.17 | 25.34 (5.79–44.89) * | 1.21 (−17.82–20.25) | 5.35 (−55.03–65.72) |
| Phenylalanine, mg/dL | 74.47 ± 12.59 | 73.07 ± 9.74 | 3.74 (−8.48–15.97) | −1.64 (−8.62–5.33) | 1.40 (−9.23–12.02) |
| Leucine, mg/dL | 136.87 ± 38.75 | 143.07 ± 27.71 | 9.26 (−15.26–33.77) | −4.64 (−28.45–19.16) | −6.21 (−38.02–25.61) |
| Isoleucine, mg/dL | 72.14 ± 24.2 | 73.36 ± 15 | 4.03 (−14.21–22.26) | −4.79 (−19.34–9.77) | −1.21 (−20.89–18.47) |

All of the study personnel and patients were blinded to the group assignment. The treatment group assignment code was disclosed at the completion of the study in April 2020. VAFS: Visual analog severity scale, GDS: Geriatric depression scale, FSS: fatigue severity scale. Values presented are Mean ± SD or Mean (95% CI). * $p < 0.05$.

### 3.2.2. Six to Twelve Months of 250 mg Niacin

At the twelve-month visit, the mean UPDRS III scores significantly decreased by 4.58 [0.85 to 8.30] points in placebo compared to the six-month visit (Table 3). In the niacin group, the mean UPDRS III scores significantly decreased by 4.63 [1.42 to 7.83] points (Table 3). Bradykinesia scores were reduced in the placebo (1.13 [0.25 to 2.02]) and niacin (1.21 [0.36 to 2.06]) groups at the twelve-month visit compared to the six-month visit (Table 3). At the twelve-month visit, rigidity scores significantly decreased in the placebo group (0.75 [−0.01 to 1.51], $p = 0.05$), while no changes were observed in the niacin group (0.008 [−0.47 to 0.49]. No significant changes were observed in resting tremor scores for placebo (0.92 [−0.12 to 1.96]) or niacin (0.1 [−0.56 to 0.76]) groups.

**Table 3.** Comparative differences in motor and cognitive scores during the open-label trial.

| Clinical Variable, Units | 6-Month Values (Mean ±SD) | | 6–12 Month Change (Open-Label Niacin Treatment) | | |
|---|---|---|---|---|---|
| | Placebo Group | Niacin Group | Placebo Group Change | Niacin Group Change | Between Group Difference |
| UPDRS III Scores | 22.4 ± 14 | 22.3 ± 16.4 | 4.58 (0.85–8.30) * | 4.63 (1.42–7.83) * | 0.12 (−12.29–12.53) |
| Rigidity | 1.5 ± 2.1 | 1.5 ± 1.9 | 0.75 (−0.01–1.51) * | 0.008 (−0.47–0.49) | 0.08 (−1.522–1.673) |
| Resting Tremor | 4.5 ± 3.3 | 3.3 ± 2.7 | 0.92 (−0.12–1.96) | 0.1 (−0.56–0.76) | 1.20 (−1.17–3.57) |
| Bradykinesia | 4.4 ± 4.4 | 4.4 ± 4.9 | 1.13 (0.25–2.02) * | 1.21 (0.36–2.06) * | 0.04 (−3.74–3.82) |
| Cognitive flexibility | 76.4 ± 63.1 | 74 ± 54.7 | −15.18 (−40.6–10.24) | 4.9 (−27.8–37.6) | 2.44 (−47.02–51.91) |
| Grip Strength, Newtons | | | | | |
| First affected hand | 299.2 ± 107.5 | 319.6 ± 118.2 | −23.58 (−79.14–31.98) | −80.3 (−176.2–15.65) | −20.38 (−167.4–126.7) |
| Non (or later) affected hand | 296.7 ± 89.4 | 315.8 ± 119.4 | −11.84 (−56.59–32.92) | −54.72 (−128.8–19.38) | −19.07 (−152.8–114.7) |
| FSS | 36.7 ± 14.2 | 38.5 ± 11 | 2.89 (−1.62–7.4) | 4.36 (1.59–7.13) * | −1.79 (−11.91–8.34) |
| VAFS | 5.6 + 2.5 | 5.6 ± 2.2 | −0.76 (−1.75–0.24) | −0.39 (−0.92–0.14) | 0.008 (−1.88–1.89) |
| REM sleep, % | 6 ± 5.9 | 6.7 ± 5.9 | 1.92 (−7.2–11.03) | −4.32 (−10.32–1.68) | 0.34 (−11.09–11.77) |
| GDS | 21.5 ±16.3 | 21.1 ± 11.6 | 1.08 (−1.12–3.28) | 1.37 (−0.5–3.23) | −0.77 (−5.53–3.99) |
| Stroop 3 trial average | 8.7 ± 6.9 | 8.4 ± 5.6 | −0.78 (−5.47–3.91) | −0.78 (−2.85–1.28) | 0.35 (−4.9–5.61) |
| Walk and Turn, s | 11 ± 3.2 | 10.2 ± 3.4 | 0.75 (−0.53–2.02) | 1.72 (0.59–2.84) * | 0.87 (−1.95–3.69) |
| Valine, mg/dL | 227.5 ± 45 | 246.4 ± 29.7 | 4.29 (−32.51–41.08) | 21.07 (−16.01–58.15) | −18.86 (−52.4–14.69) |
| Tyrosine, mg/dL | 65.1 ± 15.5 | 65.4 ± 14.4 | 1.83 (−11.66–15.31) | 4.57 (−5.33–14.47) | −0.32 (−13.74–13.11) |
| Tryptophan, mg/dL | 53.4 ± 11.6 | 53.6 ± 10.9 | −4.11 (−12.97–4.75) | 4.29 (−4.75–13.32) | −0.18 (−10.28–9.92) |
| Serotonin, mg/dL | 64.2 ± 44.5 | 83 ± 75.2 | −18.11 (−37.97–1.75) | −13.36 (−58.77–32.06) | −18.78 (−77.83–40.27) |
| Phenylalanine, mg/dL | 70.7 ± 20.6 | 74.7 ± 9.8 | −0.85 (−12–10.3) | 2.43 (−9.35–14.21) | −3.99 (−18.11–10.12) |
| Leucine, mg/dL | 127.6 ± 32.5 | 147.7 ± 21.7 | −1.75 (−29.99–26.5) | 14.86 (−9.31–39.02) | −20.1 (−44.43–4.23) |
| Isoleucine, mg/dL | 68.1 ± 20.4 | 78.1 ± 15.2 | 1.26 (−14.45–16.97) | 8.64 (−4.48–21.77) | −10.03 (−26.28–6.230) |

Six to 12 months, all the participants were given 250 mg niacin once a day. All the study personnel and patients were blinded to the group assignment. Treatment group assignment code was disclosed at the completion of the study in April 2020. Values are presented as Mean ± SD or Mean (95% CI). * $p < 0.05$.

3.2.3. Baseline to Twelve Months

Compared to baseline, a trend towards reduction in the mean UPDRS III scores was observed in the placebo (4.52 [−0.16 to 9.21]) and niacin (3.57 [−1.02 to 8.16]) groups (Table 4). At twelve months, scores for rigidity (0.90 [−0.05 to 1.84]) and resting tremor (0.97 [−0.16 to 2.09]) showed slight, non-significant decreases in the placebo group. Compared to baseline, bradykinesia scores at twelve months significantly decreased in the placebo (1.21 [0.19 to 2.23]) and niacin (0.82 [−0.004 to 1.65]) groups (Table 4).

A significant decrease occurred across both groups over a treatment period of one year ($p$ = 0.012), but no significant differences were found between treatments at any time point (Figure 2d and Table 4).

**Table 4.** Differences in motor and cognitive scores between baseline and 12-month visit.

| Clinical Variable, Units | 12-Month Values (Mean ±SD) Placebo Group | Niacin Group | 12- Month Change Placebo Group Change | Niacin Group Change | Between Group Difference |
|---|---|---|---|---|---|
| UPDRS III Scores | 17.9 ± 9.2 | 17.7 ± 13.3 | 4.52 (−0.16–9.21) | 3.57 (−1.019–8.16) | 0.17 (−10.66–11.01) |
| Rigidity | 0.8 ± 1.5 | 1.5 ± 1.9 | 0.90 (−0.05–1.84) | 0.04 (−0.43–0.5) | −0.67 (−2.25–0.91) |
| Resting Tremor | 3.6 ± 2.9 | 3.2 ± 2.7 | 0.97 (−0.16–2.09) | −0.07 (−0.94–0.81) | 0.38 (−2.18–2.94) |
| Bradykinesia | 3.3 ± 2.8 | 3.2 ± 4.3 | 1.21 (0.19–2.23) * | 0.82 (−0.004–1.65) * | 0.12 (−3.34–3.57) |
| Cognitive flexibility | 91.6 ± 72 | 69.1 ± 55.5 | 18.22 (−42.79–6.35) | 10.35 (−17.7–38.39) | 22.52 (−36.72–81.77) |
| Grip Strength, Newtons | | | | | |
| First affected hand | 322.8 ± 91.7 | 399.9 ± 54.1 | −17.71 (−62.17–26.75) | −102.9 (−218.8–13.14) | −77.1 (−186.4–32.22) |
| Non (or later) affected hand | 308.5 ± 84.6 | 370.5 ± 75.3 | −8.12 (−56.34–40.13) | −86.4 (−187.8–15.05) | −61.96 (−181.5–57.59) |
| FSS | 33.8 ± 13.6 | 34.1 ± 12 | 2.83 (−2.15–7.81) | 6.14 (−1.59–13.86) | −0.32 (−12–11.37) |
| VAFS | 6.4 ± 2.2 | 6 ± 2.5 | −0.98 (−2.2–0.25) | −0.83 (−2.16–0.49) | 0.38 (−1.84–2.59) |
| REM sleep, % | 4.9 ± 4.9 | 5.4 ± 5.3 | −4.34 (−11.45–2.76) | −2.93 (−11.11–5.26) | −5.9 (−20.57–8.78) |
| GDS | 19.5 ± 16.8 | 25.4 ± 14.1 | 1.33 (−1.01–3.66) | 2.53 (−1.56–6.62) | −0.48 (−5.24–4.28) |
| Stroop 3 trial average | 9.5 ± 7.5 | 9.2 ± 6.3 | −1.37 (−5.41–2.67) | −2.98 (−7.73–1.78) | 0.35 (−6.45–7.14) |
| Walk and Turn, s | 10.3 ± 2.8 | 8.4 ± 1.7 | 1.19 (−0.38–2.76) | 1.89 (0.55–3.23) * | 1.84 (−0.39–4.07) |
| Valine, mg/dL | 223.2 ± 37.7 | 225.3 ± 37.9 | 6.12 (−29.16–41.4) | 20.36 (−17.62–58.33) | −2.07 (−38.5–34.35) |
| Tyrosine, mg/dL | 63.3 ± 12.1 | 60.9 ± 9.2 | 10.65 (1.19–20.1) * | 4.07 (−8.28–16.42) | 2.43 (−7.98–12.84) |
| Tryptophan, mg/dL | 57.5 ± 9.3 | 49.3 ± 10.8 | 3.37 (−5.21–11.94) | 4.21 (−3.69–12.12) | 8.21 (−1.54–17.97) |
| Serotonin, mg/dL | 82.3 ± 31.6 | 96.4 ± 56.3 | 7.23 (−24.06–38.51) | −12.14 (−49.59–25.31) | −14.02 (−58.56–30.51) |
| Phenylalanine, mg/dL | 71.6 ± 11 | 72.3 ± 13.5 | 2.9 (−6.82–12.61) | 0.79 (−10.03–11.6) | −0.71 (−12.62–11.19) |
| Leucine, mg/dL | 129.4 ± 24.6 | 132.9 ± 28.9 | 7.51 (−18.63–33.65) | 10.21 (−21.1–41.53) | −3.5 (−29.45–22.45) |
| Isoleucine, mg/dL | 66.9 ± 11.2 | 69.5 ± 16 | 5.29 (−8.82–19.39) | 3.86 (−10.4–18.12) | −2.64 (−16.11–10.82) |

The study personnel were blinded to the group assignment; the randomization code was revealed at the completion of the study. Values presented are Mean ± SD or Mean (95% CI). * $p < 0.05$.

### 3.3. *Correlation with on/off Phenomenon with UPDRS III Scores*

The placebo group showed a positive correlation ($p$ = 0.031) between UPDRS III scores and the time since their most recent dose of PD medication (on/off phenomenon) (Figure 3a). Subjects in the niacin group showed a negative correlation (r = −0.15), suggesting that the on/off phenomenon has no effect on UPDRS III scores in patients taking niacin (Figure 3b).

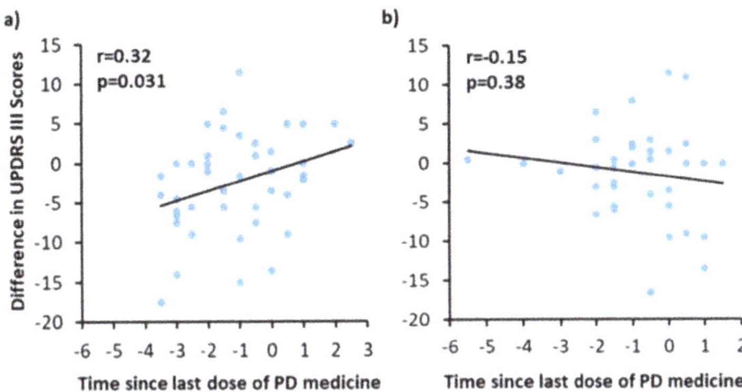


**Figure 3.** Correlation between time since last medication ($x$-axis) versus Unified Parkinson's Disease Rating Scale III (UPDRS III) scores ($y$-axis) for the (**a**) placebo and (**b**) niacin groups. The UPDRS III scores and the change in the time between the last dose of medication and the appointment were used to calculate the difference between visits; this data was used to construct dot plots and run a correlation analysis.

*3.4. Secondary Outcomes*

Grip strength, a measure of motor function and muscle energetics, showed a trending increase in the niacin group for each hand (22.56 [−53.54 to 8.43]); (31.67 [−63.74 to 0.39] PSI). However, those who took the placebo showed no change in either hand (5.88 [−14.19 to 25.94] PSI); (3.73 [−35.11 to 42.56] PSI) (Table 2). The difference between TMT-B and TMT-A is a measurement of cognitive flexibility while removing the factors of motor and visuoperceptual deficits. The change in cognitive flexibility between all the comparisons was not significant. Mean differences between the placebo and niacin groups changed from −6.04 to 22.52 over the study period (Table 2). Blood serotonin levels significantly decreased in placebo by 25.34 mg/dL [95% CI, 5.79 to 44.89] while staying relatively stable between baseline and six months of niacin supplementation (Table 2).

Rapid eye movement (REM) sleep changed significantly by 6.26% [−11.05 to −1.47] with placebo, but not with niacin (1.39% [−5.42 to 8.2]). FSS scores at twelve months decreased by 4.36 [1.59 to 7.13] points in the niacin-treated group (Table 3). No significant differences were observed for VAFS, GDS, or Stroop test (Table 2). Serum levels of amino acids valine, tyrosine, tryptophan, phenylalanine, leucine, and isoleucine were also not different between the treatment groups. Sleep efficiency or percentage of light sleep, deep sleep, or awake time did not significantly differ during the study (Table 2).

*3.5. Adverse Events*

Adverse events were similar between the niacin and placebo groups. Out of 47 recruited patients, eight patients dropped out during the first six months, and eight more dropped out before the one-year time point. The flushing effect of niacin occurred and caused discontinuation for two patients, one in each group. Unrelated injuries occurred in one patient in the niacin group and one in the placebo group, although neither resulted in the discontinuation of the study. One patient complained of leg cramps at the end of the study, but it was likely dehydration rather than supplement intake, assessed by the neurologist. No other adverse events were reported. Seven patients could not complete the study due to the SARS-CoV-2 shut-down.

## 4. Discussion

In this single-center, double-blind, placebo-controlled, randomized clinical trial comprising patients with early- and late-stage PD, supplementation of a single daily dose of niacin for twelve months improved the rigidity, bradykinesia, and overall UPDRS III scores. In a serendipitous finding, a high-dose niacin supplement was observed to reduce bradykinesia and rigidity in a PD case report [18]. Niacin supplements and agonists of the niacin receptor are shown to be neuroprotective and lead to enhanced motor function in animal models of PD (BHB, niacinamide, PINK1 fruit fly study) [19–21]. The current study demonstrated a significant decrease in UPDRS III scores from six to twelve months, in which both groups took the open-label niacin supplement. Both groups, when comparing baseline to one year, demonstrated a trend towards reduction in UPDRS III scores. There was a significant decrease in bradykinesia between baseline and twelve months and between six months and twelve months in both placebo and niacin-treated groups. A significant decrease in rigidity was observed in the placebo-treated group from six months to one year when they received niacin. Although the overall tremor score did not show any significance in the niacin-treated group, individual limb tremor scores decreased in the niacin-treated group. The placebo group showed a reduction in tremor scores from six months to twelve months after receiving niacin. Since some of the scores began higher (although insignificant) in the placebo group than niacin, such as with resting tremor, then there is more room for improvement; this may have contributed to the significant changes with only six months of niacin during the open-label portion for the placebo group opposed to the niacin group in the first six months. Taken together, small changes in these sub-scores reflect a decrease in UPDRS III scores at twelve months.

Numerous studies have attempted either raising NAD levels or directly providing NAD in PD. Niacin remains a natural source for NAD and binds to the niacin receptor, G protein-coupled receptor 109A (GPR109A), unlike other forms of vitamin B3. GPR109A is predominantly expressed in adipose tissue and immune cells, including macrophages [22]. We have previously shown that RAW264.7 macrophage cells stimulated with lipopolysaccharide express increased levels of GPR109A, and treatment with niacin reduces these levels [23]. Previously, niacin has been shown to have anti-inflammatory effects on activated macrophages in cardiovascular disease [24]. Animal and human evidence suggests that inflammation and activation of microglia in the brain are associated with the development and progression of PD [13,25,26]. Microglial cells in the brain are a modified form of macrophages that reside in the brain; we theorize that niacin supplement provides the anti-inflammatory response to these microglial cells to reduce the neuroinflammation in PD patients.

Figure 3 partially explains the effect of decreased UPDRS III scores in the placebo group during the first six months. Since Sinemet's effects are only motor, this correlation likely does not affect data involving the non-motor abilities of the subjects enrolled in the clinical trial.

We have previously shown that niacin and NAD levels in PD patients are decreased compared to age-matched controls. Fatigue, depression, strength, sleep, and quality of life indicators may be affected by the reduction in niacin levels. In this study, six months or one year of niacin reduced typical PD motor symptoms and fatigue and stabilized serotonin levels and REM sleep percentage. These effects are highly beneficial for the PD patient's quality of life. Many PD patients complain of both depression and fatigue. This study showed a halting or slowing of the drop in serotonin levels by niacin, which could potentially reduce depression or improve mood. Additionally, fatigue is likely enhanced by increasing NAD, which is low in aging populations and even lower in PD. Grip strength, although not significant, showed a trend of increasing strength bilaterally in the niacin group, but not with placebo over six months of treatment. Grip strength is well-known to correlate with longevity, so this could be a predictor of increased life expectancy by taking niacin [27]. Almost all reported secondary measures demonstrated a trend towards improvement over one year.

Most notably, serotonin levels, fatigue, and grip strength stood out in our study. Serotonin levels were significantly lowered in the placebo-treated group but not in the niacin-treated group after the first six months. The FSS scores were markedly better in the niacin-treated group but not the placebo group from six to twelve months. Both of these findings may explain the reporting of an uplift in mood reported by PD subjects who received niacin for one year.

To our knowledge, this is the first trial where niacin (a form of vitamin B3) is tested at a low dose for PD in a randomized, placebo-controlled, double-blind, prospective trial. A 250 mg daily dose of niacin produced negligible flushing symptoms when consumed after meals as instructed. Our previous preliminary studies helped us decide the low dose for niacin [12,13]. Different low-dose regimens, longer duration of intervention, multicenter trials, and inclusion of niacinamide would be pertinent future investigations.

### *4.1. Study Strengths*

The commonly used therapies for PD subjects do not currently include niacin. It is a novel approach utilizing an over-the-counter vitamin supplement at a low dose in PD. A placebo control was used for the first six months, and codes were not broken until patients completed the twelve-month study. The flushing effect of niacin was negligible and did not deter the PD patients from the study. The PD patients and caregivers were very enthusiastic after the six-month open-label niacin supplementation. Dropout rates were low. A single rater captured the motor outcome scores for all of the subjects, which extended higher confidence in the reliability of the outcomes. Since PD is a slow, progressive disease, and thus, six months may not be enough to detect all meaningful changes in symptoms and may require longer durations, such as twelve months or longer interventions (9).

### *4.2. Study Limitations*

The sample size is small. We did not titrate the dosages of niacin. The clinical trial recruited patients primarily through the Charlie Norwood VA Medical Center. Due to veterans and PD patients being predominantly men, we could only recruit seven women (four were included in the analysis). Therefore, the potential gender bias was not adequately addressed. In addition, the sample population was primarily Caucasian (three African American subjects).

Many outcome scores within the trial were self-reported surveys, including the FSS, VAFS, and GDS, although the groups were not found to be different at baseline. Furthermore, one year of niacin supplementation may be necessary to find significant differences from placebo; thus, a more extended placebo-controlled study should be performed in the future.

## 5. Conclusions

The findings presented here show that treatment with low-dose daily niacin supplementation compared to placebo resulted in significantly improved motor function outcomes. We have already demonstrated that niacin acts by polarizing the activated microglial cells in the brain and reducing GPR109A expression in white blood cells, thus reducing neuroinflammation. Our findings support the use of low-dose niacin supplementation in PD as an adjunct therapy that can reduce neuroinflammation and improve motor functions in PD patients.

**Supplementary Materials:** The following are available online at https://www.mdpi.com/article/10.3390/biomedicines9121881/s1, Table S1: Mean values for clinical variables measured for the two treatment groups at the baseline, Table S2: Comparative differences in motor and cognitive scores during randomized period (baseline vs 6months), open label trial (6 vs 12months) and baseline to study end (baseline vs 12 months).

**Author Contributions:** Conceptualization, C.W.; methodology, C.W., S.P., B.G., R.C., J.C.M. and M.S.: formal analysis, C.W., S.P. and M.S.; resources, C.W.; data curation, S.P. and M.S.; writing—original draft preparation, S.P.; writing—review and editing, S.P., M.S., R.C., B.G., J.C.M. and C.W.; visualization, S.P., M.S. and C.W.; supervision, C.W.; project administration, C.W.; funding acquisition, C.W. All authors have read and agreed to the published version of the manuscript.

**Funding:** The work was supported by Merit Review Award I01RX001613 issued by the Department of Veterans Affairs, Rehabilitation Research and Development to C.W., R.C., and J.C.M. The funder has no role in study design and conception, data acquisition and analysis, or interpretation of the data.

**Institutional Review Board Statement:** The study was conducted according to the guidelines of the Declaration of Helsinki and approved by the Institutional Review Board (or Ethics Committee) of Augusta University (protocol code 750415-33 and 27 August 2015).

**Informed Consent Statement:** Informed consent was obtained from all subjects involved in the study.

**Data Availability Statement:** Upon reasonable request, de-identified individual participant data will be available beginning 9 months and ending 36 months following the publication of this article.

**Conflicts of Interest:** The authors declare no conflict of interest. The funders had no role in the study's design, in the collection, analyses, or interpretation of data, in the writing of the manuscript, or in the decision to publish the results.

## References


1. Dorsey, E.R.; Elbaz, A.; Nichols, E.; Abbasi, N.; Abd-Allah, F.; Abdelalim, A.; Adsuar, J.C.; Ansha, M.G.; Brayne, C.; Choi, J.Y.J.; et al. Global, regional, and national burden of Parkinson's disease, 1990–2016: A systematic analysis for the Global Burden of Disease Study 2016. *Lancet Neurol.* **2018**, *17*, 939–953. [CrossRef]
2. Schrag, A.; Quinn, N. Dyskinesias and motor fluctuations in Parkinson's disease. A community-based study. *Brain* **2000**, *123*, 2297–2305. [CrossRef] [PubMed]
3. Rocha, E.M.; De Miranda, B.; Sanders, L.H. Alpha-synuclein: Pathology, mitochondrial dysfunction and neuroinflammation in Parkinson's disease. *Neurobiol. Dis.* **2018**, *109*, 249–257. [CrossRef] [PubMed]
4. Chen, C.; Turnbull, D.M.; Reeve, A.K. Mitochondrial Dysfunction in Parkinson's Disease-Cause or Consequence? *Biology* **2019**, *8*, 38. [CrossRef]
5. Giri, B.; Belanger, K.; Seamon, M.; Bradley, E.; Purohit, S.; Chong, R.; Morgan, J.C.; Baban, B.; Wakade, C. Niacin Ameliorates Neuro-Inflammation in Parkinson's Disease via GPR109A. *Int. J. Mol. Sci* **2019**, *20*, 4559. [CrossRef] [PubMed]
6. Hellenbrand, W.; Boeing, H.; Robra, B.P.; Seidler, A.; Vieregge, P.; Nischan, P.; Joerg, J.; Oertel, W.H.; Schneider, E.; Ulm, G. Diet and Parkinson's disease. II: A possible role for the past intake of specific nutrients. Results from a self-administered food-frequency questionnaire in a case-control study. *Neurology* **1996**, *47*, 644–650. [CrossRef] [PubMed]
7. Barone, P.; Antonini, A.; Colosimo, C.; Marconi, R.; Morgante, L.; Avarello, T.P.; Bottacchi, E.; Cannas, A.; Ceravolo, G.; Ceravolo, R.; et al. The PRIAMO study: A multicenter assessment of nonmotor symptoms and their impact on quality of life in Parkinson's disease. *Mov. Disord.* **2009**, *24*, 1641–1649. [CrossRef]
8. Kalia, L.V.; Lang, A.E. Parkinson's disease. *Lancet* **2015**, *386*, 896–912. [CrossRef]
9. Chong, R.; Albor, L.; Wakade, C.; Morgan, J. The dimensionality of fatigue in Parkinson's disease. *J. Transl. Med.* **2018**, *16*, 192. [CrossRef] [PubMed]
10. Schaeffer, E.; Vaterrodt, T.; Zaunbrecher, L.; Liepelt-Scarfone, I.; Emmert, K.; Roeben, B.; Elshehabi, M.; Hansen, C.; Becker, S.; Nussbaum, S.; et al. Effects of Levodopa on quality of sleep and nocturnal movements in Parkinson's Disease. *J. Neurol.* **2021**, *268*, 2506–2514. [CrossRef]
11. Bender, D.A.; Earl, C.J.; Lees, A.J. Niacin depletion in Parkinsonian patients treated with L-dopa, benserazide and carbidopa. *Clin. Sci.* **1979**, *56*, 89–93. [CrossRef] [PubMed]
12. Chong, R.; Wakade, C.; Seamon, M.; Giri, B.; Morgan, J.C.; Purohit, S. Niacin Enhancement for Parkinson's Disease: An Effectiveness Trial. *Front. Aging Neurosci.* **2021**, *13*. [CrossRef] [PubMed]
13. Wakade, C.; Chong, R.; Bradley, E.; Morgan, J.C. Low-dose niacin supplementation modulates GPR109A, niacin index and ameliorates Parkinson's disease symptoms without side effects. *Clin. Case Rep.* **2015**, *3*, 635–637. [CrossRef] [PubMed]
14. Hughes, A.J.; Daniel, S.E.; Kilford, L.; Lees, A.J. Accuracy of clinical diagnosis of idiopathic Parkinson's disease: A clinico-pathological study of 100 cases. *J. Neurol. Neurosurg. Psychiatry* **1992**, *55*, 181–184. [CrossRef] [PubMed]
15. Evans, J.R.; Mason, S.L.; Williams-Gray, C.H.; Foltynie, T.; Brayne, C.; Robbins, T.W.; Barker, R.A. The natural history of treated Parkinson's disease in an incident, community based cohort. *J. Neurol. Neurosurg. Psychiatry* **2011**, *82*, 1112–1118. [CrossRef] [PubMed]
16. Poewe, W. The natural history of Parkinson's disease. *J. Neurol.* **2006**, *253*, VII2-6. [CrossRef]
17. Kortte, K.B.; Horner, M.D.; Windham, W.K. The trail making test, part B: Cognitive flexibility or ability to maintain set? *Appl. Neuropsychol.* **2002**, *9*, 106–109. [CrossRef] [PubMed]
18. Alisky, J.M. Niacin improved rigidity and bradykinesia in a Parkinson's disease patient but also caused unacceptable nightmares and skin rash—A case report. *Nutr. Neurosci.* **2005**, *8*, 327–329. [CrossRef]
19. Schöndorf, D.C.; Ivanyuk, D.; Baden, P.; Sanchez-Martinez, A.; De Cicco, S.; Yu, C.; Giunta, I.; Schwarz, L.K.; Di Napoli, G.; Panagiotakopoulou, V.; et al. The NAD+ Precursor Nicotinamide Riboside Rescues Mitochondrial Defects and Neuronal Loss in iPSC and Fly Models of Parkinson's Disease. *Cell Rep.* **2018**, *23*, 2976–2988. [CrossRef]

20. Anderson, D.W.; Bradbury, K.A.; Schneider, J.S. Broad neuroprotective profile of nicotinamide in different mouse models of MPTP-induced parkinsonism. *Eur. J. Neurosci.* **2008**, *28*, 610–617. [CrossRef]
21. Jia, H.; Li, X.; Gao, H.; Feng, Z.; Li, X.; Zhao, L.; Jia, X.; Zhang, H.; Liu, J. High doses of nicotinamide prevent oxidative mitochondrial dysfunction in a cellular model and improve motor deficit in a Drosophila model of Parkinson's disease. *J. Neurosci. Res.* **2008**, *86*, 2083–2090. [CrossRef] [PubMed]
22. Wise, A.; Foord, S.M.; Fraser, N.J.; Barnes, A.A.; Elshourbagy, N.; Eilert, M.; Ignar, D.M.; Murdock, P.R.; Steplewski, K.; Green, A.; et al. Molecular identification of high and low affinity receptors for nicotinic acid. *J. Biol. Chem.* **2003**, *278*, 9869–9874. [CrossRef] [PubMed]
23. Wakade, C.; Giri, B.; Malik, A.; Khodadadi, H.; Morgan, J.C.; Chong, R.K.; Baban, B. Niacin modulates macrophage polarization in Parkinson's disease. *J. Neuroimmunol.* **2018**, *320*, 76–79. [CrossRef] [PubMed]
24. Chai, J.T.; Digby, J.E.; Ruparelia, N.; Jefferson, A.; Handa, A.; Choudhury, R.P. Nicotinic Acid Receptor GPR109A Is Down-Regulated in Human Macrophage-Derived Foam Cells. *PLoS ONE* **2013**, *8*, e62934. [CrossRef]
25. Gyoneva, S.; Shapiro, L.; Lazo, C.; Garnier-Amblard, E.; Smith, Y.; Miller, G.W.; Traynelis, S.F. Adenosine A2A receptor antagonism reverses inflammation-induced impairment of microglial process extension in a model of Parkinson's disease. *Neurobiol. Dis.* **2014**, *67*, 191–202. [CrossRef]
26. Hirsch, E.C.; Hunot, S.; Damier, P.; Faucheux, B. Glial cells and inflammation in Parkinson's disease: A role in neurodegeneration? *Ann. Neurol.* **1998**, *44*, S115–S120. [CrossRef] [PubMed]
27. Bohannon, R.W. Grip Strength: An Indispensable Biomarker For Older Adults. *Clin. Interv. Aging* **2019**, *14*, 1681–1691. [CrossRef] [PubMed]

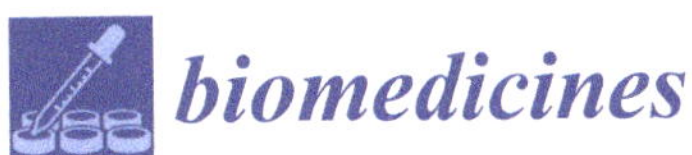

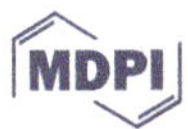

Review

# Movement Disorders in Oncology: From Clinical Features to Biomarkers

**Luca Marsili [1], Alberto Vogrig [2] and Carlo Colosimo [3,*]**

1 Gardner Family Center for Parkinson's Disease and Movement Disorders, Department of Neurology, University of Cincinnati, Cincinnati, OH 45219, USA; luca.marsili@ucmail.uc.edu
2 Clinical Neurology, Santa Maria della Misericordia University Hospital, Azienda Ospedaliero Universitaria Friuli Centrale, 33100 Udine, Italy; alberto.vogrig@gmail.com
3 Department of Neurology, Santa Maria University Hospital, 05100 Terni, Italy
* Correspondence: c.colosimo@aospterni.it; Tel.: +39-0744-205621

**Abstract:** Background: the study of movement disorders associated with oncological diseases and anticancer treatments highlights the wide range of differential diagnoses that need to be considered. In this context, the role of immune-mediated conditions is increasingly recognized and relevant, as they represent treatable disorders. Methods: we reappraise the phenomenology, pathophysiology, diagnostic testing, and treatment of movement disorders observed in the context of brain tumors, paraneoplastic conditions, and cancer immunotherapy, such as immune-checkpoint inhibitors (ICIs). Results: movement disorders secondary to brain tumors are rare and may manifest with both hyper-/hypokinetic conditions. Paraneoplastic movement disorders are caused by antineuronal antibodies targeting intracellular or neuronal surface antigens, with variable prognosis and response to treatment. ICIs promote antitumor response by the inhibition of the immune checkpoints. They are effective treatments for several malignancies, but they may cause movement disorders through an unchecked immune response. Conclusions: movement disorders due to focal neoplastic brain lesions are rare but should not be missed. Paraneoplastic movement disorders are even rarer, and their clinical-laboratory findings require focused expertise. In addition to their desired effects in cancer treatment, ICIs can induce specific neurological adverse events, sometimes manifesting with movement disorders, which often require a case-by-case, multidisciplinary, approach.

**Keywords:** movement disorders; paraneoplastic; oncology; immune-checkpoint inhibitors; autoimmune

**Citation:** Marsili, L.; Vogrig, A.; Colosimo, C. Movement Disorders in Oncology: From Clinical Features to Biomarkers. *Biomedicines* **2022**, *10*, 26. https://doi.org/10.3390/biomedicines10010026

Academic Editor: Arnab Ghosh

Received: 24 November 2021
Accepted: 18 December 2021
Published: 23 December 2021

**Publisher's Note:** MDPI stays neutral with regard to jurisdictional claims in published maps and institutional affiliations.



## 1. Introduction

The study of movement disorders occurring in the context of oncological diseases highlights the wide spectrum of differential diagnoses that need to be considered, including direct (structural or compressive) etiologies and indirect (immune-mediated or treatment-related) complications. On a mechanistic standpoint, it also sheds light on the potential role of the immune system in conditions—such as paraneoplastic neurological syndromes (PNS)—which can sometimes present similarly to neurodegenerative diseases. The link between cancer and neurodegeneration is intriguing as they represent two apparently opposite phenomena: dysregulated cell proliferation and cell death, respectively, that may be linked in some specific conditions and may be influenced by genetic, environmental, and immune system-related factors [1–3].

Movement disorders as focal manifestations of primitive and secondary brain tumors are rare [4]. Brain tumors, particularly those affecting the basal ganglia or brainstem, may often cause variegated movement disorders. There are no robust epidemiological data, but a survey of published cases shows that hyperkinetic disorders are more common than parkinsonism (60% versus 40% of cases, respectively) [4]. Paraneoplastic movement disorders are conditions associated with antineuronal antibodies targeting intracellular or neuronal surface antigens, with different prognoses and treatment response. Immune-checkpoint inhibitors (ICIs) are drugs promoting antitumor immune response by the inhibition of the immune checkpoints [5]. They are effective treatments for several tumors, but they may cause immune-mediated movement disorders as side effects.

In the present review, we critically reappraise the phenomenology, pathophysiology, diagnostic strategies, and treatment of movement disorders associated with malignancies of the brain, with paraneoplastic conditions, and finally with the intriguing new field of cancer immunotherapy such as immune-checkpoint inhibitors (ICIs).

## 2. Movement Disorders in the Context of Brain Malignancies

Movement disorders as focal manifestations of brain tumors are rare conditions and may manifest as hyperkinetic more than hypokinetic disorders [4]. Here, we will briefly summarize the main movement disorders found in association with brain tumors.

*Hemichorea-hemiballism* is a rare movement disorder characterized by high amplitude, flinging movements of an entire limb (or limbs) on one side of the body, which can be violent and stressful. The acute development of hemiballismus is usually caused by focal lesions in the contralateral basal ganglia, typically (but not exclusively) in the subthalamic nucleus. Many etiologies exist for this disorder, as for example vascular causes and nonketotic hyperglycemia, the latter representing one of the most common causes [6,7]. In rare cases, tumors localized in the brain (glioma, cavernous angioma, metastases, primary central nervous system lymphoma) can be the underlying cause of this disorder [8–10]. Prognosis is favorable for more than 60% of the patients with complete resolution without treatment [11].

*Symptomatic hemidystonia* is defined as dystonia involving the ipsilateral face, arm, and leg [12]. Rare patients with symptomatic hemidystonia due to tumor, arteriovenous malformations, stroke, or hemiatrophy were described so far [12,13]. All had typical dystonic movements and/or postures, identical to those seen in idiopathic (primary) torsion dystonia. The site(s) of the lesion responsible, as defined by CT scan or pathological examination, was in the contralateral caudate nucleus, lentiform nucleus (putamen), or thalamus, or in a combination of these structures [12,13].

*Hemifacial spasm* (HFS) is characterized by involuntary unilateral contractions of the muscles innervated by the ipsilateral facial nerve, usually starting around the eyes before progressing to the lower facial muscles [14]. Its prevalence is relatively high, 9.8 per 100,000 persons [14]. The accepted pathophysiology of HFS suggests that it affects the root entry zone of the facial nerve [15]. HFS can be divided into two types: primary and secondary. Primary HFS is triggered by vascular compression whereas secondary HFS comprises all other causes of facial nerve damage. Ponto-cerebellar angle tumors are rarely associated with HFS [14]. In a series of 214 patients with HFS by Colosimo and colleagues [14], only one case (0.47%) secondary to acoustic schwannoma was found.

*Parkinsonism* is defined as the presence of bradykinesia, in combination with at least one between resting tremor and rigidity [16]. Parkinsonism seems to be very rare in individuals with tumors located in the basal ganglia [17]. Similarly, mass lesions in the brainstem or within the posterior fossa are rarely associated with parkinsonism [17]. Conversely, supratentorial tumors sparing the basal ganglia were found to induce parkinsonism and/or rest tremor in 0.3% of the cases. Supratentorial meningioma is the most frequent cause of tumor-induced parkinsonism [17]. Bilateral thalamic tumors were also reported by a few authors to cause parkinsonism [4,17]. Basal ganglia tumors associated with parkinsonism may compress nigrostriatal neurons or their terminal axons and may induce damage to both presynaptic dopaminergic neurons and postsynaptic dopamine receptors, thus causing parkinsonian symptoms [4]. Hence, space-occupying lesions may induce similar dopaminergic nigrostriatal dysfunction as seen in idiopathic Parkinson's disease (PD) [4]. In this regard, abnormal single photon emission computed tomography (SPECT) studies were occasionally reported in parkinsonism due to brain tumors. Benincasa and colleagues [18] reported a case of hemiparkinsonism due to frontal meningioma, which, completely resolved after tumor removal, including the SPECT-related abnormalities. Secondary hemiparkinsonism (associated with a mesencephalic tumor) may respond to dopaminergic therapies, as documented by Yoshimura and colleagues [19]. Also, an abrupt change in the response to dopaminergic therapy was described in a pre-existing parkinsonism with superimposed frontal lobe tumor [20]. Again, after tumor removal (meningioma), the patient regained a marked response to levodopa treatment [20]. Extensive infiltration of the basal ganglia and thalamus by tumors may also be associated with atypical parkinsonian syndromes, particularly progressive supranuclear palsy (PSP). The distribution of neoplastic lesions in these patients is like that of PSP-tau pathology, namely in the subthalamic nucleus and brainstem, especially the midbrain tectum and the superior cerebellar peduncle [21]. The case by Posey and Spiller (1904-05), who reported a patient with progressive ophtalmoparesis and loss of balance, regarded as the earliest reported case of PSP, had in fact a midbrain sarcoma involving the right cerebral peduncle and periaqueductal area [22]. However, parkinsonism caused by mass lesion in the brainstem is rare, and there are several possible explanations to this finding. Firstly, movement disorders may be concealed by other neurological deficits, such as signs of pyramidal dysfunction or ataxia. Secondly, signs of parkinsonism may not be present until degeneration has occurred in more than 50% of the nigrostriatal fibers. Thirdly, nigrostriatal fibers are thin, and they may be more resistant to compression than well-myelinated fibers [4].

## 3. Paraneoplastic Movement Disorders

Paraneoplastic movement disorders include, by definition, any nonmetastatic, immune-mediated, hyperkinetic, or hypokinetic conditions associated with a neoplasm [23]. The spectrum of paraneoplastic movement disorders encompasses several conditions, with acute/subacute onset, rapid evolution, and multifocal localizations [24]. PNS are conditions in which autoantibodies are produced as a reaction to antigens shared by the tumor and the nervous system [25]. This phenomenon may occur for different mechanisms. PNS-associated tumors may harbor mutations in genes encoding onconeural proteins, thus leading to the production of highly immunogenic neoantigens [26]. Alternatively, in non-paraneoplastic context, autoimmunity may be due to molecular mimicry mechanisms (e.g., similarities between foreign and self-peptides causing the cross-activation of autoreactive B-cells by pathogen-derived peptides) [26]. Antibodies directed against intracellular neuronal antigens are named onconeural antibodies and are found in association to specific cytotoxic T-cells which are supposed to have a direct pathogenic role [27]. These onconeural antibodies are strong markers for an underlying malignancy and are therefore labelled "high-risk antibodies" in the updated diagnostic criteria for paraneoplastic neurologic syndromes [28]. Despite their relevant role as biomarkers, they do not have a direct pathogenic role. Conversely, antibodies against neuronal surface antigens (NSA-Ab) have a direct pathogenic role but have an intermediate or rare association with cancer ("intermediate or low-risk antibodies"). NSA-Abs are directed against receptors, ion channels, or components of neural plasma membranes [24]. The difference between onconeural and NSA-Abs is important also for therapeutic implications, in fact, immunomodulatory treatment is mainly effective in the presence of NSA-Abs, while when autoantibodies are directed against intracellular antigens, it has less marked therapeutic impact (See also Section 5).

Following a syndromic approach, paraneoplastic movement disorders may be classified in the subsequent categories: ataxia (paraneoplastic cerebellar degeneration, now labelled "rapidly progressive cerebellar syndrome" [28], chorea, dystonia, myoclonus (and opsoclonus-myoclonus ataxia syndrome—OMS), parkinsonism, paroxysmal movement disorders, stiff person spectrum disorders, and tremor. Similar disorders can develop in autoimmune (nonparaneoplastic) encephalitides, which is broad term used to indicate inflammatory brain disorders characterized by subacute onset of working memory deficits, altered mental status or psychiatric symptoms, along with new focal CNS findings (including new-onset movement disorders or seizures), with magnetic resonance imaging (MRI) or cerebrospinal fluid (CSF) evidence of inflammatory alterations, after exclusion of alternative diagnoses [27,29].

Below, we will give a brief description of each of the categories in which the paraneoplastic movement disorders are classified, the main antibodies and tumors found in association [30]. The main antibodies and tumors found in association with paraneoplastic movement disorder are displayed in the Table 1.

**Table 1.** Main antibodies and related tumors found in associations with paraneoplastic movement disorders.

| Antibody | Antigen Location | Cancer Risk | Cancer Type | Associated Movement Disorders | Other Clinical Features |
|---|---|---|---|---|---|
| Anti-Yo | I | High | Breast cancer, ovary cancer | Ataxia | Uncommon |
| Anti-Hu/ANNA1 | I | High | SCLC, NSCLC | Ataxia, chorea, OMS | SN, EM, LE |
| Anti-Ri/ANNA2 | I | High | Breast cancer in women, lung cancer in men | Ataxia, OMS, parkinsonism, jaw dystonia, laryngospasm | BE |
| Anti-Tr/DNER | I | High | Hodgkin lymphoma | Ataxia | Uncommon |
| * Anti- KLHL11 | I | High | Testicular germ cell cancer (Typically, "burned-out") | Ataxia (including paroxysmal) | BE, myelitis, LE |
| Anti-PCA2 | I | High | SCLC, NSCLC, breast cancer | Ataxia | Neuropathy, EM |
| Anti-Ma2 | I | High | Testicular cancer and NSCLC | Parkinsonism | LE, BE, diencephalitis |
| Anti-CV2/CRMP5 | I | High | SCLC and thymoma | Ataxia, chorea | SN and EM |
| Anti-Amphiphysin | I | High | SCLC and breast cancer | SPS | EM, SN, polyradiculoneuropathy |
| Anti-GABAB-R | E | Intermediate | SCLC | Ataxia, OMS | LE |
| Anti-CASPR2 | E | Intermediate | Thymoma | Ataxia (including paroxysmal), chorea | LE, Morvan syndrome, neuromyotonia |
| Anti-NMDA-R | E | Intermediate | Ovarian or extra-ovarian teratoma | Dyskinesia (orofacial and limb), chorea, dystonia, stereotypies, myoclonus, ataxia, parkinsonism | Encephalitis |
| Anti-AMPA-R | E | Intermediate | SCLC and thymoma | Tremor | LE |
| Anti-LGI1 | E | Low | Thymoma | Facio-brachial dystonic seizures, chorea, myoclonus, tremor | LE |
| Anti-GAD | S/I | Low | Rare (SCLC and thymoma) | Ataxia (including paroxysmal), SPS | LE |
| Anti-DPPX | E | Low | Lymphoma | Tremor, myoclonus, startle, ataxia, parkinsonism, PERM, SPS | Encephalitis |
| Anti-GFAP | I | Low | Ovarian teratoma and adenocarcinoma | Ataxia, tremor | Meningoencephalitis |
| Anti-Glycine-R | E | Low | Lymphoma, thymoma and lung cancer | PERM and SPS | LE |
| Anti-mGLUR-1 | E | Low | Lymphoma | Ataxia, myoclonus, dystonia, tremor | Behavioral changes |

I: intracellular; E: extracellular (Neural surface); LE: limbic encephalitis; BE: brainstem encephalitis; EM: encephalomyelitis; NHL: non-Hodgkin lymphoma; NSCLC: non-small cell lung cancer; OMS: opsoclonus-myoclonus ataxia syndrome; PERM: progressive encephalomyelitis with rigidity and myoclonus; S/I: synaptic intracellular; SN: sensory neuronopathy; SCLC: small cell lung cancer; SN: sensory neuronopathy; SPS: stiff-person syndrome. * Represents a newly described antibody associated to cerebellar syndrome [31].

*Ataxia* of paraneoplastic origin should be considered in cases showing a rapidly progressive cerebellar syndrome, particularly if involving predominantly the vermis over the cerebellar hemispheres [31]. Involvement of the cerebellum can present as predominant or isolated form, especially in patients with anti-Yo and anti-Tr/DNER antibodies, or in association with extra-cerebellar manifestations, which may in turn inform on the targeted antigen (e.g., subacute sensory neuropathy/limbic encephalitis are common in anti-Hu cases, jaw dystonia and parkinsonism can accompany anti-Ri syndrome, while diencephalitis/limbic encephalitis are the hallmarks of anti-Ma2 antibodies) [28,32].

*Chorea* of paraneoplastic origin is often accompanied by subacute cognitive decline, progressive ataxia with or without neuropathy, behavioral changes, weight loss, dysautonomic symptoms, sleep disturbances, and bulbar symptoms [24,33].

*Dystonia* of paraneoplastic origin is characterized by subacute onset with usually associated other symptoms like chorea, orofacial dyskinesia, stereotypies, and encephalopathy or psychiatric features [30,34]. Children and young adults are more frequently affected.

*Myoclonus* of paraneoplastic origin has typically a subacute onset and is associated with encephalopathy, brainstem involvement, possible seizures, dysautonomia and sleep disturbances. In some cases, myoclonus can be found in association with opsoclonus and/or ataxia, thus configuring the OMS [35].

*Parkinsonism* of paraneoplastic origin is characterized by a subacute atypical syndrome frequently due to a brainstem encephalitis with ocular abnormalities (vertical gaze palsy) and associated sleep disorders [36,37]. PSP-like symptoms with sleep disturbances are suggestive for IgLON5-related disease, which is rarely paraneoplastic [38].

*Paroxysmal movement disorders* of paraneoplastic origin are characterized by sudden and repetitive dystonic or dyskinetic movements. Dystonic posturing of the face and the limbs characterizes facio-brachial dystonic seizures (LGI1-antibodies), a condition that is rarely paraneoplastic [39]. Painful dystonic posturing was described in optic neuromyelitis and associated to the AQP4 antibodies [30].

*Stiff person spectrum disorders* of paraneoplastic origin are a spectrum of disorders characterized by stiffness, spasms, and hyperekplexia (e.g., excessive startle reaction to sudden stimuli as noise, movement, or touch) [24]. The classic form is characterized by muscle stiffness and painful spasms, involving trunk and proximal limb muscles [24]. In the stiff-limb syndrome (SLS), stiffness is more distal and confined to a limb [30]. Some variants of this condition include the so-called progressive encephalitis with rigidity and myoclonus (PERM) [40].

*Tremor* of paraneoplastic origin is usually found in association with other symptoms within the context of an autoimmune encephalitis and was described with various antibodies typically associated with widespread encephalopathy [30,34]. It is important to underline that myoclonus may be misdiagnosed as tremor.

## 4. Immune-Checkpoint Inhibitors Associated Movement Disorders

ICIs revolutionized cancer treatment, improving survivals and prognosis of several malignancies. Immune-related adverse events (irAEs) are side effects caused by ICIs. They are triggered by the inhibitions of negative regulators of the immune response with the primary aim of boosting the antitumor immunity. Therefore, ICIs may be responsible of different effects which resemble autoimmune conditions affecting several organs and systems. Indeed, endocrine, gastrointestinal, pulmonary, cardiac, renal, hematological, rheumatological and dermatological irAES were described [41]. The frequency of neurological irAEs (n-irAEs) varies from 1 to 12%, and both the CNS and peripheral nervous systems may be involved, the latter three times more [42,43]. Recently, a multi-institution group of neurologists, oncologists, and experts in irAEs developed consensus guidelines to classify the n-irAEs appropriately [42]. Seven core syndromes were defined, of which four involve the CNS and three the peripheral nervous system. IrAEs involving the CNS include immune-related (ir)-meningitis, ir-encephalitis, ir-demyelinating diseases, and ir-vasculitis [42]. The ir-encephalitis encompasses several clinical presentations of movement disorders, namely cerebellitis, OMS, and stiff person spectrum disorders/PERM [42] (Figure 1). There are clinical scenarios in which n-irAEs satisfy the criteria for the diagnosis of paraneoplastic syndromes (positive "high-risk" antibodies and compatible clinical syndrome) [44]. There is both experimental [45] and real-life experience [46] that ICIs may induce PNS. Indeed, a retrospective single-center study detected an increase (+112%) of Ma2-associated paraneoplastic syndromes diagnoses since the implementation of ICIs in France [46]. Importantly, patients with ir-encephalitis can present sometimes as movement disorders, especially in the cases linked to antiphosphodiesterase 10A-Abs [47].

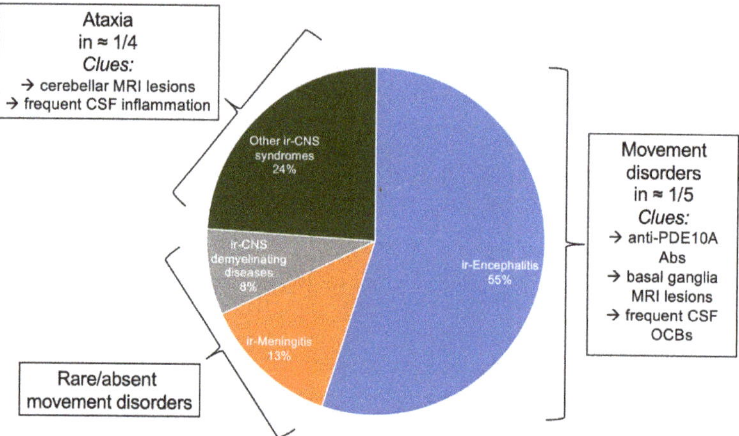


**Figure 1.** Immune-related adverse events of central nervous system associated with immune checkpoint-inhibitors. Figure is derived from observations of Marini et al. [43]. Ir-encephalitis represent 55% of cases, and movement disorders are associated in 1 out of 5 cases. Ataxia is present in 1 out of 4 cases of "Other ir-CNS syndromes". Movement disorders are rare in other ir-related conditions. MRI, magnetic resonance imaging; CSF, cerebrospinal fluid; Anti-PDE10A Abs, antibodies anti phosphodiesterase 10A; OCBs, oligoclonal bands.

## 5. Diagnostic Algorithm and Testing

When dealing with movement disorders with an acute/subacute onset, in general, once other secondary causes were ruled out, clinicians should consider oncological diagnoses according to the clinical presentation. Brain malignancies are easily individuated through neuroimaging studies. Differently, paraneoplastic syndromes are more difficult to diagnose, as the neurological syndrome typically antedates the discovery of a systemic cancer. Conversely, for the ICIs-related movement disorders, the history of a systemic cancer treated with immunotherapy is the most important clue. In the case of brain tumors and paraneoplastic syndromes, the goal is the diagnosis and treatment of the underlying tumor when possible. In PNS, prompt initiation of drugs which acutely modulate the immune system is necessary (e.g., steroids or intravenous immunoglobulin as first-line, followed by cyclophosphamide or rituximab in nonresponsive cases). When dealing with n-irAEs, the withdrawal of ICIs followed by steroid treatment are often needed. In both PNS and n-irAEs, however, the first step is always to exclude other (more common) diagnoses, including direct neoplastic involvement (as in the case of carcinomatous meningitis, which can be difficult to demonstrate) or neuro-infectious conditions. In case of paraneoplastic conditions, the likelihood for a tumor to be the underlying cause of immune-mediated process is higher for conditions associated with onconeural antibodies ("high-risk "antibodies) compared to that of conditions associated with NSA ("intermediate-" or "low-risk" antibodies) [24]. This occurrence is relevant in the clinical practice. In fact, for a given clinical phenotype (for example, limbic encephalitis), the antibody's type may suggest the possibility of having associated a cancer or not, thus directing the tumor search [28]. Typically, intracellular proteins derived from tumor apoptotic cell initiate the immune response in case of PNS and, therefore, most of the high-risk antibodies are directed towards antigens located in the nucleus or cytoplasm. A flow-chart with the main antibodies to be tested, based on the clinical picture and the related probability of having associated a neoplastic condition is proposed in Figure 2.

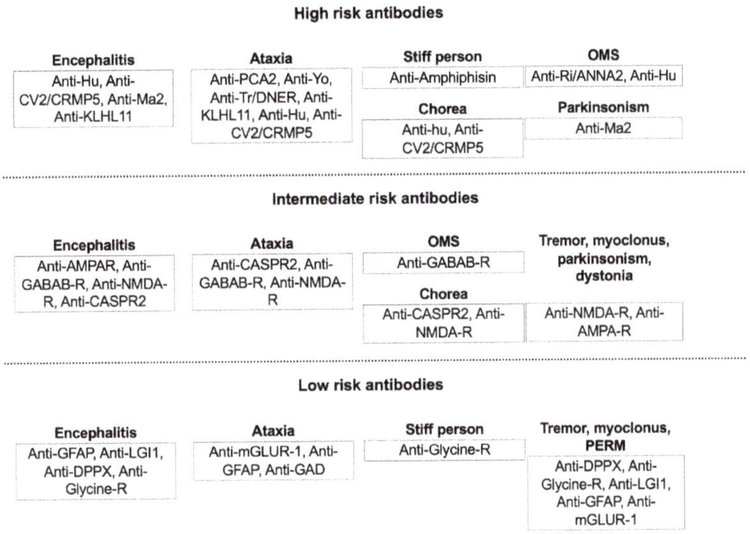

**High risk antibodies**

| Encephalitis | Ataxia | Stiff person | OMS |
|---|---|---|---|
| Anti-Hu, Anti-CV2/CRMP5, Anti-Ma2, Anti-KLHL11 | Anti-PCA2, Anti-Yo, Anti-Tr/DNER, Anti-KLHL11, Anti-Hu, Anti-CV2/CRMP5 | Anti-Amphiphisin | Anti-Ri/ANNA2, Anti-Hu |
| | | **Chorea** | **Parkinsonism** |
| | | Anti-hu, Anti-CV2/CRMP5 | Anti-Ma2 |

**Intermediate risk antibodies**

| Encephalitis | Ataxia | OMS | Tremor, myoclonus, parkinsonism, dystonia |
|---|---|---|---|
| Anti-AMPAR, Anti-GABAB-R, Anti-NMDA-R, Anti-CASPR2 | Anti-CASPR2, Anti-GABAB-R, Anti-NMDA-R | Anti-GABAB-R | |
| | | **Chorea** | |
| | | Anti-CASPR2, Anti-NMDA-R | Anti-NMDA-R, Anti-AMPA-R |

**Low risk antibodies**

| Encephalitis | Ataxia | Stiff person | Tremor, myoclonus, PERM |
|---|---|---|---|
| Anti-GFAP, Anti-LGI1, Anti-DPPX, Anti-Glycine-R | Anti-mGLUR-1, Anti-GFAP, Anti-GAD | Anti-Glycine-R | Anti-DPPX, Anti-Glycine-R, Anti-LGI1, Anti-GFAP, Anti-mGLUR-1 |

**Figure 2.** Main antibodies found in association with different paraneoplastic movement disorders, stratified per probability of having an underlying neoplastic condition. High-risk antibodies are associated with 70% probability or more of an underlying cancer. Intermediate risk antibodies with 30–70%, and low-risk antibodies with less than 30% probability of developing cancer, respectively. Each movement disorder is represented within one of three categories, together with most relevant associated antibodies. A huge overlap exists between some of these conditions, and same antibody may be found in association with different movement disorders. OMS, opsoclonus-myoclonus; OMS, opsoclonus-myoclonus ataxia syndrome; PERM, progressive encephalomyelitis with rigidity and myoclonus.

The final diagnosis of a brain tumor is mainly based on the histologic examination of the lesion [48]. Brain tumor-derived biomarkers, and in particular wet biomarkers, constitute a growing field of interest in oncological research as an alternative for invasive tumor tissue biopsy [49]. Tumor-derived biomarkers include nucleic acids, proteins, and tumor-derived extracellular vesicles that accumulate in blood or CSF and may be routinely used in the clinical diagnostic evaluation, according to the single center's experience [50]. Hematological malignancies involving the brain can be also easily individuated through biofluid analysis [51].

Paraneoplastic conditions might be diagnosed by testing the different antibodies in blood and/or CSF samples (ideally both for increasing specificity and sensitivity). The diagnosis is based on a combination of immunoblotting (used mainly for intracellular antigens), cell-based assays (CBAs) (used mainly for extracellular antigens), and tissue-based assays (TBAs) [52]. In selected cases, these tests can be supplemented by extra tests in dedicated laboratories using live cells and hippocampal rat neurons [30] or alternative tests for specific antibodies (e.g., enzyme-linked immunoassays for anti-GAD, radio-immunoassays for anti-VGCC).

Usually, the testing strategy starts with the more common antibodies, and then if they result negative, specialized TBAs and CBAs can be used in dedicated laboratories to monitor for further fewer common antibodies [30]. However, this approach for antibody detection based on commercial kits is limited by the high rate of false positive results [53], and current diagnostic criteria recommend the use of at least two distinct techniques to confirm the test results [28].

Seronegative results are common even with widespread testing. On the opposite side, incidental findings of antibodies in patients with movement disorders not due to immune-mediated conditions may be common too and may vary according to the different laboratories and techniques adopted [30]. Possible clues that may suggest a false positive/incidental finding in antibody testing are an atypical clinical presentation and the presence of antibodies only in serum and not in CSF, or at low titers. Some antibodies like anti-LGI-1 may frequently test negative in the CSF (therefore, it is important to test serum together with CSF). Regarding the n-irAEs, the diagnosis of a definite ir-encephalitis/movement disorder associated with ICIs may be challenging and requires a clinical presentation consistent with encephalitis/movement disorder, with the exclusion of secondary causes (e.g., infectious states, cancer, and radiotherapy-induced necrosis) and the presence of CNS inflammation (documented on imaging/CSF/neurophysiological studies followed by improvement with immunomodulation—steroids—and/or ICIs discontinuation, or demonstrated directly on biopsy) [42].

## 6. Therapeutic Approach

Within the context of brain malignancies, the gold standard is the complete or partial tumor removal, based on its location, and/or the prompt initiation of chemo/radiotherapy [54,55]. Again, in the case of paraneoplastic conditions, the first therapeutic step is the oncological treatment of the underlying tumor (if diagnosed), and, when necessary, the administration of first-line drugs able to suppress the immune response, such as intravenous (IV) steroids, IV high-dose immunoglobulins, and plasma-exchange [24]. Second-line drugs that can be used are rituximab (monoclonal antibody anti-CD20 receptor on the B cells surface), cyclophosphamide (alkylating agent crosslinking DNA), and other drugs including azathioprine and mycophenolate mofetil. Those immunomodulatory treatments, despite depressing/modulating the immune response, are considered safe given that they do not affect the prognosis of the cancer *per se* (e.g., they do not worsen it).

Building-up a multidisciplinary team with both neurologists and oncologists is strongly encouraged in these cases. In fact, an intensive oncological follow-up and a neurological evaluation may be required if the disease tends to relapse, or if second-line treatments are required [56]. Onconeural antibodies are more frequently associated with an underlying tumor, compared to NSA antibodies. In addition, the presence of onconeural antibodies is also associated to a lesser response to immune suppressive therapies [24,34]. Unfortunately, our knowledge and guidelines on how to manage these immune-mediated conditions is based on the single-centers' and physicians' experience, given the scarce amount of randomized clinical trials on this topic. To the best of our knowledge, only two clinical trials was conducted on the utilization of high-dose IV immunoglobulins: in one case for stiff-person syndrome [57] and in another for LGI1/CASPR2-Ab-associated epilepsy [58], with positive results in both of them. Patients with ir-encephalitis triggered by ICIs should be managed according to National Comprehensive Cancer Network guidelines [59] ICIs should be held, and steroids administered—preferentially IV methylprednisolone— followed in case of no response or worsening by intravenous immunoglobulin or plasmapheresis. Additional treatments (including second-line immunosuppression) may be considered in refractory cases.

Symptomatic therapy may be of relief for patients and may vary according to the specific underlying neurological symptoms. As an example, tumor-related or paraneoplastic forms of dystonia may benefit from botulinum toxin injections into affected muscles, according to standardized dosages [24]. Tumor-related parkinsonism may show a good response to levodopa [19]. Paraneoplastic chorea can be treated with dopamine depletory agents (caution is imperative with these compounds, to prevent tardive parkinsonism) [60]. Finally, muscle relaxants (benzodiazepines or baclofen) and gabapentin, may be used for stiffness [24].

## 7. Challenges and Future Directions

Although movement disorders due to focal neoplastic brain lesions are rare, this diagnosis should not be missed. Clinicians should be able to recognize or suspect the presence of a brain malignancy when dealing with a hyperkinetic or hypokinetic movement disorder with atypical features, suggestive of a secondary etiology. They should also consider that, other than tumor removal, there may be several symptomatic therapeutic options to ponder. Paraneoplastic movement disorders are even rarer, but their peculiar clinical and laboratory findings should always prompt the neurologist to search for occult tumors. In addition to their desired effects in cancer treatment, ICIs can break immune tolerance to self-antigens and induce specific n-irAEs, including movement disorders. What to do in those cases, must be discussed on a case-to-case basis. So far, our knowledge about movement disorders in oncology is limited due to their relative rarity and difficulty in promptly achieving the correct diagnosis. The introduction of ICIs in the clinical practice has opened a new window on possible adverse events induced by the immune system to consider when administering these life-saving treatments.

The effective role of antibodies found in PNS, and the related pathogenic mechanisms still needs some clarifications. Several studies pointed out the presence of these antibodies not only in paraneoplastic and immune-mediated neurological syndromes, but also in neurodegenerative diseases. In some cases, autoimmune-related neurodegeneration may be misdiagnosed as idiopathic PD, multiple system atrophy, PSP, frontotemporal dementia, or even Alzheimer's disease [61–63]. Interestingly, the presence of NSA-Ab was demonstrated in these neurodegenerative diseases. The percentage of positivity to NSA-Ab antibodies among neurodegenerative diseases was estimated around 14–16% according to different studies [64–66]. More importantly, NSA-Ab are usually found in patients with an atypical disease progression or with atypical clinical phenotypes [63]. Further studies are needed to clarify the role of autoantibodies in patients with neurodegenerative disorders.

Another intriguing field of intersection between movement disorders and oncology is represented by the CAR T-cell therapies, which include genetically modified T-cells expressing chimeric antigen receptors (CAR T-cell). CAR T-cell treatment is an emerging strategy for hematological malignancies, and was associated with neurotoxicity [67]. Although the characterization of movement disorders caused by CAR T-cell treatments as side effects is still underreported, it would be important to further monitor its possible occurrence with future retrospective multicentric studies, given the broader application in the future of this therapeutic option [68]. The early identification of these adverse events would be essential to optimize the functional outcome and oncologic management of patients [68].

## 8. Final Remarks

In the present review, although with some limitations as the nonsystematic approach and the relatively small number of studies analyzed, we provided a comprehensive revision of movement disorders in oncological diseases, including their clinical features, associated biomarkers, and the relationship with underlying tumors. Clinicians in general, and neurologists specialized in movement disorders in particular, should be aware of these rare but serious conditions. They should be able to diagnose and then treat these conditions. Also, when dealing with a given movement disorder that could be caused by an oncological condition, clinicians should promptly start a diagnostic and therapeutic work-up based on neuroimaging and, if needed also on antibody testing. They should also consider recommending drugs that module the immune system, as steroids, or stopping current anticancer therapies if the movement disorder is a side effect of the treatment *per se* and according to its severity.

For the next future, we envision a broader diffusion of validated kits for the detection of antibodies and other biomarkers associated with oncological conditions, a widespread knowledge of the possible CNS-associated side effects caused by ICIs (and by CAR T-cell therapy), and finally a systematic enrollment of patients in clinical trials testing putative disease-modifying drugs. Additionally, an early detection of these conditions is essential for the therapeutic success, thus increasing the patient's chance of maintaining the greatest quality of life achievable. Also, a deep understanding of immune-mediated movement disorders will help to achieve a better knowledge of the interaction between the immune and nervous system, investigating mechanisms of cell death that are frequently found in the most common neurodegenerative disorders.

**Author Contributions:** (1) research project: A. conception, B. organization, C. execution; (2) manuscript preparation: A. writing of the first draft, B. review and critique. L.M. 1 A,B,C; 2 A; A.V., 1 B; 2 B; C.C. 1 A; 2 B. All authors have read and agreed to the published version of the manuscript.

**Funding:** This research received no external funding.

**Institutional Review Board Statement:** Not applicable.

**Informed Consent Statement:** Not applicable.

**Data Availability Statement:** Not applicable.

**Conflicts of Interest:** The authors declare no conflict of interest related to the present work.

## References


1. Mahajan, A.; Chirra, M.; Dwivedi, A.K.; Sturchio, A.; Keeling, E.G.; Marsili, L.; Espay, A.J. Skin Cancer May Delay Onset but Not Progression of Parkinson's Disease: A Nested Case-Control Study. *Front. Neurol.* **2020**, *11*, 406. [CrossRef] [PubMed]
2. Sturchio, A.; Dwivedi, A.K.; Vizcarra, J.A.; Chirra, M.; Keeling, E.G.; Mata, I.F.; Kauffman, M.A.; Pandey, M.K.; Roviello, G.; Comi, C.; et al. Genetic parkinsonisms and cancer: A systematic review and meta-analysis. *Rev. Neurosci.* **2021**, *32*, 159–167. [CrossRef]
3. Magnusen, A.F.; Hatton, S.L.; Rani, R.; Pandey, M.K. Genetic Defects and Pro-inflammatory Cytokines in Parkinson's Disease. *Front. Neurol.* **2021**, *12*, 636139. [CrossRef]
4. Hatano, T.K.S.; Hattori, N.; Mizuno, Y. Movement disorders in neoplastic brain disease. In *Movement Disorders in Neurologic and Systemic Disease*; W. Poewe, J.J., Ed.; Cambridge University Press: Cambridge, UK, 2014; pp. 279–292.
5. Hoos, A. Development of immuno-oncology drugs-from CTLA4 to PD1 to the next generations. *Nat. Rev. Drug Discov.* **2016**, *15*, 235–247. [CrossRef] [PubMed]
6. Duker, A.P.; Espay, A.J. Images in clinical medicine. Hemichorea–hemiballism after diabetic ketoacidosis. *N. Engl. J. Med.* **2010**, *363*, e27. [CrossRef] [PubMed]
7. Marsili, L.; Gallerini, S.; Bartalucci, M.; Marotti, C.; Marconi, R. Paroxysmal painful spasms associated with central pontine myelinolisis in the context of nonketotic hyperglycemia. *J. Neurol. Sci.* **2018**, *388*, 37–39. [CrossRef] [PubMed]
8. Moore, F.G. Bilateral hemichorea-hemiballism caused by metastatic lung cancer. *Mov. Disord.* **2009**, *24*, 1405–1406. [CrossRef] [PubMed]
9. Patankar, A.P. Hemi-chorea: An unusual presentation of brainstem glioma. *Br. J. Neurosurg.* **2013**, *27*, 256–258. [CrossRef] [PubMed]
10. Ząbek, M.; Sobstyl, M.; Dzierzęcki, S.; Górecki, W.; Jakuciński, M. Right hemichorea treated successfully by surgical removal of a left putaminal cavernous angioma. *Clin. Neurol. Neurosurg.* **2013**, *115*, 844–846. [CrossRef] [PubMed]
11. Zagrajek, M.; Chojdak-Łukasiewicz, J. Ballism as a rare form of hyperkinetic movement disorder. *Wiad. Lek.* **2013**, *66*, 171–174.
12. Chuang, C.; Fahn, S.; Frucht, S.J. The natural history and treatment of acquired hemidystonia: Report of 33 cases and review of the literature. *J. Neurol. Neurosurg. Psychiatry* **2002**, *72*, 59–67. [CrossRef] [PubMed]
13. Lee, M.S.; Marsden, C.D. Movement disorders following lesions of the thalamus or subthalamic region. *Mov. Disord.* **1994**, *9*, 493–507. [CrossRef]
14. Colosimo, C.; Bologna, M.; Lamberti, S.; Avanzino, L.; Marinelli, L.; Fabbrini, G.; Abbruzzese, G.; Defazio, G.; Berardelli, A. A comparative study of primary and secondary hemifacial spasm. *Arch. Neurol.* **2006**, *63*, 441–444. [CrossRef] [PubMed]
15. Lefaucheur, J.P. New insights into the pathophysiology of primary hemifacial spasm. *Neurochirurgie* **2018**, *64*, 87–93. [CrossRef]
16. Marsili, L.; Rizzo, G.; Colosimo, C. Diagnostic Criteria for Parkinson's Disease: From James Parkinson to the Concept of Prodromal Disease. *Front. Neurol.* **2018**, *9*, 156. [CrossRef]
17. Krauss, J.K.; Paduch, T.; Mundinger, F.; Seeger, W. Parkinsonism and rest tremor secondary to supratentorial tumours sparing the basal ganglia. *Acta Neurochir.* **1995**, *133*, 22–29. [CrossRef] [PubMed]
18. Benincasa, D.; Romano, A.; Mastronardi, L.; Pellicano, C.; Bozzao, A.; Pontieri, F.E. Hemiparkinsonism due to frontal meningioma. *Acta Neurol. Belg.* **2008**, *108*, 29–32. [PubMed]
19. Yoshimura, M.; Yamamoto, T.; Iso-o, N.; Imafuku, I.; Momose, T.; Shirouzu, I.; Kwak, S.; Kanazawa, I. Hemiparkinsonism associated with a mesencephalic tumor. *J. Neurol. Sci.* **2002**, *197*, 89–92. [CrossRef]
20. Fabbrini, G.; Baronti, F.; Ruggieri, S.; Lenzi, G.L. Meningioma-induced loss of antiparkinsonian response to levodopa. *Mov. Disord.* **1995**, *10*, 231–232. [CrossRef] [PubMed]
21. Dickson, D.W.; Rademakers, R.; Hutton, M.L. Progressive supranuclear palsy: Pathology and genetics. *Brain Pathol.* **2007**, *17*, 74–82. [CrossRef] [PubMed]
22. Siderowf, A.D.; Galetta, S.L.; Hurtig, H.I.; Liu, G.T. Posey and Spiller and progressive supranuclear palsy: An incorrect attribution. *Mov. Disord.* **1998**, *13*, 170–174. [CrossRef] [PubMed]

23. Dalmau, J.; Rosenfeld, M.R. Paraneoplastic syndromes of the CNS. *Lancet Neurol.* **2008**, *7*, 327–340. [CrossRef]
24. Chirra, M.; Marsili, L.; Gallerini, S.; Keeling, E.G.; Marconi, R.; Colosimo, C. Paraneoplastic movement disorders: Phenomenology, diagnosis, and treatment. *Eur. J. Intern. Med.* **2019**, *67*, 14–23. [CrossRef] [PubMed]
25. Grunwald, G.B.; Klein, R.; Simmonds, M.A.; Kornguth, S.E. Autoimmune basis for visual paraneoplastic syndrome in patients with small-cell lung carcinoma. *Lancet* **1985**, *1*, 658–661. [CrossRef]
26. Vogrig, A.; Muñiz-Castrillo, S.; Desestret, V.; Joubert, B.; Honnorat, J. Pathophysiology of paraneoplastic and autoimmune encephalitis: Genes, infections, and checkpoint inhibitors. *Adv. Neurol. Disord.* **2020**, *13*, 1756286420932797. [CrossRef] [PubMed]
27. Honorat, J.A.; Komorowski, L.; Josephs, K.A.; Fechner, K.; St Louis, E.K.; Hinson, S.R.; Lederer, S.; Kumar, N.; Gadoth, A.; Lennon, V.A.; et al. IgLON5 antibody: Neurological accompaniments and outcomes in 20 patients. *Neurol. Neuroimmunol. Neuroinflamm.* **2017**, *4*, e385. [CrossRef] [PubMed]
28. Graus, F.; Vogrig, A.; Muñiz-Castrillo, S.; Antoine, J.G.; Desestret, V.; Dubey, D.; Giometto, B.; Irani, S.R.; Joubert, B.; Leypoldt, F.; et al. Updated Diagnostic Criteria for Paraneoplastic Neurologic Syndromes. *Neurol. Neuroimmunol. Neuroinflamm.* **2021**, *8*. [CrossRef] [PubMed]
29. Graus, F.; Titulaer, M.J.; Balu, R.; Benseler, S.; Bien, C.G.; Cellucci, T.; Cortese, I.; Dale, R.C.; Gelfand, J.M.; Geschwind, M.; et al. A clinical approach to diagnosis of autoimmune encephalitis. *Lancet Neurol.* **2016**, *15*, 391–404. [CrossRef]
30. Gövert, F.; Leypoldt, F.; Junker, R.; Wandinger, K.P.; Deuschl, G.; Bhatia, K.P.; Balint, B. Antibody-related movement disorders—A comprehensive review of phenotype-autoantibody correlations and a guide to testing. *Neurol. Res. Pract.* **2020**, *2*, 6. [CrossRef] [PubMed]
31. Vogrig, A.; Péricart, S.; Pinto, A.L.; Rogemond, V.; Muñiz-Castrillo, S.; Picard, G.; Selton, M.; Mittelbronn, M.; Lanoiselée, H.M.; Michenet, P.; et al. Immunopathogenesis and proposed clinical score for identifying Kelch-like protein-11 encephalitis. *Brain Commun.* **2021**, *3*, fcab185. [CrossRef]
32. Peterson, K.; Rosenblum, M.K.; Kotanides, H.; Posner, J.B. Paraneoplastic cerebellar degeneration. I. A clinical analysis of 55 anti-Yo antibody-positive patients. *Neurology* **1992**, *42*, 1931–1937. [CrossRef]
33. Yu, Z.; Kryzer, T.J.; Griesmann, G.E.; Kim, K.; Benarroch, E.E.; Lennon, V.A. CRMP-5 neuronal autoantibody: Marker of lung cancer and thymoma-related autoimmunity. *Ann. Neurol.* **2001**, *49*, 146–154. [CrossRef]
34. Balint, B.; Vincent, A.; Meinck, H.M.; Irani, S.R.; Bhatia, K.P. Movement disorders with neuronal antibodies: Syndromic approach, genetic parallels and pathophysiology. *Brain* **2018**, *141*, 13–36. [CrossRef] [PubMed]
35. Darnell, R.B.; Posner, J.B. Paraneoplastic syndromes involving the nervous system. *N. Engl. J. Med.* **2003**, *349*, 1543–1554. [CrossRef]
36. Dalmau, J.; Graus, F.; Villarejo, A.; Posner, J.B.; Blumenthal, D.; Thiessen, B.; Saiz, A.; Meneses, P.; Rosenfeld, M.R. Clinical analysis of anti-Ma2-associated encephalitis. *Brain* **2004**, *127*, 1831–1844. [CrossRef]
37. Xing, F.; Marsili, L.; Truong, D.D. Parkinsonism in Viral, Paraneoplastic, and Autoimmune Diseases. *J. Neurol. Sci.* **2021**, 120014, in press. [CrossRef]
38. Gaig, C.; Graus, F.; Compta, Y.; Högl, B.; Bataller, L.; Brüggemann, N.; Giordana, C.; Heidbreder, A.; Kotschet, K.; Lewerenz, J.; et al. Clinical manifestations of the anti-IgLON5 disease. *Neurology* **2017**, *88*, 1736–1743. [CrossRef] [PubMed]
39. Andrade, D.M.; Tai, P.; Dalmau, J.; Wennberg, R. Tonic seizures: A diagnostic clue of anti-LGI1 encephalitis? *Neurology* **2011**, *76*, 1355–1357. [CrossRef]
40. Meinck, H.M.; Thompson, P.D. Stiff man syndrome and related conditions. *Mov. Disord.* **2002**, *17*, 853–866. [CrossRef]
41. Martins, F.; Sofiya, L.; Sykiotis, G.P.; Lamine, F.; Maillard, M.; Fraga, M.; Shabafrouz, K.; Ribi, C.; Cairoli, A.; Guex-Crosier, Y.; et al. Adverse effects of immune-checkpoint inhibitors: Epidemiology, management and surveillance. *Nat. Rev. Clin. Oncol.* **2019**, *16*, 563–580. [CrossRef] [PubMed]
42. Guidon, A.C.; Burton, L.B.; Chwalisz, B.K.; Hillis, J.; Schaller, T.H.; Amato, A.A.; Betof Warner, A.; Brastianos, P.K.; Cho, T.A.; Clardy, S.L.; et al. Consensus disease definitions for Neurologic immune-related adverse events of immune checkpoint inhibitors. *J. Immunother. Cancer* **2021**, *9*, e002890. [CrossRef]
43. Marini, A.; Bernardini, A.; Gigli, G.L.; Valente, M.; Muñiz-Castrillo, S.; Honnorat, J.; Vogrig, A. Neurologic Adverse Events of Immune Checkpoint Inhibitors: A Systematic Review. *Neurology* **2021**, *96*, 754–766. [CrossRef]
44. Graus, F.; Dalmau, J. Paraneoplastic Neurological syndromes in the era of immune-checkpoint inhibitors. *Nat. Rev. Clin. Oncol.* **2019**, *16*, 535–548. [CrossRef]
45. Yshii, L.M.; Gebauer, C.M.; Pignolet, B.; Mauré, E.; Quériault, C.; Pierau, M.; Saito, H.; Suzuki, N.; Brunner-Weinzierl, M.; Bauer, J.; et al. CTLA4 blockade elicits paraneoplastic Neurological disease in a mouse model. *Brain* **2016**, *139*, 2923–2934. [CrossRef]
46. Vogrig, A.; Fouret, M.; Joubert, B.; Picard, G.; Rogemond, V.; Pinto, A.L.; Muñiz-Castrillo, S.; Roger, M.; Raimbourg, J.; Dayen, C.; et al. Increased frequency of anti-Ma2 encephalitis associated with immune checkpoint inhibitors. *Neurol. Neuroimmunol. Neuroinflamm.* **2019**, *6*, e604. [CrossRef]
47. Zekeridou, A.; Kryzer, T.; Guo, Y.; Hassan, A.; Lennon, V.; Lucchinetti, C.F.; Pittock, S.; McKeon, A. Phosphodiesterase 10A IgG: A novel biomarker of paraneoplastic Neurologic autoimmunity. *Neurology* **2019**, *93*, e815–e822. [CrossRef]
48. Louis, D.N.; Ohgaki, H.; Wiestler, O.D.; Cavenee, W.K.; Burger, P.C.; Jouvet, A.; Scheithauer, B.W.; Kleihues, P. The 2007 WHO Classification of Tumours of the Central Nervous System. *Acta Neuropathol.* **2007**, *114*, 97–109. [CrossRef]

49. Kristensen, B.W.; Priesterbach-Ackley, L.P.; Petersen, J.K.; Wesseling, P. Molecular pathology of tumors of the central nervous system. *Ann. Oncol.* **2019**, *30*, 1265–1278. [CrossRef]
50. Jelski, W.; Mroczko, B. Molecular and Circulating Biomarkers of Brain Tumors. *Int. J. Mol. Sci.* **2021**, *22*, 7039. [CrossRef] [PubMed]
51. Dunphy, K.; O'Mahoney, K.; Dowling, P.; O'Gorman, P.; Bazou, D. Clinical Proteomics of Biofluids in Haematological Malignancies. *Int. J. Mol. Sci.* **2021**, *22*, 8021. [CrossRef]
52. Mayo Foundation for Medical Education and Research. Paraneoplastic, Autoantibody Evaluation, Serum. Available online: https://Neurology.testcatalog.org/show/PAVAL (accessed on 28 September 2021).
53. Déchelotte, B.; Muñiz-Castrillo, S.; Joubert, B.; Vogrig, A.; Picard, G.; Rogemond, V.; Pinto, A.L.; Lombard, C.; Desestret, V.; Fabien, N.; et al. Diagnostic yield of commercial immunodots to diagnose paraneoplastic Neurologic syndromes. *Neurol. Neuroimmunol. Neuroinflamm.* **2020**, *7*, e701. [CrossRef]
54. Alruwaili, A.A.; De Jesus, O. Meningioma. In *StatPearls*; StatPearls Publishing LLC.: Treasure Island, FL, USA, 2021.
55. Ko, C.C.; Yeh, L.R.; Kuo, Y.T.; Chen, J.H. Imaging biomarkers for evaluating tumor response: RECIST and beyond. *Biomark Res.* **2021**, *9*, 52. [CrossRef]
56. Zoccarato, M.; Gastaldi, M.; Zuliani, L.; Biagioli, T.; Brogi, M.; Bernardi, G.; Corsini, E.; Bazzigaluppi, E.; Fazio, R.; Giannotta, C.; et al. Diagnostics of paraneoplastic Neurological syndromes. *Neurol. Sci.* **2017**, *38*, 237–242. [CrossRef]
57. Dalakas, M.C.; Fujii, M.; Li, M.; Lutfi, B.; Kyhos, J.; McElroy, B. High-dose intravenous immune globulin for stiff-person syndrome. *N. Engl. J. Med.* **2001**, *345*, 1870–1876. [CrossRef]
58. Dubey, D.; Britton, J.; McKeon, A.; Gadoth, A.; Zekeridou, A.; Lopez Chiriboga, S.A.; Devine, M.; Cerhan, J.H.; Dunlay, K.; Sagen, J.; et al. Randomized Placebo-Controlled Trial of Intravenous Immunoglobulin in Autoimmune LGI1/CASPR2 Epilepsy. *Ann. Neurol.* **2020**, *87*, 313–323. [CrossRef]
59. National Comprehensive Cancer Network. Available online: https://www.nccn.org/login?ReturnURL=https://www.nccn.org/professionals/physician_gls/pdf/immunotherapy.pdf (accessed on 29 September 2021).
60. Cardoso, F. Autoimmune choreas. *J. Neurol. Neurosurg. Psychiatry* **2017**, *88*, 412–417. [CrossRef]
61. McKeon, A.; Marnane, M.; O'Connell, M.; Stack, J.P.; Kelly, P.J.; Lynch, T. Potassium channel antibody associated encephalopathy presenting with a frontotemporal dementia like syndrome. *Arch. Neurol.* **2007**, *64*, 1528–1530. [CrossRef]
62. Sabater, L.; Gaig, C.; Gelpi, E.; Bataller, L.; Lewerenz, J.; Torres-Vega, E.; Contreras, A.; Giometto, B.; Compta, Y.; Embid, C.; et al. A novel non-rapid-eye movement and rapid-eye-movement parasomnia with sleep breathing disorder associated with antibodies to IgLON5: A case series, characterisation of the antigen, and post-mortem study. *Lancet Neurol.* **2014**, *13*, 575–586. [CrossRef]
63. Giannoccaro, M.P.; Gastaldi, M.; Rizzo, G.; Jacobson, L.; Vacchiano, V.; Perini, G.; Capellari, S.; Franciotta, D.; Costa, A.; Liguori, R.; et al. Antibodies to neuronal surface antigens in patients with a clinical diagnosis of neurodegenerative disorder. *Brain Behav. Immun.* **2021**, *96*, 106–112. [CrossRef]
64. Çoban, A.; Ismail Küçükali, C.; Bilgiç, B.; Yalçınkaya, N.; Haytural, H.; Ulusoy, C.; Turan, S.; Çakır, S.; Uçok, A.; Ünübol, H.; et al. Evaluation of incidence and clinical features of antibody-associated autoimmune encephalitis mimicking dementia. *Behav. Neurol.* **2014**, *2014*, 935379. [CrossRef]
65. Flanagan, E.P.; McKeon, A.; Lennon, V.A.; Boeve, B.F.; Trenerry, M.R.; Tan, K.M.; Drubach, D.A.; Josephs, K.A.; Britton, J.W.; Mandrekar, J.N.; et al. Autoimmune dementia: Clinical course and predictors of immunotherapy response. *Mayo Clin. Proc.* **2010**, *85*, 881–897. [CrossRef] [PubMed]
66. Doss, S.; Wandinger, K.P.; Hyman, B.T.; Panzer, J.A.; Synofzik, M.; Dickerson, B.; Mollenhauer, B.; Scherzer, C.R.; Ivinson, A.J.; Finke, C.; et al. High prevalence of NMDA receptor IgA/IgM antibodies in different dementia types. *Ann. Clin. Transl. Neurol.* **2014**, *1*, 822–832. [CrossRef] [PubMed]
67. Singh, A.K.; McGuirk, J.P. CAR T cells: Continuation in a revolution of immunotherapy. *Lancet Oncol.* **2020**, *21*, e168–e178. [CrossRef]
68. Perrinjaquet, C.; Desbaillets, N.; Hottinger, A.F. Neurotoxicity associated with cancer immunotherapy: Immune checkpoint inhibitors and chimeric antigen receptor T-cell therapy. *Curr. Opin. Neurol.* **2019**, *32*, 500–510. [CrossRef] [PubMed]

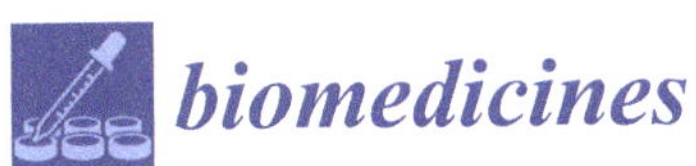 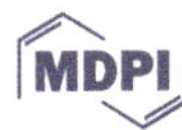

*Article*

# Phenotypic Heterogeneity among *GBA* p.R202X Carriers in Lewy Body Spectrum Disorders

**Valerio Napolioni [1,*], Carolyn A. Fredericks [1], Yongha Kim [1], Divya Channappa [2], Raiyan R. Khan [1], Lily H. Kim [1], Faria Zafar [2], Julien Couthouis [3], Guido A. Davidzon [4], Elizabeth C. Mormino [1], Aaron D. Gitler [3], Thomas J. Montine [2], Birgitt Schüle [2,†] and Michael D. Greicius [1,†]**

1 Department of Neurology and Neurological Sciences, Stanford University School of Medicine, Stanford, CA 94305, USA; carolyn.fredericks@yale.edu (C.A.F.); yonghakimis@gmail.com (Y.K.); rrk2147@columbia.edu (R.R.K.); lilyhkim@stanford.edu (L.H.K.); bmormino@stanford.edu (E.C.M.); greicius@stanford.edu (M.D.G.)
2 Department of Pathology, Stanford University School of Medicine, Stanford, CA 94305, USA; divyac2@stanford.edu (D.C.); fzafar@stanford.edu (F.Z.); tmontine@stanford.edu (T.J.M.); bschuele@stanford.edu (B.S.)
3 Department of Genetics, Stanford University School of Medicine, Stanford, CA 94305, USA; jcouthouis@ultragenyx.com (J.C.); agitler@stanford.edu (A.D.G.)
4 Department of Radiology, Stanford University School of Medicine, Stanford, CA 94305, USA; gdavidzon@stanford.edu
* Correspondence: napvale@stanford.edu; Tel.: +1-(669)-287-2586
† These authors contributed equally to this work.

**Citation:** Napolioni, V.; Fredericks, C.A.; Kim, Y.; Channappa, D.; Khan, R.R.; Kim, L.H.; Zafar, F.; Couthouis, J.; Davidzon, G.A.; Mormino, E.C.; et al. Phenotypic Heterogeneity among *GBA* p.R202X Carriers in Lewy Body Spectrum Disorders. *Biomedicines* **2022**, *10*, 160. https://doi.org/10.3390/biomedicines10010160

Academic Editors: Arnab Ghosh and Kuen-Jer Tsai

Received: 9 November 2021
Accepted: 11 January 2022
Published: 12 January 2022



**Abstract:** We describe the clinical and neuropathologic features of patients with Lewy body spectrum disorder (LBSD) carrying a nonsense variant, c.604C>T; p.R202X, in the glucocerebrosidase 1 (*GBA*) gene. While this *GBA* variant is causative for Gaucher's disease, the pathogenic role of this mutation in LBSD is unclear. Detailed neuropathologic evaluation was performed for one index case and a structured literature review of other *GBA* p.R202X carriers was conducted. Through the systematic literature search, we identified three additional reported subjects carrying the same *GBA* mutation, including one Parkinson's disease (PD) patient with early disease onset, one case with neuropathologically-verified LBSD, and one unaffected relative of a Gaucher's disease patient. Among the affected subjects carrying the *GBA* p.R202X, all males were diagnosed with Lewy body dementia, while the two females presented as PD. The clinical penetrance of *GBA* p.R202X in LBSD patients and families argues strongly for a pathogenic role for this variant, although presenting with a striking phenotypic heterogeneity of clinical and pathological features.

**Keywords:** Gaucher's disease; glucocerebrosidase; genetics; Lewy body dementia; mutation; neuropathology; Parkinson's disease; sequencing

## 1. Introduction

Intracellular aggregation of $\alpha$-synuclein is a pathological hallmark of Lewy body spectrum disorders (LBSD), a heterogeneous group of neurodegenerative diseases that includes Parkinson's disease (PD), Parkinson's disease with dementia (PDD), and dementia with Lewy bodies (DLB). Clinical manifestations of LBSD are highly diverse, with high variability in age-at-onset, disease progression, occurrence of motor symptoms, and associated cognitive impairment [1]. Genetic variants in the apolipoprotein E (*APOE*), tau (*MAPT*), $\alpha$-synuclein (*SNCA*), or glucocerebrosidase (*GBA*) genes have been associated with LBSD [1].

*GBA* variants that are causative for Gaucher's disease (GD, OMIM#230800) are a significant risk factor for PD and related $\alpha$-synucleinopathies [2,3]. Almost 500 different *GBA* variants have been associated with GD. Predominantly, recurrent or founder mutations in the *GBA* gene are present in PD patients with Ashkenazi Jewish ancestry (minor allele frequency (MAF) ranging from 10 to 31%). In contrast, *GBA* variants in non-Ashkenazi backgrounds occur at a lower MAF (ranging from 3 to 12%) and encompass a wider array of variants than the handful of founder mutations seen with Ashkenazi ancestry [4,5].

In the current work, we present detailed clinical and pathological case descriptions of two non-Ashkenazi, European-American families with LBSD who carry a rare *GBA* nonsense variant (NM_000157.3:c.604C>T, NP_000148.2:p.R202X, rs1009850780). We present other *GBA* p.R202X carriers based on a structured literature review and database search. We compare the present cases to the previously described cases and describe a pathogenic role for this mutation. Finally, considering the rapid growth of whole-exome and whole-genome sequencing in the clinical research setting, we address challenges related to identifying and interpreting *GBA* variants and considerations for clinical practice and genetic counseling.

## 2. Materials and Methods

### 2.1. Standard Protocol Approvals, Registrations, and Patient Consents

All individuals provided written informed consent before participating in this study for clinical evaluation and genetic analysis. The Stanford Institutional Review Board approved all study procedures.

### 2.2. Genetic Analysis

DNA of living subjects was collected from saliva samples, dried blood spots, or whole blood, while the DNA of the index case from Family 1 was extracted from brain-autopsy tissue.

#### 2.2.1. Family 1

The whole exome was captured using SureSelect Human All Exon (Agilent, Santa Clara, CA, USA.) and sequenced on the Illumina HiSeq2000 platform using a 2 × 100 bp Paired-End chemistry. Raw data were processed using SeqMule [6]. Variants present in the father–son pair, which the two healthy aunts did not carry, were kept, and filtered against 4449 control subjects aged 80 and older (1802 males, 2647 females) from the Alzheimer's Disease Sequencing Project (ADSP) [7]. Variants not found in any controls were annotated using the Ensembl Variant Effect Predictor toolkit [8]. Sanger sequencing of *GBA* exon 6 was performed using the long-range PCR protocol, as previously described [9]. This protocol allows the specific amplification of the *GBA* gene, avoiding the possibility of detecting false-positive variants due to the existence of the highly homologous (96%) pseudogene (*GBAP1*) located downstream from the *GBA* gene [10].

The index case's great-granddaughter and her spouse, along with their children, were tested at PerkinElmer Genomics Laboratory using an ad hoc *GBA* Gene Sequencing and Deletion/Duplication Analysis assay. Briefly, genomic DNA extracted from dried blood spots underwent long-range PCR, designed to avoid *GBAP* pseudogene contamination. A custom Agilent SureSelect enrichment kit was used to enrich the regions of interest, and NGS was performed on an Illumina system with a 2 × 100 Paired-End chemistry. NGS results were confirmed by Sanger sequence analysis.

#### 2.2.2. Family 2

Targeted sequencing of PD-related genes was conducted for the second family. Samples were tested using the PD extended NGS panel (Centogene, Rostock, Germany), which covers the entire coding region of the *ADCY5, ANO3, ATP9A, COX20, PARK7, GBA, GCH1, GNAL, GNE, KMT2B, LRRK2, MCOLN1, PRKN, PDE8B, PDGFB, PDGFRB, PINK1, PLA2G6, POLG, PRKRA, RAB12, RAB39B, SGCE, SLC20A2, SNCA, THAP1, TOR1A, VAC14, VPS13C, VPS35, XPR1,* and 3 *XDP* variants (DSC3, DSC12, and rs41438158) genes, including 10 bp of flanking intronic sequences. Raw sequence data analysis, including base calling, demultiplexing, alignment to the hg19 reference genome, and variant calling was performed using validated in-house software (Centogene, Rostock, Germany). All variants, except benign or likely benign variants, were reported.

### *2.3. Literature and Database Search*

A comprehensive literature search was carried out on PubMed using the keywords: "*GBA*", "glucocerebrosidase", "mutation", "variant", "dementia", "Parkinson" and "Lewy-body", applying the following algorithm: (*GBA* OR glucocerebrosidase) AND (dementia OR Parkinson OR Lewy-body) AND (mutation OR variant). Several publicly available genomic databases, including the Genome Aggregation Database (gnomAD) [11], the Greater Middle East (GME) Variome Project [12], and HEX (Healthy Exomes) [13], were queried to determine the frequency of *GBA* p.R202X and its ethnic stratification.

## 3. Results

### *3.1. Case Presentation*

#### 3.1.1. Family 1

The index case presented at age 73 to the Stanford Center for Memory Disorders with a three-year history of cognitive decline and parkinsonism. His wife first became concerned about him when he seemed not to understand the sequence of steps for carving a turkey at Thanksgiving. At the same time, she noted motor slowing and a shuffling in his gait. He had a history of dream enactment, an indicator for REM behavior disorder, and subsequently developed visual hallucinations, meeting the criteria for probable DLB. He died at age 74, and a brain autopsy demonstrated Lewy bodies and Lewy neurites in the midbrain, pons, and nucleus basalis of Meynert, as well as a loss of pigmented neurons in the substantia nigra, consistent with a pathologic diagnosis of diffuse Lewy body disease (Braak 6/6, NIA-AA Alzheimer's disease neuropathologic change 3/3) (Figure 1). Neurofibrillary tangles were confined to the hippocampus, with the presence of mild arteriolosclerosis. There were no signs of hippocampal sclerosis or TDP-43 inclusions.

A few years after his death, his son, then aged 60, presented to the Stanford Center for Memory Disorders, reporting a two-year history of visual hallucinations and a slow, shuffling gait, with a recent onset of dream enactment. Though he described mild difficulties with executive function, word-finding difficulties, and being less comfortable with driving, he was functionally unimpaired at the time of examination. His symptoms continued to progress slowly, so that at age 62, he was still driving locally, but dressing himself had become difficult due to bradykinesia. He made occasional errors in managing his finances and medications. He enrolled in the Stanford Alzheimer's Disease Research Center (ADRC) where he underwent research amyloid and tau PET scans. The amyloid scan was read as negative, and the tau scan showed limited tracer uptake in the medial temporal lobes that was consistent with healthy controls at this age. Quantitative PET data for this patient are shown in Figure 2.

These two individuals belong to a large Irish American family with a documented history of dementia and PD across three generations (Figure 3A). The index case had three living sisters (ages 72, 75, and 77) who were contacted to assess their neurologic status. The oldest sister was cognitively healthy following clinical and neuropsychological evaluations at the Stanford ADRC. The youngest sister was presumed unaffected based on a Clinical Dementia Rating [14] score of 0 obtained by a telephone interview. A precise clinical diagnosis for the middle sister was not possible due to a history of developmental delay (presumed secondary to scarlet fever) and confounding severe arthritis symptoms with associated immobility.

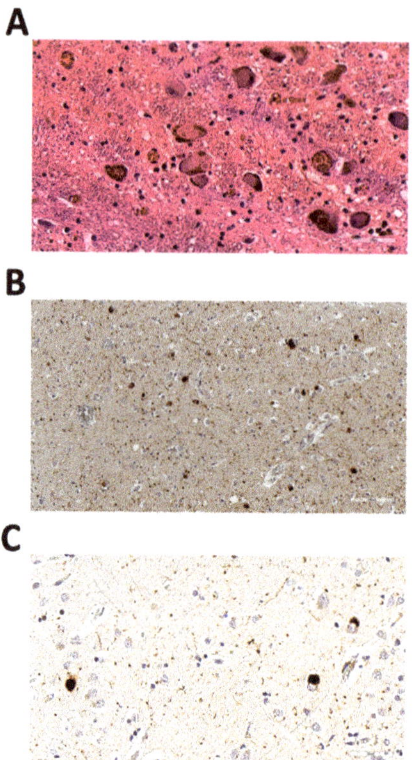


**Figure 1.** Neuropathologic examination of the index case from Family 1 showing diffuse Lewy body disease. (**A**) Hematoxylin and eosin (HE)-stained section from the locus coeruleus, 40× magnification; (**B**) phosphorylated α-synuclein [pS129]-stained section from the left amygdala, 20× magnification; (**C**) phosphorylated α-synuclein [pS129]-stained section from the right frontal cortex, 40× magnification.

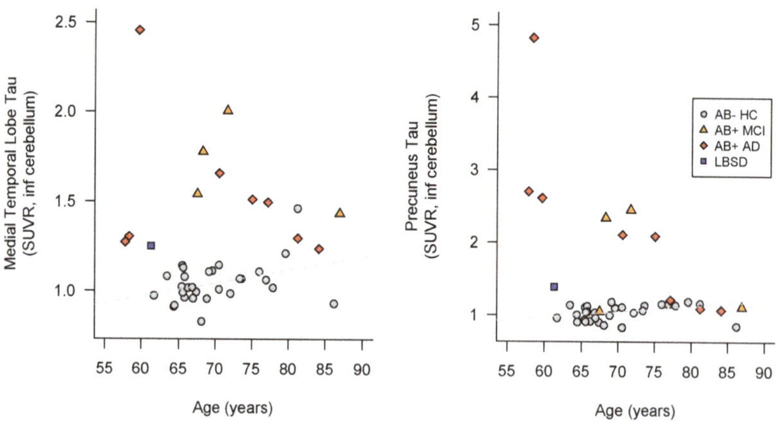


**Figure 2.** Age and tau PET scans, according to amyloid deposition positivity, in Stanford ADRC participants. Family 1: affected son of the index case is reported as a blue square (LBSD). AB = beta-amyloid; AD = Alzheimer's disease; HC = healthy control; MCI = mild cognitive impairment.

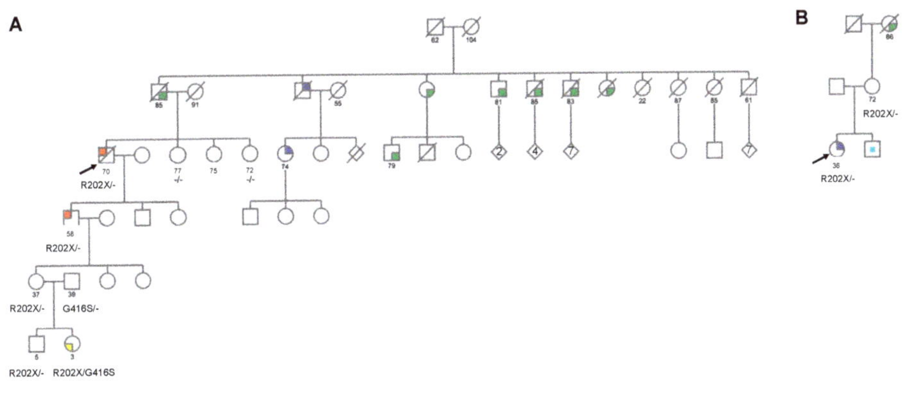


**Figure 3.** Pedigree of the reported LBSD families. Family 1 (**panel** (**A**)) and Family 2 (**panel** (**B**)). Arrows indicate the index cases.

Notably, since the initial evaluation of the index case, his granddaughter gave birth to a girl who was diagnosed with neuronopathic-type GD Type III at age 3 (Figure 3A). Genetic testing disclosed the presence of compound heterozygous *GBA* genotype (p.R202X/p.G416S), with the p.G416S mutation (NM_000157.3:c.1246G>A, rs121908311) inherited from the father. Both the mother and the unaffected brother (age 5) were found to be carriers of *GBA* p.R202X (Figure 3A).

#### 3.1.2. Family 2

At 36 years of age, the index case, of British-American ancestry, developed a left arm tremor, reduced left-arm swing, and balance problems. She was diagnosed with early-onset, tremor-predominant PD at age 38. Additional symptoms included anxiety and depression, constipation, and urinary urgency. She was responsive to dopaminergic therapy. She scored a 27/30 (normal range) on the Montreal Cognitive Assessment [15] at age 43. She underwent deep brain stimulation at age 45. Her mother is a carrier of the *GBA* p.R202X variant but did not show symptoms at age 72. Her younger brother has reported tremors, but he has not been formally evaluated. Her maternal grandmother developed unspecified dementia in her late 70s, with family noting that her "conversations went in circles". In the end, she could neither prepare meals, nor understand dates or holidays. She died at age 86.

### *3.2. Identification of GBA p.R202X Variant*

Whole-exome (WES) and targeted sequencing of PD genes in two unrelated European-American families with index cases presenting with LBSD revealed the presence of a rare *GBA* stop-gain variant (NM_000157.3:c.604C>T, NP_000148.2:p.Arg202Ter, rs1009850780, gnomAD [11] v.2.1.1, global MAF = $9.02 \times 10^{-6}$) in all affected subjects, the granddaughter of the index case in Family 1, along with her children, and the unaffected mother of the index case in Family 2 (Figure 3). The variant was not found among the two unaffected sisters of the Family 1 index case, nor in any Alzheimer's Disease Sequencing Project (ADSP) [7] controls aged 80 and above.

Family 1 members were sequenced using both WES and targeted-sequencing approaches since the diagnosis of GD in the 3-year-old great-granddaughter of the index case prompted independent clinical genetic testing.

WES of the four Family 1 members (the index case and three of his first-degree relatives, including the affected son) yielded 252 million reads for a total of approximatively 25.2 Gbps, resulting in an average depth of target coverage of 68X per sample. The joint variant calling by SeqMule [6] yielded 54,104 variants that were filtered according to their presence in both affected subjects and their absence in the two healthy sisters. We retained only the non-synonymous (missense, frameshift, and nonsense) variants with a minor allele frequency (MAF) < 0.05 that were not present in healthy ADSP [7] controls over 80 years of age. The final list included 32 candidate variants, with the *GBA* p.R202X being the only variant predicted to have a high-impact consequence. A literature search for the other 31 candidate variants did not suggest any possible biological link with the affected subjects' phenotype. Sanger sequencing confirmed *GBA* p.R202X in the affected son of the index case and its absence from the two unaffected siblings (Figure 4). No DNA was available for *GBA* p.R202X Sanger sequencing of the index case.

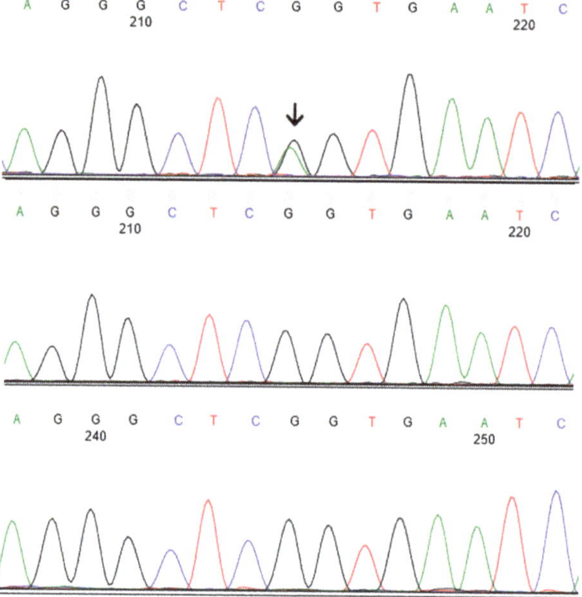


**Figure 4.** Sanger sequencing results of *GBA* p.R202X in Family 1. The top panel shows the presence of the G/A (heterozygote) genotype in the affected son of the index case and its absence from the two unaffected sisters. No DNA was available for *GBA* p.R202X Sanger sequencing of the index case.

Targeted sequencing of PD genes revealed the presence of *GBA* p.R202X in both Family 2 members.

### 3.3. Literature Search of GBA p.R202X Variant Carriers

The systematic literature search for other *GBA* p.R202X carriers, carried out in June 2021, yielded 812 articles published between 1993 and 2021, 190 of which were review articles. We adopted the *GBA* mutation nomenclature according to the Human Genome Variation Society (http://hgvs.org, accessed on 11 October 2021); the old nomenclature was based on amino-acid residue numbering, which excludes the first 39 amino acids of the leader sequence, thus defining the mutation as p.Arg163Ter (p.R163X).

We identified three additional reported subjects carrying the same *GBA* mutation, including one PD patient with early-onset illness beginning at 47 years [16–19], one case with neuropathologically-verified LBSD [1], and one unaffected relative of a GD patient [20]. Only two non-Finnish European subjects (one Swedish and one Estonian) from gnomAD v.2.1.1 were reported to be heterozygote carriers of *GBA* p.R202X (gnomAD reports the age, between 55 and 60, for one of the two carriers). We did not find additional *GBA* p.R202X carriers in the Greater Middle East (GME) Variome Project [12] or the Healthy Exomes (HEX) database [13].

We describe the clinical and demographic characteristics of the seven *GBA* p.R202X carriers in Table 1.

**Table 1.** Clinical and demographic characteristics of *GBA* p.R202X heterozygote carriers.

| Study | Diagnosis | Sex | Age-at-Onset | Age-at-Death or Last Assessed Normal | Autopsy-Confirmed | *APOE* Genotype | Ancestry |
|---|---|---|---|---|---|---|---|
| Present—Family 1 | LBD | M | 70 | 74 | Y | 3/3 | Irish-American |
| Present—Family 1 | LBSD | M | 58 | - | - | 3/4 | Irish-American |
| Present—Family 2 | PD | F | 36 | - | - | 3/3 | British-American |
| Present—Family 2 | Unaffected | F | - | 72 | - | - | British-American |
| Irwin, D.J., et al. [1] | LBSD | M | 50 | 57 | Y | 3/3 | NA |
| Mata, I.F., et al.[16], Sidransky, E., et al. [17], Chahine, L.M., et al. [18], Davis, M.Y., et al. [19] | PD | F | 47 | - | - | - | African-American |
| Barrett, M.J., et al. [20] | - | - | - | - | - | - | NA |

M = Male; F = Female; Y = Yes; LBD = Lewy body dementia; LBSD = Lewy body spectrum disorder; NA = not available; PD = Parkinson's disease.

## 4. Discussion

The presence of the *GBA* p.R202X mutation in both LBSD families argues strongly for a pathogenic role for this variant in LBSD, although with phenotypic heterogeneity. *GBA* p.R202X is a loss-of-function variant that leads to haploinsufficiency, and we would anticipate high penetrance for disease. However, we found profound phenotypic variability among affected family members in the two families, demonstrating rather heterogeneous effects of this *GBA* variant on LBSD. The clinical presentation in the affected *GBA* p.R202X carriers ranged from early-onset PD for the index case of Family 2 (age-at-onset 37 years) to neuropathologically confirmed late-onset DLB for the index case of Family 1 (age-at-onset 70 years). Moreover, the cognitively healthy, 72-year-old mother of the index case in Family 2 also carries the mutation. Such phenotypic heterogeneity provides strong support for the idea that other genetic modifier loci strongly impact the phenotypic presentation of LBSD. For instance, we can speculate that the significant difference in age-at-onset for the two male cases in Family 1 (70 years vs. 58 years) could be attributable to the presence of *APOE**4 allele in the earlier onset subject. *APOE**4 is now a confirmed risk factor for DLB, independent of any co-morbid Alzheimer's disease pathology [21]. Nevertheless, we cannot exclude the possibility of other biological factors, not detectable by targeted NGS, as the basis of the phenotypic heterogeneity characterizing the affected members of the two families described here. Indeed, it has been shown that telomere length may influence the occurrence of dementia in PD patients [22]. Additionally, several studies have argued for the existence of genetic modifiers of PD clinical presentation, such as *TMEM106B* [23], *SCNA* [24], and *COMT* [25].

Similarly, sex may play a role. Among the affected subjects carrying the *GBA* p.R202X variant, all males were diagnosed with LBD, while the two affected females presented as PD. This is not entirely surprising, as previous studies have highlighted sex-specific differences in the phenotype of *GBA* mutation carriers. While most men presented with DLB, most women presented with PD [26]; moreover, males with *GBA*-associated PD have a higher burden of trait anxiety and depression than females [27].

Undoubtedly, a deeper biological characterization of the two families described here, obtained by performing a wider genomic investigation (e.g., by whole-genome sequencing and structural variation typing), eventually coupled with the analysis of epigenomic changes (e.g., telomere length and methylation profiling), would help to identify new modifiers of clinical phenotypes in LBSD.

Despite the association of recurrent *GBA* mutations with PD predominantly in the Ashkenazi Jewish population [4], the presented results and literature search both point to a non-Ashkenazi origin for this mutation. However, the *GBA* locus is characterized by frequent recombination events involving both gene conversion and reciprocal recombination [10]. As a result, it is difficult to attribute *GBA* p.R202X to a specific ethnic background. Notably, most studies and clinical tests are based on the genotyping of a limited number of mutations that are most relevant for the Ashkenazi Jewish population. The sequencing of the whole gene will be of paramount relevance in determining *GBA* variants in other ethnic groups that otherwise would be missed.

In this context, special attention must be paid when choosing the genotyping method of *GBA*. Since the coding region of the *GBA* gene is 96% homologous to *GBAP*, long amplicons are generally needed to ensure that only the *GBA* gene is being targeted when genotyping. Moreover, the frequency of *GBA-GBAP1* complex rearrangements makes next-generation sequencing (NGS) analysis of *GBA* challenging [28], and adequate strategies (such as *GBA*-specific long-range PCR for library preparation, followed by *GBA*-specific alignment) must be adopted to avoid misdetection of *GBA* recombinant mutations. Because of these challenges, we suspect that the impact of *GBA* mutations on LBSD may have been underestimated in large genetic studies that employed NGS (whole-exome and whole-genome sequencing) and SNP-array-based techniques. Targeted *GBA*-specific sequencing in patients reporting LBSD in the future will help to clarify the prevalence of this highly significant class of pathogenic mutations.

In clinical practice, clinical genetic testing is often performed as a genotyping panel for the most common *GBA* variants (e.g., Invitae GBA carrier screening). In this clinical context, we expect that *GBA* variants that are not commonly present in the Ashkenazi population will be undetected, meaning that clinicians may miss rarer, causal variants in other ethnic backgrounds, including the *GBA* p.R202X described here.

The cases described in the present study represent the first clinical–genetic report on the rare *GBA* p.R202X variant in LBSD. The phenotypic heterogeneity seen in individuals carrying this variant, even within a single family, is striking. Our report also raises the possibility of incomplete penetrance, as the mother of the index case in Family 2 carries the variant but has thus far remained clinically unaffected. These cases emphasize the need for targeted *GBA*-specific sequencing in patients with family histories of LBSD or PD to capture all disease-relevant variants.

**Author Contributions:** Conceptualization, V.N., B.S. and M.D.G.; methodology, V.N., B.S. and M.D.G.; formal analysis, V.N., Y.K., D.C., R.R.K., F.Z., J.C. and T.J.M.; investigation, V.N., Y.K., D.C., R.R.K., L.H.K., F.Z. and J.C.; resources, E.C.M., T.J.M., B.S. and M.D.G.; data curation, V.N., Y.K., R.R.K., F.Z. and G.A.D.; writing—original draft preparation, V.N.; writing—review and editing, C.A.F., E.C.M., T.J.M., B.S. and M.D.G.; supervision, V.N., E.C.M., A.D.G., T.J.M., B.S. and M.D.G.; funding acquisition, B.S. and M.D.G. All authors have read and agreed to the published version of the manuscript.

**Funding:** This research was funded by The Iqbal Farrukh and Asad Jamal Fund; NIH-P30 AG066515; NIH-R01 AG060747.

**Institutional Review Board Statement:** The study was conducted according to the guidelines of the Declaration of Helsinki and approved by the Stanford Institutional Review Board.

**Informed Consent Statement:** Informed consent was obtained from all subjects involved in the study.

**Data Availability Statement:** The data presented in this study are available on request from the corresponding author. The data are not publicly available due to privacy policies and Terms and Conditions agreements.

**Conflicts of Interest:** The authors declare no conflict of interest.

## References

1. Irwin, D.J.; Grossman, M.; Weintraub, D.; Hurtig, H.I.; Duda, J.E.; Xie, S.X.; Lee, E.B.; Van Deerlin, V.M.; Lopez, O.L.; Kofler, J.K.; et al. Neuropathological and genetic correlates of survival and dementia onset in synucleinopathies: A retrospective analysis. *Lancet Neurol.* **2017**, *16*, 55–65. [CrossRef]
2. Riboldi, G.M.; Di Fonzo, A.B. Gaucher Disease, and Parkinson's Disease: From Genetic to Clinic to New Therapeutic Approaches. *Cells* **2019**, *8*, 364. [CrossRef]
3. Do, J.; McKinney, C.; Sharma, P.; Sidransky, E. Glucocerebrosidase and its relevance to Parkinson disease. *Mol. Neurodegener.* **2019**, *14*, 36. [CrossRef] [PubMed]
4. Zhang, Y.; Shu, L.; Sun, Q.; Zhou, X.; Pan, H.; Guo, J.; Tang, B. Integrated Genetic Analysis of Racial Differences of Common GBA Variants in Parkinson's Disease: A Meta-Analysis. *Front. Mol. Neurosci.* **2018**, *11*, 43. [CrossRef] [PubMed]
5. Pastores, G.M.; Hughes, D.A. Gaucher disease. In *GeneReviews™*; Pagon, R.A., Adam, M.P., Bird, T.D., Dolan, C.R., Fong, C.T., Stephens, K., Eds.; University of Washington: Seattle, WA, USA, 2000.
6. Guo, Y.; Ding, X.; Shen, Y.; Lyon, G.J.; Wang, K. SeqMule: Automated pipeline for analysis of human exome/genome sequencing data. *Sci. Rep.* **2015**, *5*, 14283. [CrossRef] [PubMed]
7. Beecham, G.W.; Bis, J.; Martin, E.; Choi, S.-H.; DeStefano, A.L.; van Duijn, C.; Fornage, M.; Gabriel, S.; Koboldt, D.; Larson, D.; et al. The Alzheimer's Disease Sequencing Project: Study design and sample selection. *Neurol. Genet.* **2017**, *3*, e194. [CrossRef] [PubMed]
8. McLaren, W.; Gil, L.; Hunt, S.E.; Riat, H.S.; Ritchie, G.R.S.; Thormann, A.; Flicek, P.; Cunningham, F. The Ensembl Variant Effect Predictor. *Genome Biol.* **2016**, *17*, 122. [CrossRef] [PubMed]
9. Finckh, U.; Seeman, P.; Von Widdern, O.C.; Rolfs, A. Simple PCR amplification of the entire glucocerebrosidase gene (GBA) coding region for diagnostic sequence analysis. *DNA Seq.* **1998**, *8*, 349–356. [CrossRef] [PubMed]
10. Tayebi, N.; Stubblefield, B.K.; Park, J.; Orvisky, E.; Walker, J.M.; LaMarca, M.E.; Sidransky, E. Reciprocal and Nonreciprocal Recombination at the Glucocerebrosidase Gene Region: Implications for Complexity in Gaucher Disease. *Am. J. Hum. Genet.* **2003**, *72*, 519–534. [CrossRef] [PubMed]
11. Karczewski, K.J.; Francioli, L.C.; Tiao, G.; Cummings, B.B.; Alföldi, J.; Wang, Q.; Collins, R.L.; Laricchia, K.M.; Ganna, A.; Birnbaum, D.P.; et al. The mutational constraint spectrum quantified from variation in 141,456 humans. *Nature* **2020**, *581*, 434–443. [CrossRef] [PubMed]
12. Scott, E.M.; Halees, A.; Itan, Y.; Spencer, E.G.; He, Y.; Azab, M.A.; Gabriel, S.B.; Belkadi, A.; Boisson, B.; Abel, L.; et al. Characterization of Greater Middle Eastern genetic variation for enhanced disease gene discovery. *Nat. Genet.* **2016**, *48*, 1071–1076. [CrossRef]
13. Guerreiro, R.; Sassi, C.; Gibbs, J.R.; Edsall, C.; Hernandez, D.; Brown, K.; Lupton, M.K.; Parkinnen, L.; Ansorge, O.; Hodges, A.; et al. A comprehensive assessment of benign genetic variability for neurodegenerative disorders. *bioRxiv* **2018**, 270686. [CrossRef]
14. Hughes, C.P.; Berg, L.; Danziger, W.L.; Coben, L.A.; Martin, R.L. A New Clinical Scale for the Staging of Dementia. *Br. J. Psychiatry* **1982**, *140*, 566–572. [CrossRef] [PubMed]
15. Nasreddine, Z.S.; Phillips, N.A.; Bédirian, V.; Charbonneau, S.; Whitehead, V.; Collin, I.; Cummings, J.L.; Chertkow, H. The Montreal Cognitive Assessment, MoCA: A Brief Screening Tool For Mild Cognitive Impairment. *J. Am. Geriatr. Soc.* **2005**, *53*, 695–699. [CrossRef] [PubMed]
16. Mata, I.F.; Leverenz, J.; Weintraub, D.; Trojanowski, J.Q.; Chen-Plotkin, A.; Van Deerlin, V.M.; Ritz, B.; Rausch, R.; Do, S.A.F.; Wood-Siverio, C.; et al. GBA Variants are associated with a distinct pattern of cognitive deficits in Parkinson's disease. *Mov. Disord.* **2016**, *31*, 95–102. [CrossRef] [PubMed]
17. Sidransky, E.; Nalls, M.A.; Aasly, J.O.; Aharon-Peretz, J.; Annesi, G.; Barbosa, E.R.; Bar-Shira, A.; Berg, D.; Bras, J.; Brice, A.; et al. Multicenter Analysis of Glucocerebrosidase Mutations in Parkinson's Disease. *N. Engl. J. Med.* **2009**, *361*, 1651–1661. [CrossRef]
18. Chahine, L.M.; Qiang, J.; Ashbridge, E.; Minger, J.; Yearout, D.; Horn, S.; Colcher, A.; Hurtig, H.I.; Lee, V.M.-Y.; Van Deerlin, V.M.; et al. Clinical and Biochemical Differences in Patients Having Parkinson Disease with vs WithoutGBAMutations. *JAMA Neurol.* **2013**, *70*, 852–858. [CrossRef]
19. Davis, M.Y.; Johnson, C.O.; Leverenz, J.B.; Weintraub, D.; Trojanowski, J.Q.; Chen-Plotkin, A.; Van Deerlin, V.M.; Quinn, J.F.; Chung, K.A.; Peterson-Hiller, A.L.; et al. Association of GBA Mutations and the E326K Polymorphism with Motor and Cognitive Progression in Parkinson Disease. *JAMA Neurol.* **2016**, *73*, 1217–1224. [CrossRef]
20. Barrett, M.J.; Giraldo, P.; Capablo, J.L.; Alfonso, P.; Irun, P.; Garcia-Rodriguez, B.; Pocovi, M.; Pastores, G.M. Greater risk of parkinsonism associated with non-N370S GBA1 mutations. *J. Inherit. Metab. Dis.* **2013**, *36*, 575–580. [CrossRef]

21. Tsuang, D.; Leverenz, J.B.; Lopez, O.L.; Hamilton, R.L.; Bennett, D.A.; Schneider, J.A.; Buchman, A.S.; Larson, E.B.; Crane, P.K.; Kaye, J.A.; et al. APOE ε4 increases risk for dementia in pure synucleinopathies. *JAMA Neurol.* **2013**, *70*, 223–228. [CrossRef]
22. Levstek, T.; Redenšek, S.; Trošt, M.; Dolžan, V.; Podkrajšek, K. Assessment of the Telomere Length and Its Effect on the Symptomatology of Parkinson's Disease. *Antioxidants* **2021**, *10*, 137. [CrossRef] [PubMed]
23. Tropea, T.F.; Mak, J.; Guo, M.H.; Xie, S.X.; Suh, E.; Rick, J.; Siderowf, A.; Weintraub, D.; Grossman, M.; Irwin, D.; et al. TMEM106B Effect on cognition in Parkinson disease and frontotemporal dementia. *Ann. Neurol.* **2019**, *85*, 801–811. [CrossRef] [PubMed]
24. Sampedro, F.; Marin-Lahoz, J.; Martinez-Horta, S.; Pagonabarraga, J.; Kulisevsky, J. Cortical Thinning Associated with Age and CSF Biomarkers in Early Parkinson's Disease is Modified by the SCNA rs356181 Polymorphism. *Neurodegener. Dis.* **2018**, *18*, 233–238. [CrossRef] [PubMed]
25. Chung, J.; Ushakova, A.; Doitsidou, M.; Tzoulis, C.; Tysnes, O.-B.; Dalen, I.; Pedersen, K.F.; Alves, G.; Maple-Grødem, J. The impact of common genetic variants in cognitive decline in the first seven years of Parkinson's disease: A longitudinal observational study. *Neurosci. Lett.* **2021**, *764*, 136243. [CrossRef]
26. Gámez-Valero, A.; Prada-Dacasa, P.; Santos, C.; Adame-Castillo, C.; Campdelacreu, J.; Reñé, R.; Gascón-Bayarri, J.; Ispierto, L.; Álvarez, R.; Ariza, A.; et al. GBA Mutations Are Associated with Earlier Onset and Male Sex in Dementia with Lewy Bodies. *Mov. Disord.* **2016**, *31*, 1066–1070. [CrossRef] [PubMed]
27. Swan, M.; Doan, N.; Ortega, R.A.; Barrett, M.; Nichols, W.; Ozelius, L.; Soto-Valencia, J.; Boschung, S.; Deik, A.; Sarva, H.; et al. Neuropsychiatric characteristics of GBA-associated Parkinson disease. *J. Neurol. Sci.* **2016**, *370*, 63–69. [CrossRef]
28. Zampieri, S.; Cattarossi, S.; Bembi, B.; Dardis, A. GBA Analysis in Next-Generation Era: Pitfalls, Challenges, and Possible Solutions. *J. Mol. Diagn.* **2017**, *19*, 733–741. [CrossRef]

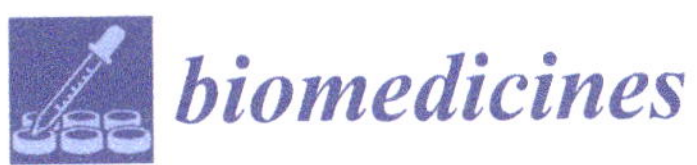

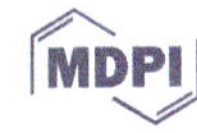

*Article*

# Biomarkers Analysis and Clinical Manifestations in Comorbid Creutzfeldt–Jakob Disease: A Retrospective Study in 215 Autopsy Cases

**Nikol Jankovska [1], Robert Rusina [2], Jiri Keller [3,4], Jaromir Kukal [5], Magdalena Bruzova [1], Eva Parobkova [1], Tomas Olejar [1] and Radoslav Matej [1,6,7,*]**

1 Department of Pathology and Molecular Medicine, Third Faculty of Medicine, Charles University and Thomayer University Hospital, 140 59 Prague, Czech Republic; nikol.jankovska@ftn.cz (N.J.); magdalena.bruzova@ftn.cz (M.B.); eva.parobkova@ftn.cz (E.P.); tomas.olejar@ftn.cz (T.O.)
2 Department of Neurology, Third Faculty of Medicine, Charles University and Thomayer University Hospital, 140 59 Prague, Czech Republic; robert.rusina@lf3.cuni.cz
3 Department of Neurology, Third Faculty of Medicine, Charles University and University Hospital Kralovske Vinohrady, 100 34 Prague, Czech Republic; jiri.keller@lf3.cuni.cz
4 Department of Radiology, Na Homolce Hospital, 150 00 Prague, Czech Republic
5 Faculty of Nuclear Sciences and Physical Engineering, Czech Technical University, 115 19 Prague, Czech Republic; jaromir.kukal@fjfi.cvut.cz
6 Department of Pathology, First Faculty of Medicine, Charles University and General University Hospital, 128 00 Prague, Czech Republic
7 Department of Pathology, Third Faculty of Medicine, Charles University and University Hospital Kralovske Vinohrady, 100 34 Prague, Czech Republic
* Correspondence: radoslav.matej@ftn.cz; Tel.: +420-261-083-741

**Citation:** Jankovska, N.; Rusina, R.; Keller, J.; Kukal, J.; Bruzova, M.; Parobkova, E.; Olejar, T.; Matej, R. Biomarkers Analysis and Clinical Manifestations in Comorbid Creutzfeldt–Jakob Disease: A Retrospective Study in 215 Autopsy Cases. *Biomedicines* **2022**, *10*, 680. https://doi.org/10.3390/biomedicines10030680

Academic Editor: Arnab Ghosh

Received: 8 February 2022
Accepted: 14 March 2022
Published: 16 March 2022



**Abstract:** Creutzfeldt–Jakob disease (CJD), the most common human prion disorder, may occur as "pure" neurodegeneration with isolated prion deposits in the brain tissue; however, comorbid cases with different concomitant neurodegenerative diseases have been reported. This retrospective study examined correlations of clinical, neuropathological, molecular-genetic, immunological, and neuroimaging biomarkers in pure and comorbid CJD. A total of 215 patients have been diagnosed with CJD during the last ten years by the Czech National Center for Prion Disorder Surveillance. Data were collected from all patients with respect to diagnostic criteria for probable CJD, including clinical description, EEG, MRI, and CSF findings. A detailed neuropathological analysis uncovered that only 11.16% were "pure" CJD, while 62.79% had comorbid tauopathy, 20.47% had Alzheimer's disease, 3.26% had frontotemporal lobar degeneration, and 2.33% had synucleinopathy. The comorbid subgroup analysis revealed that tauopathy was linked to putaminal hyperintensity on MRIs, and AD mainly impacted the age of onset, hippocampal atrophy on MRIs, and beta-amyloid levels in the CSF. The retrospective data analysis found a surprisingly high proportion of comorbid neuropathologies; only 11% of cases were verified as "pure" CJD, i.e., lacking hallmarks of other neurodegenerations. Comorbid neuropathologies can impact disease manifestation and can complicate the clinical diagnosis of CJD.

**Keywords:** Creutzfeldt–Jakob disease; comorbid neuropathology; Alzheimer's disease; tauopathy; MRI; beta-amyloid

## 1. Introduction

Creutzfeldt-Jakob disease (CJD), the most common human prion disorder [1], is neuropathologically characterized by spongiform encephalopathy involving the subcortical grey matter of the cerebral and cerebellar cortex [2]. It can also be described as encephalopathy with protease-resistant prion protein (PrP) immunoreactivity in the form of plaques, diffuse synaptic, and a patchy/perivacuolar pattern [2].

Three types of CJD are distinguished based on different etiologies [3]: in most countries, sporadic (sCJD) is the dominant form, followed by genetic (gCJD) and acquired CJD, which has two additional subtypes, i.e., iatrogenic (iCJD) [4] and variant (vCJD) [5]. A worldwide incidence of 1–2 cases of sCJD per million inhabitants is commonly reported [6]. The situation in the Czech Republic is similar, but with a slightly higher proportion of genetic cases [7].

Clinical manifestation (criteria for possible CJD) typically includes dementia with pyramidal and/or extrapyramidal signs, cerebellar ataxia, visuospatial dysfunction, myoclonus, and akinetic mutism [8]. Typical biomarkers can help establish the final clinical diagnosis: positive 14-3-3 protein in the cerebrospinal fluid (CSF), generalized periodic EEG patterns, MRI hyperintensities on FLAIR/DWI sequences in the basal ganglia (putamen and caudate) or cortical areas, i.e., cortical ribboning (criteria for probable CJD) and positive results from CSF real-time quaking-induced conversion (RT-QuIC) analysis [8]. Definite CJD is confirmed by neuropathological and immunohistochemistry examination of brain tissue [8].

CJD has long been considered a homogeneous clinical-neuropathological entity. There is, however, increasing evidence of a frequent co-occurrence of other neurodegenerative diseases in CJD cases. Kovacs et al. already published data on the relatively high incidence of tau co-pathology in CJD [9], while Rossi et al. monitored comorbid cases of CJD and Alzheimer's disease (CJD/AD) and CJD with primary age-related tauopathy (CJD/PART) [10].

The aim of our study was to retrospectively analyse neuropathological findings from autopsy specimens in a large nationwide study of definite CJD cases collected over ten years by the Czech National Center for Human Prion Disorder Surveillance and compare them to clinical, radiological, genetic, and biochemical data. We hypothesised that neuropathological comorbidities could be more frequent than previously thought and could impact disease manifestation or neuroimaging/biochemical results. To our best knowledge, this is the first comprehensive study comparing non-comorbid to comorbid CJD cases based on clinical-neuropathological correlations.

## 2. Materials and Methods

Postmortem confirmed CJD cases resulting from ten years of systematic prion surveillance and available clinical data, neuroimaging findings, and results of neuropathological, molecular-genetic, and immunological investigations were analysed with statistical comparison of non-comorbid versus comorbid cases.

### 2.1. Patients

A total of 215 patients diagnosed with definite CJD (age range 40–87 years, median 66 years) using current diagnostic criteria were neuropathologically examined, and the presence of $PrP^{Sc}$ in brain tissue was confirmed by both western-blot and immunohistochemical methods. The genetic screening revealed 193 sporadic and 22 genetic cases that mostly had the E200K mutation in the *PRNP* gene, but the *D178* and *P102L* mutations and five octapeptide repeat insertions were also found. Clinical as well as neuroimaging data (CT or MRI) from all patients were analysed; moreover, in most cases, EEG and CSF findings were also available.

Characteristics of individual subgroups of pure or comorbid CJD are summarised in Table 1. The table contains detailed information on age, gender, codon 129 methionine and/or valine polymorphism, eventual *PRNP* mutation, specification of the type (type 1 or 2) of abnormal $PrP^{Sc}$ isoform, protein 14-3-3 positivity, CSF neurodegenerative biomarkers (h-tau, p-tau, and Aβ), clinical data regarding dementia, pyramidal and/or extrapyramidal signs, visuospatial or cerebellar dysfunction, myoclonus, and akinetic mutism. Supplementary Material also contains EEG and MRI findings. The data were analysed with respect for patient privacy and with the consent of the local Ethics Committee of the Institute of Clinical and Experimental Medicine in Prague and Thomayer University Hospital, No G-19-18, obtained 26 June 2017.

**Table 1.** Summary of available epidemiological, neuropathological, immunological and genetic data in non-comorbid vs. comorbid CJD cases. The first column shows the neuropathological diagnosis of patients, second shows the total number of cases in each group, third indicate the gender distribution (female/male). In the fourth column is age range with median age (in years) and the last two columns show methionine/valine polymorphism and presence of 14-3-3 protein in cerebrospinal fluid examinated by western blot.

| Diagnosis | No. of Cases | Sex | Age (Years) | Etiology | Genotype | 14-3-3 Protein in CSF |
|---|---|---|---|---|---|---|
| CJD | 24 | 24× F | 40–78 (median 60) | 21× sCJD<br>3× gCJD | 17× MM<br>4× MV<br>3× VV | 17× positive<br>7× negative |
| CJD/tau | 135 | 73× F<br>62× M | 49–87 (median 65) | 119× sCJD<br>16× gCJD | 85× MM<br>34× MV<br>16× VV | 106× positive<br>29× negative |
| CJD/AD | 44 | 24× F<br>20× M | 56–85 (median 71) | 41× sCJD<br>3× gCJD | 27× MM<br>8× MV<br>9× VV | 38× positive<br>6× negative |
| CJD/FTLD | 7 | 5× F<br>2× M | 55–78 (median 67) | 7× sCJD | 4× MM<br>3× VV | 6× positive<br>1× negative |
| CJD/synuclein | 5 | 3× F<br>2× M | 59–76 (median 71) | 5× sCJD | 3× MM<br>2× VV | 4× positive<br>1× negative |

F—female, M—male, MM—Methionine/Methionine polymorphism, MV—Methionine/Valine polymorphism, VV—Valine/Valine polymorphism.

### 2.2. *Tissue Samples*

Brain tissue samples were fixed for 3–4 weeks in buffered 10% formalin. Selected tissue blocks, using a standardized protocol [11], were then embedded in paraffin using an automatic tissue processor. Five-µm-thick sections were prepared and stained with hematoxylin-eosin, Klüver-Barrera, and silver impregnation methods. Thirty-six representative blocks from standardized regions were chosen for analysis.

### 2.3. *Immunofluorescence and Immunohistochemistry*

Briefly, 5-µm-thick sections of formalin-fixed and paraffin-embedded tissue samples were deparaffinized and then incubated with primary antibodies for 20 min at room temperature. For Aβ and $PrP^{Sc}$ antibody staining, 96% formic acid was applied prior to the primary antibody. A second layer for light microscopy visualization, consisting of secondary horseradish peroxidase-conjugated antibody (EnVision FLEX/HRP, Dako M822, Glostrup, Denmark), was applied for 20 min at room temperature. The samples were then incubated with DAB (Substrate-Chromogen Solution, Dako K3468, Glostrup, Denmark) for 10 min to visualize the reaction. Mayer's Hematoxylin Solution was used as a counterstain.

For confocal microscopy, secondary antibodies conjugated to Alexa Fluor® (see below) were used. Paraffin sections were also treated with 20× TrueBlack® (Biotium 23007, Fremont, CA, USA) diluted in 1× 70% alcohol to quench lipofuscin autofluorescence.

#### 2.3.1. Primary Antibodies

For immunohistochemistry, 5-µm-thick sections of formalin-fixed and paraffin-embedded tissue were selected from the hippocampal region, including the entorhinal and transentorhinal cortex. These were incubated with primary antibodies against the following antigens: (1) PrP (1:8000, mouse monoclonal, clone 12F10; Bertin Pharma A03221, Bordeaux, France), (2) PrP (1:3000, mouse monoclonal, clone 6H8; Prionics 7500996, Schlieren, Switzerland), (3) Aβ (1:1000, mouse monoclonal, clone 6F/3D; Dako M0872, Glostrup, Denmark),

(4) Phospho-Tau (Ser202, Thr205) Monoclonal Antibody (1:500, mouse monoclonal, clone AT8; Thermo Fisher Scientific MN1020, Waltham, ME, USA), (5) Ubiquitin (1:500, rabbit polyclonal; Dako Z0458, Lakeside, UK), (6) Phospho TDP-43 (1:4000, mouse monoclonal, clone 11-9; Cosmo Bio TIP-PTD-M01, Carlsbad, CA, USA), (7) Alpha-Synuclein (1:1000, mouse monoclonal, clone 5G4; Dianova NDG-76506, Barcelona, Spain).

#### 2.3.2. Secondary Antibodies

Detection of immunostaining was carried out using horseradish peroxidase–diaminobenzidine (see above) for immunohistochemistry and secondary antibodies conjugated with Alexa Fluor® 488 (1:1000, donkey anti-rabbit, H + L IgG, Thermo Fischer Scientific, Waltham, ME, USA) and Alexa Fluor® 568 (1:1000, donkey anti-mouse, H + L IgG, Thermo Fischer Scientific, Waltham, ME, USA) for immunofluorescence staining. Slides incubated with only the secondary antibody were used as specificity controls.

### *2.4. Microscopy Evaluation*

#### 2.4.1. Light Microscopy

Samples were examined, and the results of immunohistochemical methods were classified according to currently valid neuropathological criteria for individual neurodegenerative diseases. Moreover, Alzheimer's disease was subsequently scored using the National Institute on Aging–Alzheimer's Association (NIA-AA) consensus scheme [12,13], and dementia with Lewy bodies (DLB) using the DLB consensus criteria [14] with a determination of the Braak stage [15].

#### 2.4.2. Confocal Microscopy

Co-expression of pathogenic protein aggregates was imaged using a Leica TCS SP5 confocal fluorescent laser scanning microscope (Leica Microsystems Inc., Wetzlar, Germany). The HCX PL APO objective was chosen with 60× magnification and an oil immersion pinhole of 1 AU. Anti-rabbit donkey IgG secondary antibody was conjugated to Alexa Fluor® 488 and excited at 488 nm from a 65 mW multi-line argon laser, whereas anti-mouse donkey IgG conjugated to Alexa Fluor® 568 donkey was excited at 561 nm from a 20 mW DPSS laser.

### *2.5. Immunological Methods*

#### 2.5.1. CSF Analysis

After a single lumbar puncture and collection, CSF samples were centrifuged at 5000 RPM for 5 min and stored in polypropylene tubes at −80 °C in aliquots to avoid thawing and refreezing until the analysis.

The presence of protein 14-3-3 beta (14-3-3β) was determined using a standardized western blot protocol (adapted from Green et al. [16]) and EURO-CJD standards, with stringent control quality. Briefly, samples in doublets were separated using sodium-dodecyl sulfate-polyacrylamide gel electrophoresis (SDS-PAGE) and blotted onto nitrocellulose membranes. For detection of the 14-3-3β, polyclonal antibody K-19 (1:1000, cat. #sc-629; Santa Cruz Biotechnology, Santa Cruz, CA, USA), and after being discontinued (in 2017), monoclonal antibody B-8 (1:1000, cat. #sc-133233; Santa Cruz Biotechnology) were used. Incubation with an appropriate secondary antibody (1:1000, cat. #sc-2004; Santa Cruz Biotechnology, later with the change of primary antibody cat. #sc-516102; Santa Cruz Biotechnology) was followed by chemiluminescent detection (Pierce ECL Plus Western Blotting Substrate; cat. #32132; Thermo Scientific). A weak positive test was interpreted to mean that one sample load was positive and the other negative (the positive control was always positive). CSF levels of t-tau, p-tau, and $A\beta_{42}$ were measured during routine diagnostic testing using commercially available enzyme-linked immunoassay (ELISA) kits (INNOTEST hTAU Ag, cat. #80323/81572, INNOTEST PHOSPHO-TAU (181P), cat. #80317/81574, INNOTEST β-AMYLOID (1–42), cat. #80324/81576, all Innogenetics/FUJIREBIO); all testing was conducted according to the manufacturer's protocol. Although the individual values of analytes in the CSF are not entirely decisive and combinations of their ratios would be more accurate [17], the values are as follows. For t-tau, the cut-off was assessed to be 1160 pg/mL with sensitivity of 90.3 % and specificity of 90.7% (AUC: 0.926, $p < 0.0001$). For p-tau and $A\beta_{42}$, the indicative normative values were determined. The values of p-tau levels > 60 pg/mL and $A\beta_{42}$ levels < 430 pg/mL were considered as abnormal. Our laboratory has extensive experience determining CSF biomarkers and successfully participates in the Alzheimer's Association's external quality control program.

#### 2.5.2. Brain Tissue Analysis

Native brain tissue samples were frozen at −80 °C until analysis. The presence of PrPSc was determined using a standardized western blot protocol (adapted from Collinge et al. [18]). Briefly, brain homogenates were treated with Proteinase K (Proteinase K from Tritirachium album, cat. #SRE0005; Sigma-Aldrich, St. Louis, MI, USA). Samples were separated using SDS-PAGE and blotted onto nitrocellulose membranes. For detection of the PrPSc, two different monoclonal antibodies: 12F10 (1:1667, cat. #A03221.200; Bertin Bioreagent, Montigny le Bretonneux, France), and 6H4 (1:5000, cat. #01-010 and since 2017 cat. #7500996, Prionics, Zürich, Switzerland) were used. Incubation with an appropriate secondary antibody (1:2500 and 1:7500, respectively, cat. #P0447; Dako) was followed by chemiluminescent detection (Pierce ECL Plus Western Blotting Substrate, cat. #32132; Thermo Scientific, Waltham, MA, USA). After limited proteolysis, three PrPSc glycoforms were detected.

### 2.6. *Molecular-Genetic Methods*

*PRNP* (NC-000020.11) is a 16 kb long gene located on chromosome 20 (4686151–4701588). It contains two exons, and exon 2 carries the open reading frame, which encodes the 253 amino acids (AA) PrP protein. Exon 1 is a noncoding exon, which may serve as a transcription initiation site. Post-translational modifications result in removing the first 22 AA N-terminal fragments (NTF) and the last 23 AA C-terminal fragments (CTF).

#### 2.6.1. Study Population

Our study was designed as a retrospective. We analysed data from 215 patients (n = 215), age range 40–87 years, median 66 years. No family history of CJD was retraced. We included patients with postmortem confirmed sCJD and then collected data regarding clinical presentation, biochemical analysis, EEG, and neuroimaging.

Gene analysis was performed at the level of genomic DNA, assuming an effect on the protein sequence. Only the coding part of the *PRNP* (NM_000311) gene and the adjacent intronic region were evaluated. Genetic analysis of genes was performed from autoptic samples of definitively confirmed cases. DNA was isolated from bone marrow (QIAamp DNA Kits).

#### 2.6.2. Genetic Screen

Mutation analyses by *PRNP* gene sequencing were performed on genomic DNA extracted from bone marrow. The targeted gene captured all exons and the flanking intronic regions of the *PRNP* gene to cover the splice sites.

Genomic DNA was amplified using two pairs of specific PCR primers (*PRNP* 1F: 5′ TACCATTGCTATGCACTCATT 3′, *PRNP* 1R: 5′GTCACTGCCCGAAATGTATGA 3′ *PRNP*, 2F: 5′AGGTGGCACCCACAGTCAGT 3′ PRNP 2R: 5′ CCTATCCGGGACAAA-GAGAGA 3′). Primers were designed using mPCR software, and specific target regions were amplified using PCR (temperature profile in the *PRNP* 1: 95 °C/12 min, 29× (95 °C/30″, 53.1 °C/30″, 72 °C/40″), 72 °C/5′, 4 °C/∞. Temperature profile in the *PRNP* 2: 95 °C/12 min, 30× (95 °C/30″, 60.5 °C/30″, 72 °C/70″), 72 °C/5′, 4 °C/∞). PCR products were enzymatically purified using recombinant Shrimp Alkaline Phosphatase (rSAP) and Exonuclease I (Exo I). The purified products were amplified in a sequencing reaction (temperature profile: 96 °C/60″, 25× (96 °C/10″, 50 °C, 5″, 60 °C/30″), 4 °C/∞) using BigDye Terminator v3.1 Cycle Sequencing Kit's (Applied Biosystems™). Cleanup PCR products were sequenced on an Applied Biosystems® 3130 Genetic Analyser (using the DNA sequencing Standard Operating Protocol SOPV. We use Sequencing Analysis 5.3.1 software (Applied Biosystems, Waltham, MA, USA—Life Technologies), SeqScape v.2.6 (Applied Biosystems, Waltham, MA, USA—Life Technologies) to evaluate electrophoretic sequencing data.

Results are summarised in Table 2. In our CJD samples, we present an analysis of codon 129 distribution in 215 cases. Methionine homozygotes represented 63.25%, valine homozygotes 15.35%, and methionine/valine 21.40%.

**Table 2.** Distribution of MV polymorphisms in pure and comorbid CJD cases.

| Polymorphism | Pure CJD | CJD/tau | CJD/AD | CJD/FTLD | CJD/Synuclein |
|---|---|---|---|---|---|
| MM | 17 | 85 | 27 | 4 | 3 |
| VV | 3 | 16 | 9 | 3 | 2 |
| MV | 4 | 34 | 8 | 0 | 0 |
| TOTAL | 24 | 135 | 44 | 7 | 5 |

VV—Valine/Valine, MM—Methionine/Methionine, MV—Methionine/Valine, total stands for total number of cases in each group.

Although the cohort of 215 patients is limited, we noticed that the ratio of valine homozygotes varied from group to group. In pure CJD, VV homozygotes form 11.00% of cases, in CJD/tau 12.50%, in CJD/AD 20.45%, in AD/FTLD 43.00%, and in CJD with comorbid synucleinopathy 40.00% of cases.

### 2.7. Clinical Data

This study was conceived as a retrospective data analysis. Medical records from different hospitals across the Czech Republic were assessed; in cases with insufficient data, the concerned hospitals were directly contacted to retrieve complete data. For this study, we focused on the presence/absence of key features mentioned by the current WHO diagnostic criteria for probable CJD, i.e., dementia, pyramidal or extrapyramidal signs, visuospatial or cerebellar dysfunction, myoclonus, and akinetic mutism (see Supplementary Material).

### 2.8. Magnetic Resonance Imaging

Available MRI scans were assessed independently by two investigators (J.K. and R.R.) to confirm typical MRI findings listed in the WHO diagnostic criteria for probable CJD, i.e., cortical hyperintensities (typically in the frontal and periinsular areas) and basal ganglia hyperintensities (putamen and caudate) in FLAIR and DWI sequences. DWI data included in all cases an acquisition with a b value equal to 1000. Hyperintensities were evaluated qualitatively, ADC maps were used only to confirm the restriction of the diffusion. No fixed windowing was used as it has been reported to have a lower area under the receiver operating characteristic curves when used by radiologists [19]. Moreover, we used semiquantitative scales for detecting focal atrophy in temporal areas (including the hippocampi) and parietal cortices—for this purpose, we used the MTA scale [20] (measuring mesial temporal atrophy) and the Koedam score [21] (assessing parieto-occipital atrophy). Furthermore, cerebrovascular lesions were coded using the Fazekas scale [22]. All available results are summarised in the Supplementary Material section.

### 2.9. Statistical METHODS

The data set was split into two groups using additional diagnoses; hypothesis testing was performed at $p = 0.05$. Logical explanatory variables were processed using the Fisher exact test of variable independence in 2 × 2 contingency tables to obtain significant Odds Ratios (OR). Real explanatory variables were processed using the two-sampled Wilcoxon–

Mann–Whitney test of median equity. All the calculations were performed in the MATLAB 2019 Statistical Toolbox.

## 3. Results

### 3.1. Neuropathological Results

#### 3.1.1. "Pure" CJD

Immunohistochemical methods revealed the presence of several comorbidities in neuropathological examinations. Of the 215 patients, only 24 cases (11.16%) had pure CJD, i.e., lacking any other pathological intra- or extracellular aggregates. The age range of the pure CJD cases was 40–78 years, and the median age was 60 years, which is statistically significantly younger than in the comorbid subgroups.

#### 3.1.2. Comorbid CJD + Tauopathy

Based on clinical data, patients with neuropathological signs of tauopathy lacking clinical correlate were included in this group. The criteria met one hundred thirty-five patients (62.79%), of which 99 (46.05% of 215 cases) had primary age-related tauopathy (CJD/PART). Another 34 cases (15.81%) suffered from CJD/AGD; one patient had CJD/ARTAG (0.47%). Eighteen cases (8.37%) had a combination of CJD/PART and another tauopathy: 13 cases (6.04%) had argyrophilic grain disease (CJD/PART + AGD), and five cases (2.33%) had ageing-related tau astrogliopathy (CJD/PART + ARTAG). Two patients (0.93%) had a combination CJD/ARTAG+AGD, and finally, there was one case (0.47%) with CJD/PART + ARTAG + AGD. The age range of CJD/tau comorbid cases ranged from 49 to 87 years, and the median age was 65 years.

#### 3.1.3. Comorbid CJD/AD

The cohort contained 44 comorbid cases (20.47%) of CJD/AD with possible additional co-pathology. According to the revised "ABC" classification of the National Institute on Aging–Alzheimer's Association (NIA-AA) [13], changes were classified as level "none" (1 case; 0.47%), "low" (23 cases; 10.70%), or "intermediate" (19 cases; 8.84%), no patients in the "high" category were found. The presence of tauopathies was relatively common with the Alzheimer's pathology—ARTAG was diagnosed in 10 cases (4.65%), AGD in four cases (1.86%); in one of these cases (0.47%), the criteria for ARTAG + AGD was met. The age range for this group was aged 56–85 years, and the median age was 71 years.

#### 3.1.4. Comorbid CJD/FTLD

Considering comorbid cases of CJD and frontotemporal lobar degeneration (CJD/FTLD) with characteristic frontotemporal clinical symptomatology, seven cases (3.26%) were found, of which six cases (2.80%) had FTLD/tau, and one (0.47%) had frontotemporal lobar degeneration with positive inclusions for ubiquitin-proteasome system markers (FTLD/UPS). The age range was 55–78 years, and the median age was 67 years.

#### 3.1.5. Comorbid CJD + Synucleinopathy

Finally, five patients (2.33%) suffered from CJD with comorbid synucleinopathy; four patients (1.86%) met the criteria for DLB, and one (0.47%) had Parkinson's disease (PD). The age ranged from 59 to 76 years, with a median age of 71 years.

### 3.2. CSF Analysis Results

CSF analysis was performed antemortem in about 80% of cases: 174 (80.93%) patients were tested for the presence of 14-3-3β, 168 (78.14%) patients were tested for levels of t-tau, p-tau, and $A\beta_{42}$. For CJD, the cut-off level for t-tau was set at 1200 pg/mL [17].

Results of the 14-3-3 analysis are summarised in Table 3 (full details are available in the Supplementary Material). In all groups, 14-3-3β positivity, which is one of the diagnostic criteria for probable CJD (CDC, 2018), was less common than very high t-tau levels (Table 3).

**Table 3.** Numbers (n) and percentage (%) of positive, low positive, negative and unanalysed results of the presence of 14-3-3β, t-tau levels and the combined presence of 14-3-3β and t-tau protein levels in CSF. Percentage is related to the whole cohort.

| | | 14-3-3β (n) | 14-3-3β (%) | t-tau (n) | t-tau (%) | 14-3-3β + t-tau (n) | 14-3-3β + t-tau (%) |
|---|---|---|---|---|---|---|---|
| pure CJD | pos | 12 | 5.58 | 17 | 7.91 | 11 | 5.12 |
| | low pos | 1 | 0.47 | N/A | N/A | 8 | 3.72 |
| | neg | 8 | 3.72 | 3 | 1.40 | 2 | 0.93 |
| | no | 3 | 1.40 | 4 | 1.86 | 3 | 1.40 |
| CJD/tau | pos | 67 | 31.16 | 92 | 42.79 | 74 | 34.42 |
| | low pos | 16 | 7.44 | N/A | N/A | 27 | 12.56 |
| | neg | 27 | 12.56 | 13 | 6.05 | 9 | 4.19 |
| | no | 25 | 11.63 | 30 | 13.95 | 25 | 11.63 |
| CJD/AD | pos | 24 | 11.16 | 31 | 14.42 | 27 | 12.56 |
| | low pos | 5 | 2.33 | N/A | N/A | 6 | 2.79 |
| | neg | 4 | 1.86 | 2 | 0.93 | 0 | 0.00 |
| | no | 11 | 5.12 | 11 | 5.12 | 11 | 5.12 |
| CJD/FTLD | pos | 6 | 2.79 | 7 | 3.26 | 6 | 2.79 |
| | low pos | 0 | 0.00 | N/A | N/A | 1 | 0.47 |
| | neg | 1 | 0.47 | 0 | 0.00 | 0 | 0.00 |
| | no | 0 | 0.00 | 0 | 0.00 | 0 | 0.00 |
| CJD/synuclein | pos | 2 | 0.93 | 3 | 1.40 | 2 | 0.93 |
| | low pos | 0 | 0.00 | N/A | N/A | 1 | 0.47 |
| | neg | 1 | 0.47 | 0 | 0.00 | 0 | 0.00 |
| | no | 2 | 0.93 | 2 | 0.93 | 2 | 0.93 |

pos = positive; low pos = low positive; neg = negative; no = unanalysed; N/A = not applicable. T-tau cut-off: 1200 pg/mL; lower negative. For the combination of 14-3-3β + t-tau, "pos" means both variables are positive, "low pos" means that one of the variables is positive, and the other is negative.

When every group was tested separately, the lowest frequency of 14-3-3β positivity was found in the pure CJD subgroup (12 out of 21, 57.14%). The 14-3-3 positivity was much higher in the comorbidity subgroups (CJD/tau 67 out of 110, 60.91%; CJD/AD 24 out of 33, 72.73%; CJD/FTLD 6 out of 7, 85.71%; and CJD/others 2 out of 3; 66.67%). In pure CJD, t-tau was positive in 17 out of 20 (85.00%). T-tau positivity was higher (CJD/tau 92 out of 105, 87.62% and CJD/AD 31 out of 33, 93.94%) in the comorbidity subgroups.

### 3.3. Clinical Analysis Results

Clinical data were available from all patients and are summarised in Table 1. Diagnostic criteria for possible sCJD [23] were fulfilled in all 215 cases, i.e., all had dementia, and at least two of the four needed signs, i.e., (1) pyramidal or extrapyramidal signs, (2) visuospatial or cerebellar dysfunction, (3) myoclonus, and (4) akinetic mutism. The distribution was as follows: pyramidal or extrapyramidal signs 189 cases (87.90%), visuospatial signs 159 cases (73.95%), myoclonus 133 cases (61.86%), and akinetic mutism 99 cases (46.05%).

### 3.4. MRI Results

MRIs were available in 206 cases (95.81%), and FLAIR/DWI sequences were available in 188 of these (87.44%; for detailed information, see Table 1). Typical FLAIR and DWI findings meeting the WHO diagnostic criteria for probable CJD were found as follows: cortical hyperintensities in 146 of 188 cases (77.66%), basal ganglia (caudate and putaminal) hyperintensities in 122 of 188 cases (64.89%), and both cortical plus basal ganglia hyperintensities in 109 of 188 cases (57.98%). Manifest mesial temporal atrophy (Scheltens MTA score 2) was present in 32 of 206 cases (15.53%), severe parieto-occipital atrophy (Koedam score 2) was present in 22 of 206 cases (10.68%), and potentially clinically relevant ischemic subcortical white matter lesions (Fazekas score 2 and 3) were present in 32 of 188 cases (17.02%). For detail see Figure 1.

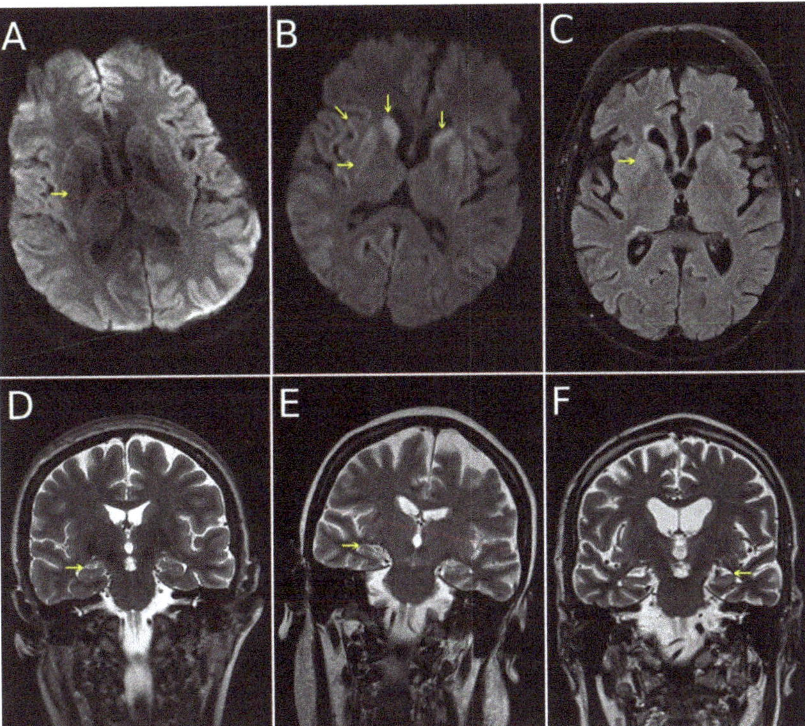


**Figure 1.** MRI in CJD subjects performed at 1.5T field strength: diffusion-weighed images ((**A**,**B**), DWI) with b-factor 1000, FLAIR image (**C**), coronal T2-weighted images (**D**–**F**). In the first column (**A**,**D**) data from subject with pure CJD—no DWI hyperintensity in putamina (arrow) is present and MTA is 0 (read as normal). In the second column (**B**,**E**) subject with tau comorbidity with mild hippocampal atrophy (MTA 1, arrow on (**E**)) and DWI (**B**) hyperintensity in putamina (horizontal arrow), caudates (vertical arrows) and with cortical ribboning (oblique arrow). In the third column (**C**,**F**) subject with CJD and AD comorbidity is shown. A moderate hyperintensity is visible not only on DWI (not shown), but as well on FLAIR image (**C**). Hippocampal atrophy is well pronounced, MTA 2 (arrow from right side of the (**F**), pointing to the left hippocampus which manifests clear atrophy).

### *3.5. Confocal Microscopy Colocalization Results*

Multichannel fluorescence confocal microscopy was used in comorbid CJD case examinations to monitor the colocalization of individual pathological aggregates. We devoted our previous publication [24] to the morphology of colocalizing pathological prion protein and amyloid-beta, as well as pathological tau-positive inclusions. Compound plaques with either Aβ or hyperphosphorylated tau protein (h-tau) in colocalization with $PrP^{Sc}$ were sparse. In contrast, $PrP^{Sc}$ aggregates colocalized predominantly with the non-compact (diffuse) regions of Aβ plaques, and colocalization of h-tau with $PrP^{Sc}$ had a dotted pattern. According to the NIA-Alzheimer's association guidelines, no association between the micromorphology of plaques and type of colocalization with polymorphism at codon 129, type of $PrP^{Sc}$, and the AD ABC score was found. See Figures 2–4.

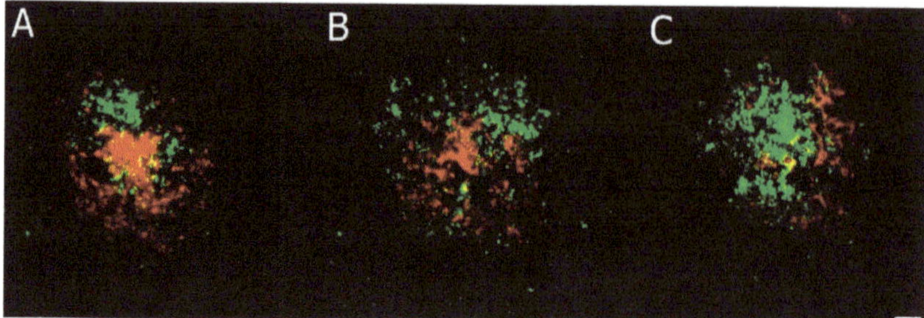


**Figure 2.** (**A–C**) Immunofluorescence illustration of different patterns of amyloid β (Aβ; red) and prion protein ($PrP^{Sc}$; green) colocalization in compound plaques in comorbid Alzheimer's (AD) and Creutzfeldt–Jakob diseases (CJD) cases. Primary antibodies: anti-PrP (rabbit recombinant monoclonal antibody) + anti-amyloid β-protein (mouse monoclonal antibody). The secondary antibody was conjugated with either Alexa Fluor® 488 (anti-rabbit IgG; green) or Alexa Fluor® 568 (anti-mouse IgG; red). Scale bar indicates 10 μm. Images come from the hippocampal region (archicortical parts).

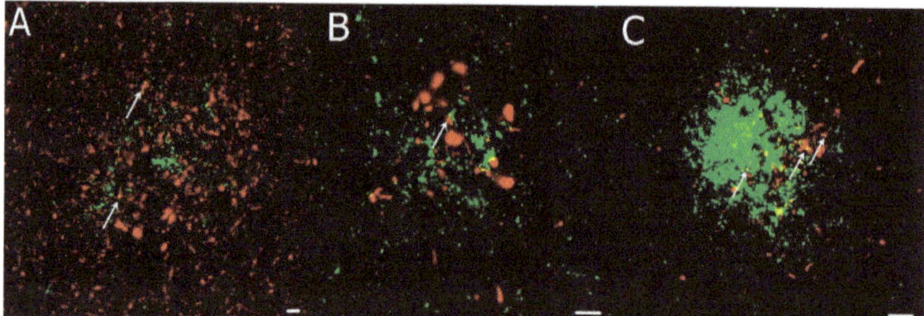


**Figure 3.** (**A–C**) Immunofluorescence illustrates h-tau-positive (red) dystrophic neurites colocalizing with $PrP^{Sc}$ (green) extracellular deposits in comorbid CJD/AD cases. Primary antibodies: PrP (rabbit recombinant monoclonal antibody) + AT8 (mouse monoclonal antibody). The secondary antibody was conjugated with either Alexa Fluor® 488 (anti-rabbit IgG, green) or Alexa Fluor® 568 (anti-mouse IgG, red). Scale bars indicate 10 μm. Arrows indicate minor colocalization of AT8 with PrP. Images come from the hippocampal region (archicortical parts).

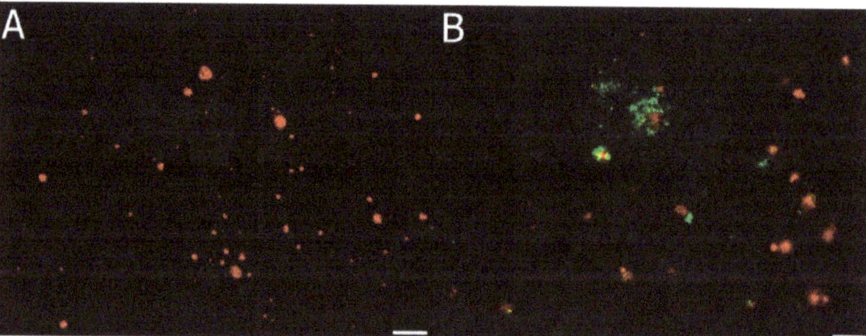


**Figure 4.** (**A,B**) Immunofluorescence illustration of the predominance of non-compound or minimal-compound plaques with minimal colocalization of Aβ (red) and $PrP^{Sc}$ (green) in the majority of plaques. Primary antibodies: anti-PrP (rabbit recombinant monoclonal antibody) + anti-amyloid β-protein (mouse monoclonal antibody). The secondary antibody was conjugated with either Alexa Fluor® 488 (anti-rabbit IgG; green) or Alexa Fluor® 568 (anti-mouse IgG; red). Scale bars indicate 100 μm. Images come from the hippocampal region (archicortical parts).

## 4. Discussion

The main findings from comparing pure CJD with different comorbid subgroups were as follows: (1) pure CJD had a significantly lower age of onset; (2) tau comorbidity was associated with a higher probability of putaminal hyperintensities and had a lower MTA score on MRI; (3) AD comorbidity was associated with a higher age of onset, a lower probability for developing putaminal hyperintensities on MRI, and had significantly lower beta-amyloid levels in the CSF; (4) pure CJD compared to CJD/AD had a lower age at onset and a lower MTA score on MRI; (5) comorbid CJD/tau differed from comorbid CJD/AD by having a lower age of onset, lower MTA scores, and higher beta-amyloid CSF levels, and (6) comorbid co-pathology is not dependent on codon 129 homo/heterozygosity nor the genetic background of CJD.

First, the lower age of onset in "pure" CJD cases could be explained by the absence of age-related changes in the brain tissue. In this subgroup, early-onset prion pathology with rapid disease progression probably leads to death before the development of other comorbidities.

Second, comorbid tauopathies were more likely than in other subgroups associated with putaminal DWI hyperintensities on MRI. It is known that changes in these signals correlate roughly equally with vacuolation and the amount of $PrP^{Sc}$ deposition (and less with astrocytic gliosis) [25]. The reason why this hypersignal is more pronounced in CJD subjects with comorbid tauopathy remains unclear since isolated tauopathies are not associated with similar MRI findings, and putaminal deposition of tau protein is not typical; however, it has been reported [26]. We can, therefore, only hypothesise that in subjects with comorbid CJD and tauopathy, the presence of tau facilitates signal increases on DWI either by tau and prion protein co-occurrence or by putaminal microstructure changes, since no micromorphological differences were visible. Lower MTA scores in the CJD/tau subgroup are even more difficult to understand, as in tau positive FTLD, pronounced frontal and temporal lobe atrophy is a frequent finding, as well as in AD, for which higher MTA scores are characteristic [27].

Third, comorbid AD was linked to a higher age of onset. Again, this is a rather surprising finding; as already discussed above, one would expect neurodegenerative comorbidities to have a significant impact relative to the destruction of brain tissue and thus lead to the earlier onset and faster disease progression. Nevertheless, CJD/AD can be viewed from different angles. Pre-existing AD development is more likely to be present at older ages, and from this point of view, it would not be unexpected that comorbid CJD/AD cases are older on average. In one of our previous publications, based on morphological findings using a multichannel fluorescent confocal microscope, we speculated that $A\beta_{42}$ might be acting as $PrP^{Sc}$ seeds within the brain [24] since PrP-Aβ colocalization predominates in the periphery of plaques where $A\beta_{42}$ is more abundant.

Nevertheless, it is important to emphasise that compound plaques represent only a minority of plaques since PrP and Aβ plaques tended to be, in most cases, located separately or formed "minimal compound" plaques. However, even this view of CJD/AD assumes faster progression in CJD/AD comorbid cases than in "pure" CJD, although the data obtained from our 10-year surveillance did not support such a tendency. MRI findings of putaminal sparing can be hypothesised by reduced basal ganglia involvement and fewer parkinsonian features in non-comorbid AD patients compared to pure FTLD patients. The observed low beta-amyloid levels in CSF were concordant with current biomarker findings in pure AD.

A recently published Italian study [10] showed data similar to our observations: the mean age of the CJD/AD cases (71.07 years for our cohort versus 76.1 years for the Italian patients) is strikingly higher than in pure CJD cases; no link was found between the existence of comorbid AD and disease subtype, prion strain, or *PRNP* genotype; in both cohorts, there were no patients in the "high" level of AD; data from both cohorts showed low Aβ levels in the CSF. There was, however, a surprising difference in the percentage of cases in which AD was reported: 61.5% of cases with CJD/AD reported in Italy compared to only 20.47% in our study.

Fourth, some of the previous findings became more obvious when we compared pure CJD to only comorbid CJD/AD. The difference in age of onset and MTA scores were larger between pure CJD and CJD/AD than when comparing pure CJD to all subgroups. The MTA scale is a widely used scoring system for assessing hippocampal atrophy in AD patients and may also monitor disease progression over time [28,29]. We thus suggest that AD could be present before prion disease in older patients.

Fifth, the role of AD on clinical manifestations and biomarkers in our cases was visible when comparing CJD/tau to CJD/AD subgroups. In line with previously discussed points, higher age of onset, higher MTA scores, and lower beta-amyloid CSF levels were key features of the impact of AD on our cohort.

Sixth, from the genetic point of view, we found no differences between codon 129 status of the *PRNP* gene or between genetic and sporadic CJD; in line with our pilot study, no prominent abnormalities in the deep genetic analysis of "pure" CJD cases and CJD cases in comorbidity with AD and tauopathies, respectively were seen, nor in the analysis of 15 genes related to the most important neurodegenerative diseases [30]. It has been suggested that increased expression of *Syntaxin-6* (*Stx6*) in the basal ganglia could raise the risk of prion disease, and *Stx-6* deposits have been identified as a risk factor for a 4R-tauopathy and progressive supranuclear palsy. The same study also suggests a possible role for *GAL3ST1* [31] in encoding galactose-3-O-sulfotransferase 1, which affects myelin maintenance. This would be consistent with the finding that sphingolipid metabolism is disrupted early in the pathogenesis of prion disorders in mouse models [32].

Finally, compared to a study by Kovacs et al. [9] that focused on tau pathology in CJD and identified 69.3% of cases with prominent tau co-pathology and an additional 16.0% of cases with discrete non-significant tau-immunoreactive neurites, our percentage (11.16%) of "pure" cases was surprisingly low. A possible explanation for the difference in the percentage of "pure" cases by Kovacs et al. is that they did not discuss other pathological deposits. By contrast, our study revealed cases of rare comorbidities such as CJD/FTLD or CJD/synucleinopathies; some correlations between imaging findings and co-pathologies were also found.

The main limitations of our study were the single-center expertise and the very uneven extent of neuroimaging and clinical data from patients examined in different hospitals. These factors made a more robust analysis of the data and clinical correlations difficult.

## 5. Conclusions

We present results from a large cohort of postmortem confirmed CJD patients (with pure CJD and neurodegenerative comorbidities) with clinical, MRI, CSF, neuropathological, and immunohistochemical data. Our retrospective data analysis found a surprisingly high proportion of comorbid neuropathologies, with only 11% of our cases being pure non-comorbid CJD. These patients were found to have the lowest age of disease onset.

The most interesting findings from our comorbid subgroup analysis were that tauopathy is linked to putaminal hyperintensity one MRIs and that AD is associated with the age of disease onset, the degree of hippocampal atrophy seen on MRIs (low MTA scores), and the low beta-amyloid levels in the CSF. However, further investigation on a broader spectrum of comorbid neuropathologies is needed before evidence of their impact on the clinical presentation can enter routine practice, especially when new biological and potentially targeted therapies become available for treating specific proteinopathies.

**Supplementary Materials:** The following supporting information can be downloaded at: https://www.mdpi.com/article/10.3390/biomedicines10030680/s1.

**Author Contributions:** The authors confirm contribution to the paper as follows: study conception and design, R.M. and R.R.; data collection, N.J., R.R., M.B. and E.P.; analysis and interpretation of results, N.J., T.O., R.R., J.K. (Jiri Keller), J.K. (Jaromir Kukal), M.B. and E.P.; draft manuscript preparation, N.J. All authors have read and agreed to the published version of the manuscript.

**Funding:** This study was supported by the MH CZ–DRO: Conceptual Development of Research Organization, the General University Hospital, Prague (VFN, 00064165); the Thomayer University Hospital, Prague (TUH, 00064190); the Grants Agency of the Ministry of Health (NV19-04-00090); and by Charles University (Project Cooperatio and GAUK 142120) and by the Czech Ministry of Education: NPO Program Exceles-Neuroscience.

**Institutional Review Board Statement:** The study was conducted according to the guidelines of the Declaration of Helsinki approved in advance by the Ethics Committee of the Institute for Clinical and Experimental Medicine and Thomayer University Hospital No G-19-18, obtained 26 June 2017. Cerebrospinal fluid was processed in accordance with F-IS-TN-2302012, Version No. 4. No informed consent obtained as only archival tissue of dead subjects was investigated retrospectively in anonymous setting with respect to their privacy, no treatment or diagnostic intervention was performed.

**Informed Consent Statement:** Not applicable.

**Data Availability Statement:** The authors confirm that all data underlying the findings are fully available without restriction. All data are included within the manuscript.

**Acknowledgments:** The authors wish to thank Tom Secrest for the revision of the English version of this article.

**Conflicts of Interest:** The authors declare no conflict of interest.

## References

1. Sikorska, B.; Knight, R.; Ironside, J.W.; Liberski, P.P. Creutzfeldt-Jakob Disease. *Retin. Degener. Dis.* **2012**, *724*, 76–90. [CrossRef]
2. Budka, H.; Aguzzi, A.; Brown, P.; Brucher, J.-M.; Bugiani, O.; Gullotta, F.; Haltia, M.; Hauw, J.-J.; Ironside, J.W.; Jellinger, K.; et al. Neuropathological Diagnostic Criteria for Creutzfeldt-Jakob Disease (CJD) and Other Human Spongiform Encephalopathies (Prion Diseases). *Brain Pathol.* **1995**, *5*, 459–466. [CrossRef] [PubMed]
3. Hill, A.F.; Joiner, S.; Wadsworth, J.D.F.; Sidle, K.C.L.; Bell, J.E.; Budka, H.; Ironside, J.W.; Collinge, J. Molecular classification of sporadic Creutzfeldt–Jakob disease. *Brain* **2003**, *126*, 1333–1346. [CrossRef] [PubMed]
4. E Bell, J.; Ironside, J.W. Neuropathology of spongiform encephalopathies in humans. *Br. Med. Bull.* **1993**, *49*, 738–777. [CrossRef]
5. Collinge, J. Variant Creutzfeldt-Jakob disease. *Lancet* **1999**, *354*, 317–323. [CrossRef]
6. Uttley, L.; Carroll, C.; Wong, R.; Hilton, D.A.; Stevenson, M. Creutzfeldt-Jakob disease: A systematic review of global incidence, prevalence, infectivity, and incubation. *Lancet Infect. Dis.* **2020**, *20*, e2–e10. [CrossRef]
7. Jankovska, N.; Rusina, R.; Bruzova, M.; Parobkova, E.; Olejar, T.; Matej, R. Human Prion Disorders: Review of the Current Literature and a Twenty-Year Experience of the National Surveillance Center in the Czech Republic. *Diagnostics* **2021**, *11*, 1821. [CrossRef] [PubMed]
8. Watson, N.; Brandel, J.-P.; Green, A.; Hermann, P.; Ladogana, A.; Lindsay, T.; Mackenzie, J.; Pocchiari, M.; Smith, C.; Zerr, I.; et al. The importance of ongoing international surveillance for Creutzfeldt–Jakob disease. *Nat. Rev. Neurol.* **2021**, *17*, 362–379. [CrossRef] [PubMed]
9. Kovacs, G.G.; Rahimi, J.; Ströbel, T.; Lutz, M.I.; Regelsberger, G.; Streichenberger, N.; Perret-Liaudet, A.; Höftberger, R.; Liberski, P.P.; Budka, H.; et al. Tau pathology in Creutzfeldt-Jakob disease revisited. *Brain Pathol.* **2016**, *27*, 332–344. [CrossRef]
10. Rossi, M.; Kai, H.; Baiardi, S.; Bartoletti-Stella, A.; Carlà, B.; Zenesini, C.; Capellari, S.; Kitamoto, T.; Parchi, P. The characterization of AD/PART co-pathology in CJD suggests independent pathogenic mechanisms and no cross-seeding between misfolded Aβ; and prion proteins. *Acta Neuropathol. Commun.* **2019**, *7*, 53. [CrossRef]
11. Autopsy. Netherlands Brain Bank. Available online: https://www.brainbank.nl/brain-tissue/autopsy/ (accessed on 14 February 2021).
12. Montine, T.J.; Phelps, C.H.; Beach, T.G.; Bigio, E.H.; Cairns, N.J.; Dickson, D.W.; Duyckaerts, C.; Frosch, M.P.; Masliah, E.; Mirra, S.S.; et al. National Institute on Aging–Alzheimer's Association guidelines for the neuropathologic assessment of Alzheimer's disease: A practical approach. *Acta Neuropathol.* **2011**, *123*, 1–11. [CrossRef] [PubMed]
13. Hyman, B.T.; Phelps, C.H.; Beach, T.G.; Bigio, E.H.; Cairns, N.J.; Carrillo, M.C.; Dickson, D.W.; Duyckaerts, C.; Frosch, M.P.; Masliah, E.; et al. National Institute on Aging-Alzheimer's Association guidelines for the neuropathologic assessment of Alzheimer's disease. *Alzheimer Dement.* **2012**, *8*, 1–13. [CrossRef]
14. McKeith, I.G.; Boeve, B.F.; Dickson, D.W.; Halliday, G.; Taylor, J.-P.; Weintraub, D.; Aarsland, D.; Galvin, J.; Attems, J.; Ballard, C.G.; et al. Diagnosis and management of dementia with Lewy bodies. *Neurology* **2017**, *89*, 88–100. [CrossRef] [PubMed]

15. Weisman, D.; Cho, M.; Taylor, C.; Adame, A.; Thal, L.J.; Hansen, L.A. In dementia with Lewy bodies, Braak stage determines phenotype, not Lewy body distribution. *Neurology* **2007**, *69*, 356–359. [CrossRef] [PubMed]
16. E Green, A.J.; Thompson, E.J.; E Stewart, G.; Zeidler, M.; McKenzie, J.M.; MacLeod, M.-A.; Ironside, J.W.; Will, R.G.; Knight, R.S.G. Use of 14-3-3 and other brain-specific proteins in CSF in the diagnosis of variant Creutzfeldt-Jakob disease. *J. Neurol. Neurosurg. Psychiatry* **2001**, *70*, 744–748. [CrossRef] [PubMed]
17. Bruzova, M.; Rusina, R.; Stejskalova, Z.; Matej, R. Autopsy-diagnosed neurodegenerative dementia cases support the use of cerebrospinal fluid protein biomarkers in the diagnostic work-up. *Sci. Rep.* **2021**, *11*, 10837. [CrossRef]
18. Collinge, J.; Sidle, K.C.L.; Meads, J.; Ironside, J.; Hill, A.F. Molecular analysis of prion strain variation and the aetiology of 'new variant' CJD. *Nature* **1996**, *383*, 685–690. [CrossRef] [PubMed]
19. Fujita, K.; Harada, M.; Sasaki, M.; Yuasa, T.; Sakai, K.; Hamaguchi, T.; Sanjo, N.; Shiga, Y.; Satoh, K.; Atarashi, R.; et al. Multicentre multiobserver study of diffusion-weighted and fluid-attenuated inversion recovery MRI for the diagnosis of sporadic Creutzfeldt–Jakob disease: A reliability and agreement study. *BMJ Open* **2012**, *2*, e000649. [CrossRef]
20. Scheltens, P.; Leys, D.; Barkhof, F.; Huglo, D.; Weinstein, H.C.; Vermersch, P.; Kuiper, M.; Steinling, M.; Wolters, E.C.; Valk, J. Atrophy of medial temporal lobes on MRI in probable Alzheimer's disease and normal ageing: Diagnostic value and neuropsychological correlates. *J. Neurol. Neurosurg. Psychiatry* **1992**, *55*, 967–972. [CrossRef] [PubMed]
21. Koedam, E.L.G.E.; Lehmann, M.; Van Der Flier, W.M.; Scheltens, P.; Pijnenburg, Y.A.L.; Fox, N.; Barkhof, F.; Wattjes, M.P. Visual assessment of posterior atrophy development of a MRI rating scale. *Eur. Radiol.* **2011**, *21*, 2618–2625. [CrossRef]
22. Fazekas, F.; Kleinert, R.; Offenbacher, H.; Schmidt, R.; Payer, F.; Radner, H.; Lechner, H. Pathologic correlates of incidental MRI white matter signal hyperintensities. *Neurology* **1993**, *43*, 1683. [CrossRef] [PubMed]
23. Zerr, I.; Kallenberg, K.; Summers, D.M.; Romero, C.; Taratuto, A.; Heinemann, U.; Breithaupt, M.; Varges, D.; Meissner, B.; Ladogana, A.; et al. Updated clinical diagnostic criteria for sporadic Creutzfeldt-Jakob disease. *Brain* **2009**, *132*, 2659–2668. [CrossRef] [PubMed]
24. Jankovska, N.; Olejar, T.; Matej, R. Extracellular Protein Aggregates Colocalization and Neuronal Dystrophy in Comorbid Alzheimer's and Creutzfeldt–Jakob Disease: A Micromorphological Pilot Study on 20 Brains. *Int. J. Mol. Sci.* **2021**, *22*, 2099. [CrossRef] [PubMed]
25. Geschwind, M.D.; Potter, C.A.; Sattavat, M.; Garcia, P.A.; Rosen, H.J.; Miller, B.L.; DeArmond, S.J. Correlating DWI MRI With Pathologic and Other Features of Jakob-Creutzfeldt Disease. *Alzheimer Dis. Assoc. Disord.* **2009**, *23*, 82–87. [CrossRef] [PubMed]
26. Zhou, Y.; Bai, B. Tau and Pet/Mri Imaging Biomarkers for Detecting and Diagnosing Early Dementia. *Jacobs J. Med. Diagn. Med. Imaging* **2017**, *2*, 17.
27. Claus, J.J.; Staekenborg, S.S.; Holl, D.C.; Roorda, J.J.; Schuur, J.; Koster, P.; Tielkes, C.E.M.; Scheltens, P. Practical use of visual medial temporal lobe atrophy cut-off scores in Alzheimer's disease: Validation in a large memory clinic population. *Eur. Radiol.* **2017**, *27*, 3147–3155. [CrossRef] [PubMed]
28. Korf, E.S.; Wahlund, L.O.; Visser, P.J.; Scheltens, P. Medial temporal lobe atrophy on MRI predicts dementia in patients with mild cognitive impairment. *Neurology* **2004**, *63*, 94–100. [CrossRef] [PubMed]
29. Geroldi, C.; Rossi, R.; Calvagna, C.; Testa, C.; Bresciani, L.; Binetti, G.; Zanetti, O.; Frisoni, G.B. Medial temporal atrophy but not memory deficit predicts progression to dementia in patients with mild cognitive impairment. *J. Neurol. Neurosurg. Psychiatry* **2006**, *77*, 1219–1222. [CrossRef]
30. Parobkova, E.; Van Der Zee, J.; Dillen, L.; Van Broeckhoven, C.; Rusina, R.; Matej, R. Sporadic Creutzfeldt-Jakob Disease and Other Proteinopathies in Comorbidity. *Front. Neurol.* **2020**, *11*, 596108. [CrossRef]
31. Jones, E.; Hummerich, H.; Viré, E.; Uphill, J.; Dimitriadis, A.; Speedy, H.; Campbell, T.; Norsworthy, P.; Quinn, L.; Whitfield, J.; et al. Identification of novel risk loci and causal insights for sporadic Creutzfeldt-Jakob disease: A genome-wide association study. *Lancet Neurol.* **2020**, *19*, 840–848. [CrossRef]
32. Hwang, D.; Lee, I.Y.; Yoo, H.; Gehlenborg, N.; Cho, J.; Petritis, B.; Baxter, D.; Pitstick, R.; Young, R.; Spicer, D.; et al. A systems approach to prion disease. *Mol. Syst. Biol.* **2009**, *5*, 252. [CrossRef] [PubMed]

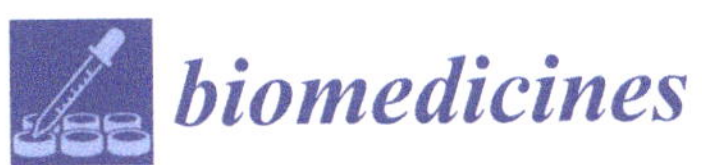 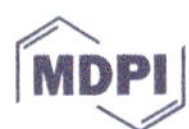

*Review*

# Serum-Based Biomarkers in Neurodegeneration and Multiple Sclerosis

**Patrizia LoPresti**

Department of Psychology, The University of Illinois at Chicago, 1007 West Harrison Street, Chicago, IL 60607, USA; patrizia.lopresti.22@gmail.com

**Abstract:** Multiple Sclerosis (MS) is a debilitating disease with typical onset between 20 and 40 years of age, so the disability associated with this disease, unfortunately, occurs in the prime of life. At a very early stage of MS, the relapsing-remitting mobility impairment occurs in parallel with a progressive decline in cognition, which is subclinical. This stage of the disease is considered the beginning of progressive MS. Understanding where a patient is along such a subclinical phase could be critical for therapeutic efficacy and enrollment in clinical trials to test drugs targeted at neurodegeneration. Since the disease course is uneven among patients, biomarkers are needed to provide insights into pathogenesis, diagnosis, and prognosis of events that affect neurons during this subclinical phase that shapes neurodegeneration and disability. Thus, subclinical cognitive decline must be better understood. One approach to this problem is to follow known biomarkers of neurodegeneration over time. These biomarkers include Neurofilament, Tau and phosphotau protein, amyloid-peptide-β, Brl2 and Brl2-23, N-Acetylaspartate, and 14-3-3 family proteins. A composite set of these serum-based biomarkers of neurodegeneration might provide a distinct signature in early vs. late subclinical cognitive decline, thus offering additional diagnostic criteria for progressive neurodegeneration and response to treatment. Studies on serum-based biomarkers are described together with selective studies on CSF-based biomarkers and MRI-based biomarkers.

**Keywords:** neurodegeneration; cognition; progressive multiple sclerosis; biomarkers; diagnosis; treatment; prognosis; personalized medicine; cytoskeleton; synapse

**Citation:** LoPresti, P. Serum-Based Biomarkers in Neurodegeneration and Multiple Sclerosis. *Biomedicines* **2022**, *10*, 1077. https://doi.org/10.3390/biomedicines10051077

Academic Editor: Arnab Ghosh

Received: 9 February 2022
Accepted: 29 April 2022
Published: 6 May 2022



## 1. Introduction

Multiple Sclerosis (MS) affects approximately 2.2 million people worldwide, with prevalence in white northern European descendants, and affecting more women than men [1–3]. The onset of this debilitating disease is usually between 20 and 40 years, so the disability associated with MS, unfortunately, occurs in the prime of life, making MS the most common neurological disability in young adults. While the cause of MS has not been determined, combinations of epidemiology, genetics, and environment are thought to contribute.

The risk of developing MS increases with low exposure to the sun, viral infections, smoking, genetic susceptibility, and location north of the equator. Recent work has shown that the high prevalence of Epstein-Barr virus is associated with MS [4,5]. Overall MS disease results from multiple agents priming the immune system over time until the immune system starts to attack and damage the central nervous system (CNS) [3,5]. Each patient has unique inflammatory responses as well as interactions between the innate and acquired immune systems. The involvement of inflammation and complex interactions between innate and acquired immunity makes the disease unique in each patient with different impacts on the CNS.

The symptoms of MS include fatigue, depression, vertigo, visual problems, cognitive dysfunction, muscle-related symptoms, bowel and bladder symptoms, and sexual dysfunctions. The diagnosis of MS is made using a combination of tests, such as magnetic resonance imaging, spinal tap, and evoked potential analysis. In addition, the expanded disability status scale is widely used to measure the degree of disability [6,7]. The use of diagnostic tools to detect subclinical neuronal functional decline is imperative; a new MS classification should address the degree of neurodegeneration, which would facilitate correct enrollment into clinical trials.

MS is a complex disease, having independent and interconnected components [8]. The subclinical mobility defect detected with the highly sensitive glove test [9] was not included in the definition of relapsing-remitting (RR)-MS, whereas Benedict et al. [10] described some recovery of cognitive function throughout the disease; however, that recovery was partial, which inevitably would result in a progressive decline of cognitive functions.

The main therapeutic challenge is that within an apparent clinically homogenous group of MS patients, the underlying neurodegeneration might be at earlier or later stages. Indeed, detecting such subclinical (silent) progression would aid in MS diagnosis, treatment with new therapeutics, and prognosis [11,12]. Neurons damaged during MS release molecules into the extracellular CNS compartments where they can be re-internalized and/or destroyed [13]. The extent of re-internalization and/or destruction would determine the levels of biomarkers detected in cerebrospinal fluid (CSF) and blood samples. CSF sampling offers a more accurate analysis [13,14]; however, CSF sampling is not easy for patients. In contrast, blood samples can be obtained from patients with little stress or discomfort, and serum-based biomarkers are a less expensive means to assess neuronal degeneration. These tests can be easily repeated at a low cost. In contrast, Magnetic Resonance Imaging (MRI)-based biomarkers can only be performed at select clinical medical centers, in addition to being expensive and time-consuming.

A personalized medicine approach is greatly needed as a set of biomarkers could flag each patient affected by MS before and after treatment [15,16]. Biomarkers provide a platform for identifying disease mechanisms and pharmacological targets. Exploratory analysis and validation are some of the steps required to validate biomarkers for routine clinical practice [13,14]. The combined use of several biomarkers could better elucidate the underlying mechanisms during neurodegeneration. Biomarkers of axonal and neuronal degeneration could include NFL, tau, P-tau, β-amyloid 1-42, Bri2 (Integral membrane protein 2B), Bri2-23 (generated from Bri2), the neuronal mitochondrial metabolite NAA (N-acetyl aspartate), and 14-3-3. At the same time, a biomarker of T-cell-mediated autoimmunity such as Osteopontin could be added to further analyze disease activity [17–29]. In addition to the enzyme-linked immunosorbent assay (ELISA), new technologies with increased sensitivity and accuracy have been developed, including electrochemiluminescence (ECL), single-molecule array (SIMOA) technology, immunomagnetic reduction, immunoprecipitation/mass spectrometry, and dried plasma spot [30].

It is important to determine the ratio of CSF/plasma of selective biomarkers in disease models and upon treatment with various therapeutics. The widely used experimental autoimmune encephalomyelitis (EAE) mice should be used in parallel with additional models, including the model of MS where oligodendrocyte death results in immune-mediated CNS demyelination [31]. In addition, the Non-Obese Diabetic (NOD)-EAE model could also be useful since this model mimics RR-MS becoming Secondary Progressive (SP)-MS [32].

Synapses are believed to be an early target of MS disease, driving processes that lead to permanent neuronal loss [33–42]. Such an insidious foe for the synapses and neurons at the beginning of disease requires insight and targeted therapeutics. The United States Food and Drug Administration (FDA) has approved drugs that regulate immune-mediated inflammation. However, subclinical synaptic alterations are largely unmodified by current approaches, and a set of biomarkers could be used to characterize early vs. late neurodegeneration. Understanding where a patient is along the subclinical neurodegeneration pathway could be a critical tool for guiding drug enrollment in clinical studies (Figure 1).

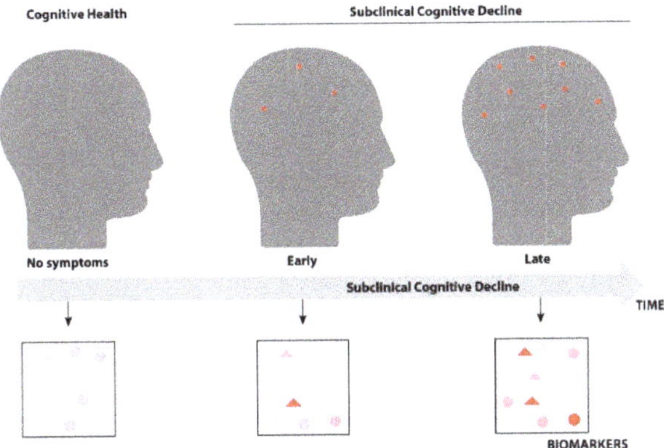


**Figure 1.** Biomarkers during Subclinical Cognitive Decline. During the subclinical cognitive decline preceding progressive multiple sclerosis, the patients are in early or late subclinical decline, i.e., far from, or closer to, developing progressive multiple sclerosis. A set of distinct biomarkers at these two-time points can provide insight into both diagnosis and treatment. The red dots represent synaptic dysfunction and neurodegeneration, whereas the panels with biomarkers indicate representative differences in biomarkers and distinctive signatures.

It is crucial to determine normal and pathological values of biomarkers (Figure 2) along with their specific fold-increase over longitudinal patient analysis [13,27,43]. Kappos et al. [44] have proposed using a roving reference value in prospective studies rather than a fixed value. Further, the distinction between biomarker expression during disease activity and progression must be understood in the context of underlying events, such as increased protein turnover vs. increased protein levels due, for example, to cytoskeletal disruption.

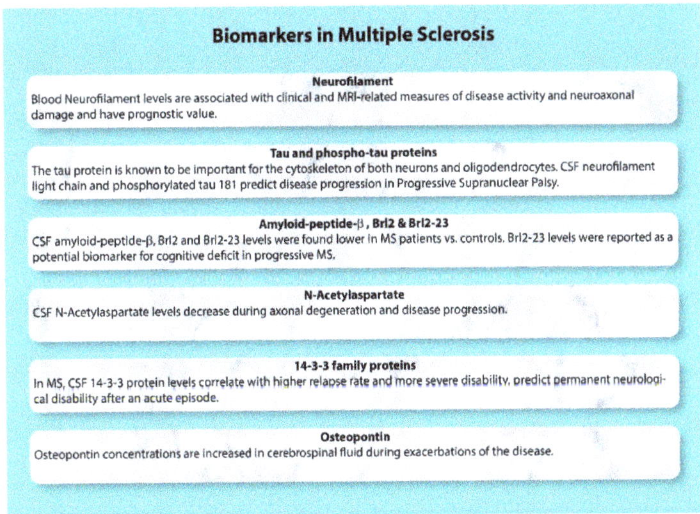


**Figure 2.** Biomarkers in Multiple Sclerosis. Biomarkers of neurodegeneration and inflammation are indicated. Neurodegeneration biomarkers include Neurofilament, Tau and phosphotau protein, amyloid-peptide-β, Brl2 and Brl2-23, N-Acetylaspartate, and 14-3-3 family proteins, whereas Osteopontin is an inflammation biomarker.

## 2. Neurofilaments

Neurofilaments (NFs) are proteins of the axonal cytoskeleton that are critical for intracellular transport and the health of the axons [45–47]. Neurofilaments consist of NF-light (L), -middle (M), and heavy (H) chains [48,49]. NF-L is a soluble and abundant component of neuronal axons.

NF-L is the most abundant and soluble, whereas NF-H is the largest [13]. Both NF-H and NF-M regulate axonal diameter based on their phosphorylation levels. Highly phosphorylated NF-H is believed to indicate an axonal injury and may also increase during the progression of neurological diseases [50,51]. Healthy individuals have low levels of NF-L in the blood, whereas high levels of NF-L are detected in degenerative diseases, including Amyotrophic lateral sclerosis (ALS), MS, and Alzheimer's disease (AD) [52–54].

NF-L levels correlate with axonal damage and with cognitive performance [55,56]. Studies on NF-L in AD could offer insight into approaches to neurodegeneration in MS because elevated NF-L levels in CSF and plasma indicate a neuronal injury and appear to be promising markers of AD severity and progression [57,58]. Of note, NF-L levels are increased in pre-symptomatic and early symptomatic stages of AD and correlate with cognitive decline, progression of brain atrophy, and decreased survival. Furthermore, the use of ultrasensitive biomarker assays such as SIMOA has allowed the quantitation of low NF-L levels in blood samples. Plasma or serum NF-L levels differentiate pre-symptomatic and early symptomatic AD from controls in studies of familial and sporadic AD, accurately predicting rates of disease progression over time [46,59].

NF-L increases during the acute phase of MS and high N-FL levels correlate with disease progression and/or conversion of RR-MS to SP-MS [60–66]. In contrast, the concentration of NF-L did not correlate with gender, age, or disease duration [13,67]. Blood NF-L levels are associated with clinical and MRI-related measures of disease activity and neuroaxonal damage and have prognostic value. Work by Kuhle et al. [68] supports the utility of blood NF-L as an easily accessible biomarker of disease evolution and treatment response. Of interest, the CSF NF-L chain predicts 10-year clinical and radiologic worsening in multiple sclerosis [69,70]. Lycke et al. [70] also showed that the CSF NF-L protein is a potential marker of activity in multiple sclerosis. Immunosuppressive therapy reduces axonal damage, and NF-L levels in CSF are a potential marker for treatment efficacy [68,71]. Further, diffusely abnormal white matter in clinically isolated syndrome, a first clinical episode compatible with MS, is associated with parenchymal loss and elevated neurofilament levels [72], and NF-L levels are associated with chronic white matter inflammation [73]. Recent important work has shown that antibodies to NF-L are potential MS biomarkers [74], and new MRI activity and NF-L levels effectively monitor MS patients [75]. In summary, NF-L is recognized as having an important value in both research and clinical trial settings [76]. Barro et al. [53] showed that CFLs predict disease worsening and brain and spinal cord atrophy in MS. Further, NF-L in CSF and serum is a sensitive marker for axonal white matter injury [77]. Bridel et al. [78] showed that NF-L is associated with progression in Natalizumab-treated patients with RR-MS, whereas Kuhle et al. [79] showed a reduction in sNF-L following early alemtuzumab treatment in RR-MS patients. Cantó et al. [80] showed an association between sNF levels and long-term disease course, and Kuhle et al. [81] demonstrated a correlation between high NF-L levels and long-term outcomes. Additional work is required to investigate whether selected drugs aimed at neuroprotection decrease NF-L levels in MS patients. Table 1 summarizes neurofilament detection in various types of human samples using a variety of assays, including ELISA, ECL, and SIMOA.

**Table 1.** Neurofilament light is detected in various types of MS patient samples. Neurofilament light is detected in various types of human samples. The detection methods use a variety of assays as indicated, including ELISA, ECL, and SIMOA [65,68,82–113].

| Sample | Detection | References |
| --- | --- | --- |
| Serum | ELISA | [65] |
| | ECL | [82,83] |
| | SIMOA | [84–86] |
| Blood | SIMOA | [68] |
| CSF | ELISA | [87–103] |
| Plasma | SIMOA | [104] |
| Serum + CSF | ELISA | [105,106] |
| | ECL | [107] |
| | SIMOA | [108–113] |

## 3. Total and Phosphorylated Tau

Tau protein is important for the cytoskeleton of both neurons and oligodendrocytes [114–117]. Neurons and oligodendrocytes depend on efficient intracellular transport to accomplish tasks such as synaptic transmission and myelination, which are both essential for CNS health. Abnormally phosphorylated (P-)tau, a hallmark of CNS degenerative diseases, was found in chronic EAE and progressive MS [118,119].

Abnormally phosphorylated P-tau in neurons and/or oligodendrocytes causes cells to deteriorate, which would enhance disease progression [115–117,120,121]. Histological studies have clearly shown increased levels of P-tau in progressive MS [117–119]. Surprisingly, studies on total tau and P-tau as MS biomarkers have yielded contradictory data, perhaps due to a high sensitivity to tau protein degradation during improper samplings [13]. Indeed, some studies have reported higher levels of tau/P-tau in MS than in controls; however, others could not confirm this finding. Similar contradictions were reported regarding the correlation between a disability, inflammation, and age or MS disease duration [13,122]. Prednisolone effectively reduces plasma tau and P-tau in EAE rats [123]. Of interest, Rojas et al. [124] showed that CSF NF-L and tau phosphorylated at threonine 181 (P-tau181) predict disease progression in Progressive Supranuclear Palsy. It is imperative to investigate whether drugs aimed at neuroprotection in MS decrease NF-L levels in association with decreased tau phosphorylated at a specific site. Because cerebrospinal Tau levels predict early disability in MS [21], NF-L and tau have been proposed as biomarkers to monitor prognosis and treatment response, distinguishing different MS subtypes [125].

## 4. Amyloid-Peptide-β, Bri2, and Bri2-23

Amyloid precursor protein (APP) functions as cargo transported by fast anterograde axonal transport, whereas APP builds up in the cell body during diseases of axons [43]. APP, an integral membrane protein, is cleaved by the integral membrane aspartyl protease BACE1 (β-site APP-cleaving enzyme 1) into three fragments (α-sAPP, β-sAPP, and Aβ42) [13]. CSF levels of these fragments were lower in MS patients than in controls. Interestingly, the Bri2 and Bri2-23 molecules interact with APP and regulate amyloid-peptide-β (Aβ)42 cleavage and aggregation in vivo. Bri2 is a transmembrane protein and Bri2-23 is a peptide cleaved from Bri2. Because Bri2-23 levels have been suggested as a potential biomarker for cognitive deficit in progressive MS, studies should assess the effect of drugs aimed at neuroprotection on APP-derived proteins and on Bri2 and Bri2-23. Finally, Aβ42 does not correlate with age or disease duration [13,126,127].

The extent of APP expression appears to correlate with histopathological lesions, suggesting that APP detection is a sensitive marker for MS disease progression [126,128]. Insight from studies in AD could help to better tackle the challenges of MS biomarkers. High levels of CSF tau and/or P-tau181, and low levels of CSF Aβ42, are detected in the pre-symptomatic stages of AD disease [129]. Importantly, the ratio of CSF tau/Aβ42 or

CSF P-tau181/Aβ42 indicates the progression of AD pathology, which could also predict cognitive impairment in cognitively normal individuals [130–132]. The utility of the ratio of CSF levels Aβ42/Aβ40 or Aβ42/Aβ38 provides a better diagnostic value than the total levels of CSF Aβ42 [131]. Tau phosphorylation at selective sites, in particular, levels of CSF P-tau231 (threonine 231) and P-tau181, but not CSF P-tau199 (serine tau 199), differentiate AD from non-AD dementias [131]. CSF P-tau231 aids in differentiating AD from frontotemporal dementia and CSF P-tau181 differentiates AD from Lewy body dementia (LBD) [131]. In addition, the levels of CSF P-tau217 (threonine tau 217) increase in AD and provide a better diagnostic performance in differentiating AD from non-AD dementias than CSF P-tau181 [133]. The levels of CSF P-tau217 had a stronger correlation with CSF and positron emission tomography (PET) measures of cortical amyloid deposition than did CSF P-tau181 [131].

Levels of the blood-based biomarker, plasma P-tau181, increase early in AD, differentiating AD from cognitively normal controls and other dementias [131]. Plasma P-tau181 levels also increase with AD disease progression over time and predict progression to AD dementia in individuals with mild cognitive impairment (MCI). Plasma P-tau217 has received attention as a blood-based biomarker for AD [134].

In contrast to AD, MS affects the entire CNS, without predictable insight into which region of the CNS will be affected in each MS patient. Thus, a form of tau phosphorylated at a specific site might not be found.

Novel assays, using immunoprecipitation coupled with mass spectrometry or SIMOA, allow the measurement of plasma Aβ with high precision and demonstrate the ability of plasma Aβ40/Aβ42 levels to accurately predict amyloid-positive PET scans in cognitively normal or impaired individuals. The SIMOA platform has also been used successfully for plasma P-tau181 measurements, demonstrating the ability of plasma P-tau181 to accurately predict increased brain amyloid and tau on PET scans [30]. For subclinical neurodegeneration in MS, ideally, biomarkers would also need to correlate with changes at the CNS level, indicating neurodegenerative events.

## 5. N-Acetylaspartate

N-Acetylaspartate (NAA) is an abundant amino acid (AA) synthesized in neurons [13,135]. Several functions for this AA have been postulated, including working as an osmolyte important for the removal of water from neurons. Acetate is also important for myelin synthesis and is a mitochondrial energy source. Acetate is a precursor for N-acetyl aspartyl glutamate and a ligand for glutamate receptors [13]. Reduced acetate levels have been found in MS lesions. Of interest, glatiramer acetate, widely used to treat MS, increases NAA levels in MS lesions [136]. CSF NAA levels decrease during axonal degeneration and disease progression [13,135–137]. In addition, Narayanan et al. [137] showed that NAA increases in interferon (IFN) treated vs. untreated groups, suggesting that IFN reverses, in part, axonal injury during MS. It is imperative to investigate whether drugs aimed at neuroprotection increase NAA. Of interest, NAA is a marker of disability in secondary progressive MS as shown in a proton MR spectroscopic imaging study [138].

## 6. 14-3-3 Family Proteins

14-3-3 family proteins are highly concentrated in the brain and are expressed in the cytoplasmic and nuclear regions of neurons and glia [13]. These proteins regulate a variety of intracellular processes by interacting with hundreds of target proteins. 14-3-3 proteins are also molecular chaperones with anti-apoptotic effects. The presence of 14-3-3 protein in the CSF establishes Creutzfeldt-Jakob disease, but 14-3-3 protein is also detected in the CSF during other prion-unrelated conditions associated with CNS tissue damage. In MS, CSF, 14-3-3 protein levels correlate with a higher relapse rate and more severe disability, predicting permanent neurological disability after an acute episode [13,139–142]. No study to date has studied how neuroprotective drugs regulate 14-3-3 protein levels.

## 7. Additional Biomarkers of Neurodegeneration

Contactin-1 and contactin-2 in cerebrospinal fluid are potential biomarkers for axonal dysfunction in MS [143,144]. Contactin 1, a cell adhesion molecule, is a glycosylphosphatidy linositol-anchored neuronal membrane protein [145], and Contactin-2 is a cell adhesion molecule critical for neuronal patterning and ion channel clustering [146]. Recent evidence has shown the importance of MiR-142-3p for synaptopathy-driven disease progression in MS [147]. Previous studies have also shown glial activation markers in CSF and serum from patients with PP-MS. The authors suggested that serum glial fibrillary acidic protein (GFAP) is a potential marker for disease severity progression [148,149]. Further, monitoring reactive chemical species, oxidative enzymes, antioxidative enzymes, and degradation products might identify the redox status of MS patients [150], and thiol homeostasis may be useful to monitor disease activity [151]. The role of low levels of vitamin D in MS progression is an area of intense research, thus, serum levels of 25-hydroxyvitamin D should also be monitored during MS disease [152].

## 8. Osteopontin

Osteopontin (OPN) is an extracellular matrix glycol-phosphoprotein with a role in autoimmune-mediated demyelinating diseases during multiple sclerosis. OPN regulates inflammatory and regenerative processes during various diseases of the nervous system. OPN concentrations are increased in CSF during active multiple sclerosis [153,154].

## 9. Future Directions

The perspective of serum-based biomarkers described in this review must be combined with additional diagnostics. Work by LoPresti [33,155] indicated that an early defect at the level of HDAC6 is present in an animal model of MS. Serum-biomarkers should be added to in vivo HDAC6 changes. HDAC6 human brain mapping with [$^{18}$F] Bavarostat as a radiotracer has been proposed [156] and could be added to serum-based biomarkers to define MS types based on neurodegeneration, subgrouping MS into those patients with early or late neurodegeneration.

This review offers a new approach to elucidate a set of neurodegeneration biomarkers at two distinct time points. The aim is to identify distinct biomarker signatures in early and late subclinical cognitive decline. Newly identified biomarkers could identify the transition between early and late subclinical cognitive decline. For example, recent evidence pointed to GFAP as an important biomarker for progressive MS [148,149], as increased GFAP levels could help to delineate the transition into the late phase of subclinical cognitive decline, preceding progressive MS. Another approach could be the analysis of non-coding RNAs (ncRNAs). Joilin et al. [157] identified a potential ncRNA biomarker signature for ALS. In MS, a potential area of interest could include ncRNAs that distinguish disease activity from cytoskeletal disruption.

The biggest challenges in MS are two-fold; first, immune-inflammatory alterations during the disease are specific to each patient. Second, any area of the CNS can be a target of the disease. Therefore, by extending the concept of personalized medicine, we propose that the biomarker signature must be personalized for each patient. For example, standard assays should establish the baseline signature of selective biomarkers for each patient, and the evolution of such signature over time would be monitored. The signature shift could indicate progression along with subclinical cognitive decline, bringing that specific patient closer to developing progressive MS.

## 10. Summary

Focusing on neurons in MS patients, synaptic dysfunction and neurodegeneration should be measured so therapeutics can be planned to target each of these problems. Since tau protein is present at the synapses, a specific change in tau posttranslational modification might reveal a synaptic dysfunction, whereas large amounts of tau could indicate tau release due to neurodegeneration. Initial studies in mouse models of MS will highlight the relative importance of a set of serum-based biomarkers that characterizes synaptic dysfunction and neurodegeneration at early, mid, and late stages. In human samples, we expect distinct biomarker profiles to be identified in apparently similar types of MS. In particular, analysis of the blood of MS patients will show that each patient has a unique pattern, irrespective of their apparent clinical type, providing an educated rationale for intervention with selective therapeutics to modify the synaptic or neurodegeneration component. As the ability to distinguish synaptic dysfunction and neurodegeneration is established in each patient, a new understanding of the disease and therapeutic horizons can be envisioned.

## 11. Outstanding Questions

a. Would a new classification of MS types have to include silent progression?

b. Within clinically similar MS types, could we identify separate entities based on biomarkers of synaptic dysfunction and neurodegeneration?

c. Can a biomarker-based diagnostic test determine 1. The rate of subclinical memory decline, and 2. The time before the transition from subclinical to clinically apparent neurodegeneration?

**Funding:** This research received no external funding.

**Acknowledgments:** The author thanks Vieri Failli for assistance in preparing the Figures.

**Conflicts of Interest:** The author declares no conflict of interest.

## Abbreviations

| | |
|---|---|
| AA: | Amino acid |
| AD: | Alzheimer's disease |
| ALS: | Amyotrophic lateral sclerosis |
| APP: | Amyloid precursor protein |
| CNS: | Central nervous system |
| CSF: | Cerebrospinal fluid |
| EAE: | Experimental autoimmune encephalomyelitis |
| ECL: | Electro chemi luminescence |
| ELISA: | Enzyme-linked immunosorbent assay |
| GFAP: | Glial fibrillary acidic protein |
| IFN: | Interferon |
| LBD: | Lewy body dementia |
| MCI: | Mild cognitive impairment |
| MRI: | Magnetic resonance imaging |
| MS: | Multiple sclerosis |
| NAA: | N-Acetylaspartate |
| NFs: | Neurofilaments |
| NFL: | Neurofilament light |
| PET: | Positron emission tomography |
| PP-MS: | Primary progressive multiple sclerosis |
| RR-MS: | Relapsing-remitting multiple sclerosis |
| SIMOA: | Single-molecule array |
| sNF: | Serum neurofilament |
| SP-MS: | Secondary progressive multiple sclerosis |

## References

1. GBD 2016 Multiple Sclerosis Collaborators. Global, regional, and national burden of multiple sclerosis 1990–2016: A systematic analysis for the Global Burden of Disease Study 2016. *Lancet Neurol.* **2019**, *18*, 269–285. [CrossRef]
2. Hogancamp, W.E.; Rodriguez, M.; Weinshenker, B.G. The epidemiology of multiple sclerosis. *Mayo Clin. Proc.* **1997**, *72*, 871–878. [CrossRef] [PubMed]
3. Compston, A.; Coles, A. Multiple sclerosis. *Lancet* **2002**, *359*, 1221–1231. [CrossRef]

4. Bjornevik, K.; Cortese, M.; Healy, B.C.; Kuhle, J.; Mina, M.J.; Leng, Y.; Elledge, S.J.; Niebuhr, D.W.; Scher, A.I.; Munger, K.L.; et al. Longitudinal analysis reveals a high prevalence of Epstein-Barr virus-associated with multiple sclerosis. *Science* **2022**, *375*, 296–301. [CrossRef]
5. Kuchroo, V.K.; Weiner, H.L. How does Epstein-Barr virus trigger MS? *Immunity* **2022**, *55*, 390–392. [CrossRef]
6. Kurtzke, J.F. Rating neurologic impairment in multiple sclerosis: An expanded disability status scale (EDSS). *Neurology* **1983**, *33*, 1444–1452. [CrossRef]
7. Tsang, B.K.; Macdonell, R. Multiple sclerosis- diagnosis, management and prognosis. *Aust. Fam. Physician* **2011**, *40*, 948–955.
8. Banwell, B.; Giovannoni, G.; Hawkes, C.; Lublin, F. Multiple Sclerosis is a multifaceted disease. *Mult. Scler. Relat. Disord.* **2014**, *3*, 553–554. [CrossRef]
9. Bonzano, L.; Bove, M.; Sormani, M.P.; Stromillo, M.L.; Giorgio, A.; Amato, M.P.; Tacchino, A.; Mancardi, G.L.; De Stefano, N. Subclinical motor impairment assessed with an engineered glove correlates with magnetic resonance imaging tissue damage in radiologically isolated syndrome. *Eur. J. Neurol.* **2019**, *26*, 162–167. [CrossRef]
10. Benedict, R.H.; Pol, J.; Yasin, F.; Hojnacki, D.; Kolb, C.; Eckert, S.; Tacca, B.; Drake, A.; Wojcik, C.; Morrow, S.A.; et al. Recovery of cognitive function after relapse in multiple sclerosis. *Mult. Scler. J.* **2021**, *27*, 71–78. [CrossRef]
11. LoPresti, P. Silent Free Fall at Disease Onset: A Perspective on Therapeutics for Progressive Multiple Sclerosis. *Front. Neurol.* **2018**, *9*, 973. [CrossRef] [PubMed]
12. Cree, B.A.C.; Hollenbach, J.A.; Bove, R.; Kirkish, G.; Sacco, S.; Caverzasi, E.; Bischof, A.; Gundel, T.; Zhu, A.H.; Papinutto, N.; et al. Silent progression in disease activity-free relapsing multiple sclerosis. *Ann. Neurol.* **2019**, *85*, 653–666. [PubMed]
13. Dujmovic, I. Cerebrospinal fluid and blood biomarkers of neuroaxonal damage in multiple sclerosis. *Mult. Scler. Int.* **2011**, *2011*, 767083. [CrossRef] [PubMed]
14. Comabella, M.; Montalban, X. Body fluid biomarkers in multiple sclerosis. *Lancet Neurol.* **2014**, *13*, 113–126. [CrossRef]
15. Gafson, A.; Craner, M.J.; Matthews, P.M. Personalised medicine for multiple sclerosis care. *Mult. Scler. J.* **2017**, *23*, 362–369. [CrossRef]
16. Fox, R.J. Tissue Markers for Acute Multiple Sclerosis Treatment Response-A Step toward Personalized Medicine. *JAMA Neurol.* **2018**, *75*, 406–407. [CrossRef]
17. Shinomoto, M.; Kasai, T.; Tatebe, H.; Kondo, M.; Ohmichi, T.; Morimoto, M.; Chiyonobu, T.; Terada, N.; Allsop, D.; Yokota, I.; et al. Plasma neurofilament light chain: A potential prognostic biomarker of dementia in adult Down syndrome patients. *PLoS ONE* **2019**, *14*, e0211575. [CrossRef]
18. Preische, O.; Schultz, S.A.; Apel, A.; Kuhle, J.; Kaeser, S.A.; Barro, C.; Gräber, S.; Kuder-Buletta, E.; LaFougere, C.; Laske, C.; et al. Serum neurofilament dynamics predicts neurodegeneration and clinical progression in presymptomatic Alzheimer's disease. *Nat. Med.* **2019**, *25*, 277–283. [CrossRef]
19. Lee, J.Y.; Taghian, K.; Petratos, S. Axonal degeneration in multiple sclerosis: Can we predict and prevent permanent disability? *Acta Neuropathol. Commun.* **2014**, *2*, 97. [CrossRef]
20. Cree, B.A.; Gourraud, P.A.; Oksenberg, J.R.; Bevan, C.; Crabtree-Hartman, E.; Gelfand, J.; Goodin, D.; Graves, J.; Green, A.; Mowry, E.; et al. Long-term evolution of multiple sclerosis disability in the treatment era. *Ann. Neurol.* **2016**, *80*, 499–510.
21. Virgilio, E.; Vecchio, D.; Crespi, I.; Serino, R.; Cantello, R.; Dianzani, U.; Comi, C. Cerebrospinal Tau levels as a predictor of early disability in multiple sclerosis. *Mult. Scler. Relat. Disord.* **2021**, *56*, 103231. [CrossRef] [PubMed]
22. Kapoor, R.; Smith, K.E.; Allegretta, M.; Arnold, D.L.; Carroll, W.; Comabella, M.; Furlan, R.; Harp, C.; Kuhle, J.; Leppert, D.; et al. Serum neurofilament light as a biomarker in progressive multiple sclerosis. *Neurology* **2020**, *95*, 436–444. [CrossRef] [PubMed]
23. Hein Née Maier, K.; Köhler, A.; Diem, R.; Sättler, M.B.; Demmer, I.; Lange, P.; Bähr, M.; Otto, M. Biological markers for axonal degeneration in CSF and blood of patients with the first event indicative for multiple sclerosis. *Neurosci. Lett.* **2008**, *436*, 72–76. [CrossRef]
24. Spitzer, P.; Lang, R.; Oberstein, T.J.; Lewczuk, P.; Ermann, N.; Huttner, H.B.; Masouris, I.; Kornhuber, J.; Ködel, U.; Maler, J.M. A Specific Reduction in Aβ1-42 vs. a Universal Loss of Aβ Peptides in CSF Differentiates Alzheimer's Disease From Meningitis and Multiple Sclerosis. *Front. Aging Neurosci.* **2018**, *10*, 152. [CrossRef] [PubMed]
25. Harris, V.K.; Diamanduros, A.; Good, P.; Zakin, E.; Chalivendra, V.; Sadiq, S.A. Bri2-23 is a potential cerebrospinal fluid biomarker in multiple sclerosis. *Neurobiol. Dis.* **2010**, *40*, 331–339. [CrossRef] [PubMed]
26. Harris, V.K.; Sadiq, S.A. Disease biomarkers in multiple sclerosis: Potential for use in therapeutic decision making. *Mol. Diagn. Ther.* **2009**, *13*, 225–244. [CrossRef]
27. Miller, D.H. Biomarkers and surrogate outcomes in neurodegenerative disease: Lessons from multiple sclerosis. *NeuroRx* **2004**, *1*, 284–294. [CrossRef]
28. Agah, E.; Zardoui, A.; Saghazadeh, A.; Ahmadi, M.; Tafakhori, A.; Rezaei, N. Osteopontin (OPN) as a CSF and blood biomarker for multiple sclerosis: A systematic review and meta-analysis. *PLoS ONE* **2018**, *13*, e0190252. [CrossRef]
29. Housley, W.J.; Pitt, D.; Hafler, D.A. Biomarkers in multiple sclerosis. *Clin. Immunol.* **2015**, *161*, 51–58. [CrossRef]
30. Ferreira-Atuesta, C.; Reyes, S.; Giovanonni, G.; Gnanapavan, S. The Evolution of Neurofilament Light Chain in Multiple Sclerosis. *Front. Neurosci.* **2021**, *15*, 642384. [CrossRef]
31. Traka, M.; Podojil, J.R.; Mccarthy, D.P.; Miller, S.D.; Popko, B. Oligodendrocyte death results in immune-mediated CNS demyelination. *Nat. Neurosci.* **2016**, *19*, 65–74. [CrossRef] [PubMed]

32. Basso, A.S.; Frenkel, D.; Quintana, F.J.; Costa-Pinto, F.A.; Petrovic-Stojkovic, S.; Puckett, L.; Monsonego, A.; Bar-Shir, A.; Engel, Y.; Gozin, M.; et al. Reversal of axonal loss and disability in a mouse model of progressive multiple sclerosis. *J. Clin. Investig.* **2008**, *118*, 1532–1543. [CrossRef]
33. LoPresti, P. The Selective HDAC6 Inhibitor ACY-738 Impacts Memory and Disease Regulation in an Animal Model of Multiple Sclerosis. *Front. Neurol.* **2019**, *10*, 519. [CrossRef] [PubMed]
34. Trapp, B.D.; Nave, K.A. Multiple sclerosis: An immune or neurodegenerative disorder? *Annu. Rev. Neurosci.* **2008**, *31*, 247–269. [CrossRef]
35. Di Filippo, M.; Mancini, A.; Bellingacci, L.; Gaetani, L.; Mazzocchetti, P.; Zelante, T.; La Barbera, L.; De Luca, A.; Tantucci, M.; Tozzi, A.; et al. Interleukin-17 affects synaptic plasticity and cognition in an experimental model of multiple sclerosis. *Cell Rep.* **2021**, *37*, 110094. [CrossRef] [PubMed]
36. Bourel, J.; Planche, V.; Dubourdieu, N.; Oliveira, A.; Séré, A.; Ducourneau, E.G.; Tible, M.; Maitre, M.; Lesté-Lasserre, T.; Nadjar, A.; et al. Complement C3 mediates early hippocampal neurodegeneration and memory impairment in experimental multiple sclerosis. *Neurobiol. Dis.* **2021**, *160*, 105533. [CrossRef] [PubMed]
37. Mandolesi, G.; Gentile, A.; Musella, A.; Fresegna, D.; De Vito, F.; Bullitta, S.; Sepman, H.; Marfia, G.A.; Centonze, D. Synaptopathy connects inflammation and neurodegeneration in multiple sclerosis. *Nat. Rev. Neurol.* **2015**, *11*, 711–724. [CrossRef]
38. LoPresti, P. Glatiramer acetate guards against rapid memory decline during relapsing-remitting experimental autoimmune encephalomyelitis. *Neurochem. Res.* **2015**, *40*, 473–479. [CrossRef]
39. Buffolo, F.; Petrosino, V.; Albini, M.; Moschetta, M.; Carlini, F.; Floss, T.; Kerlero de Rosbo, N.; Cesca, F.; Rocchi, A.; Uccelli, A.; et al. Neuroinflammation induces synaptic scaling through IL-1β-mediated activation of the transcriptional repressor REST/NRSF. *Cell Death Dis.* **2021**, *12*, 180. [CrossRef]
40. Bruno, A.; Dolcetti, E.; Rizzo, F.R.; Fresegna, D.; Musella, A.; Gentile, A.; De Vito, F.; Caioli, S.; Guadalupi, L.; Bullitta, S.; et al. Inflammation-Associated Synaptic Alterations as Shared Threads in Depression and Multiple Sclerosis. *Front. Cell. Neurosci.* **2020**, *14*, 169. [CrossRef]
41. Nasios, G.; Bakirtzis, C.; Messinis, L. Cognitive Impairment and Brain Reorganization in MS: Underlying Mechanisms and the Role of Neurorehabilitation. *Front. Neurol.* **2020**, *11*, 147. [CrossRef] [PubMed]
42. Rizzo, F.R.; Musella, A.; De Vito, F.; Fresegna, D.; Bullitta, S.; Vanni, V.; Guadalupi, L.; Stampanoni Bassi, M.; Buttari, F.; Mandolesi, G.; et al. Tumor Necrosis Factor and Interleukin-1β Modulate Synaptic Plasticity during Neuroinflammation. *Neural. Plast.* **2018**, *10*, 1–12. [CrossRef]
43. Teunissen, C.E.; Dijkstra, C.; Polman, C. Biological markers in CSF and blood for axonal degeneration in multiple sclerosis. *Lancet Neurol.* **2005**, *4*, 32–41. [CrossRef]
44. Kappos, L.; Butzkueven, H.; Wiendl, H.; Spelman, T.; Pellegrini, F.; Chen, Y.; Dong, Q.; Koendgen, H.; Belachew, S.; Trojano, M.; et al. Greater sensitivity to multiple sclerosis disability worsening and progression events using a roving versus a fixed reference value in a prospective cohort study. *Mult. Scler. J.* **2018**, *24*, 963–973. [CrossRef] [PubMed]
45. Brady, S.T. Motor neurons and neurofilaments in sickness and in health. *Cell* **1993**, *73*, 1–3. [CrossRef]
46. Yuan, A.; Nixon, R.A. Neurofilament Proteins as Biomarkers to Monitor Neurological Diseases and the Efficacy of Therapies. *Front. Neurosci.* **2021**, *15*, 689938. [CrossRef]
47. Khalil, M.; Teunissen, C.E.; Otto, M.; Piehl, F.; Sormani, M.P.; Gattringer, T.; Barro, C.; Kappos, L.; Comabella, M.; Fazekas, F.; et al. Neurofilaments as biomarkers in neurological disorders. *Nat. Rev. Neurol.* **2018**, *14*, 577–589. [CrossRef]
48. Teunissen, C.E.; Petzold, A.; Bennett, J.L.; Berven, F.S.; Brundin, L.; Comabella, M.; Franciotta, D.; Frederiksen, J.L.; Fleming, J.O.; Furlan, R.; et al. A consensus protocol for the standardization of cerebrospinal fluid collection and biobanking. *Neurology* **2009**, *73*, 1914–1922. [CrossRef] [PubMed]
49. Lee, M.K.; Cleveland, D.W. Neuronal intermediate filaments. *Ann. Rev. Neurosci.* **1996**, *19*, 187–217. [CrossRef]
50. Semra, Y.K.; Seidi, O.A.; Sharief, M.K. Heightened intrathecal release of axonal cytoskeletal proteins in multiple sclerosis is associated with progressive disease and clinical disability. *J. Neuroimmunol.* **2002**, *122*, 132–139. [CrossRef]
51. Malmestrom, C.; Haghighi, S.; Rosengren, L.; Andersen, O.; Lycke, J. Neurofilament light protein and glial fibrillary acidic protein as biological markers in MS. *Neurology* **2003**, *61*, 1720–1725. [CrossRef] [PubMed]
52. Feneberg, E.; Oeckl, P.; Steinacker, P.; Verde, F.; Barro, C.; Van Damme, P.; Gray, E.; Grosskreutz, J.; Jardel, C.; Kuhle, J.; et al. Multicenter evaluation of neurofilaments in early symptom onset amyotrophic lateral sclerosis. *Neurology* **2018**, *90*, e22–e30. [CrossRef] [PubMed]
53. Barro, C.; Benkert, P.; Disanto, G.; Tsagkas, C.; Amann, M.; Naegelin, Y.; Leppert, D.; Gobbi, C.; Granziera, C.; Yaldizli, Ö.; et al. Serum neurofilament as a predictor of disease worsening and brain and spinal cord atrophy in multiple sclerosis. *Brain* **2018**, *141*, 2382–2391. [CrossRef] [PubMed]
54. Budelier, M.M.; He, Y.; Barthelemy, N.R.; Jiang, H.; Li, Y.; Park, E.; Henson, R.L.; Schindler, S.E.; Holtzman, D.M.; Bateman, R.J. A map of neurofilament light chain species in brain and cerebrospinal fluid and alterations in Alzheimer's disease. *Brain Commun.* **2022**, *4*, fcac045. [CrossRef] [PubMed]
55. Gunnarsson, M.; Malmeström, C.; Axelsson, M.; Sundström, P.; Dahle, C.; Vrethem, M.; Olsson, T.; Piehl, F.; Norgren, N.; Rosengren, L.; et al. Axonal damage in relapsing multiple sclerosis is markedly reduced by natalizumab. *Ann. Neurol.* **2011**, *69*, 83–89. [CrossRef]

56. Jakimovski, D.; Zivadinov, R.; Ramanthan, M.; Hagemeier, J.; Weinstock-Guttman, B.; Tomic, D.; Kropshofer, H.; Fuchs, T.A.; Barro, C.; Leppert, D.; et al. Serum neurofilament light chain level associations with clinical and cognitive performance in multiple sclerosis: A longitudinal retrospective 5-year study. *Mult. Scler. J.* **2020**, *26*, 1670–1681. [CrossRef] [PubMed]
57. Chen, Y.; Therriault, J.; Luo, J.; Ba, M.; Zhang, H.; Initiative, A. Neurofilament light as a biomarker of axonal degeneration in patients with mild cognitive impairment and Alzheimer's disease. *J. Integr. Neurosci.* **2021**, *20*, 861–870. [CrossRef]
58. Lee, E.H.; Kwon, H.S.; Koh, S.H.; Choi, S.H.; Jin, J.H.; Jeong, J.H.; Jang, J.W.; Park, K.W.; Kim, E.J.; Kim, H.J.; et al. Serum neurofilament light chain level as a predictor of cognitive stage transition. *Alzheimer's Res. Ther.* **2022**, *14*, 6. [CrossRef]
59. Silva-Spínola, A.; Lima, M.; Leitão, M.J.; Durães, J.; Tábuas-Pereira, M.; Almeida, M.R.; Santana, I.; Baldeiras, I. Serum neurofilament light chain as a surrogate of cognitive decline in sporadic and familial frontotemporal dementia. *Eur. J. Neurol.* **2022**, *29*, 36–46. [CrossRef]
60. Fialová, L.; Bartos, A.; Švarcová, J.; Zimova, D.; Kotoucova, J. Serum and cerebrospinal fluid heavy neurofilaments and antibodies against them in early multiple sclerosis. *J. Neuroimmunol.* **2013**, *259*, 81–87. [CrossRef]
61. Disanto, G.; Barro, C.; Benkert, P.; Naegelin, Y.; Schädelin, S.; Giardiello, A.; Zecca, C.; Blennow, K.; Zetterberg, H.; Leppert, D.; et al. Serum Neurofilament light: A biomarker of neuronal damage in multiple sclerosis. *Ann. Neurol.* **2017**, *81*, 857–870. [CrossRef]
62. Kuhle, J.; Nourbakhsh, B.; Grant, D.; Morant, S.; Barro, C.; Yaldizli, Ö.; Pelletier, D.; Giovannoni, G.; Waubant, E.; Gnanapavan, S. Serum neurofilament is associated with progression of brain atrophy and disability in early MS. *Neurology* **2017**, *88*, 826–831. [CrossRef]
63. Brureau, A.; Blanchard-Bregeon, V.; Pech, C.; Hamon, S.; Chaillou, P.; Guillemot, J.C.; Barneoud, P.; Bertrand, P.; Pradier, L.; Rooney, T.; et al. NF-L in cerebrospinal fluid and serum is a biomarker of neuronal damage in an inducible mouse model of neurodegeneration. *Neurobiol. Dis.* **2017**, *104*, 73–84. [CrossRef]
64. Martin, S.J.; McGlasson, S.; Hunt, D.; Overell, J. Cerebrospinal fluid neurofilament light chain in multiple sclerosis and its subtypes: A meta-analysis of case-control studies. *J. Neurol. Neurosurg. Psychiatry* **2019**, *90*, 1059–1067. [CrossRef]
65. Siller, N.; Kuhle, J.; Muthuraman, M.; Barro, C.; Uphaus, T.; Groppa, S.; Kappos, L.; Zipp, F.; Bittner, S. Serum neurofilament light chain is a biomarker of acute and chronic neuronal damage in early multiple sclerosis. *Mult. Scler. J.* **2019**, *25*, 678–686. [CrossRef]
66. Sellebjerg, F.; Royen, L.; Soelberg Sørensen, P.; Oturai, A.B.; Jensen, P. Prognostic value of cerebrospinal fluid neurofilament light chain and chitinase-3-like-1 in newly diagnosed patients with multiple sclerosis. *Mult. Scler. J.* **2019**, *25*, 1444–1451. [CrossRef]
67. Norgren, N.; Sundström, P.; Svenningsson, A.; Rosengren, L.; Stigbrand, T.; Gunnarsson, M. Neurofilament and glial fibrillary acidic protein in multiple sclerosis. *Neurology* **2004**, *63*, 1586–1590. [CrossRef]
68. Kuhle, J.; Kropshofer, H.; Hearing, D.A.; Kundu, U.; Meinert, R.; Barro, C.; Dahlke, F.; Tomic, D.; Leppert, D.; Kappos, L. Blood neurofilament light chain as a biomarker of MS disease activity and treatment response. *Neurology* **2019**, *92*, e1007–e1015. [CrossRef]
69. Bhan, A.; Jacobsen, C.; Dalen, I.; Bergsland, N.; Zivadinov, R.; Alves, G.; Myhr, K.M.; Farbu, E. CSF neurofilament light chain predicts 10-year clinical and radiologic worsening in multiple sclerosis. *Mult. Scler. J. Exp. Transl. Clin.* **2021**, *7*, 20552173211060337. [CrossRef]
70. Lycke, J.N.; Karlsson, J.E.; Andersen, O.; Rosengren, L.E. Neurofilament protein in cerebrospinal fluid: A potential marker of activity in multiple sclerosis. *J. Neurol. Neurosurg. Psychiatry* **1998**, *64*, 402–404. [CrossRef]
71. Cai, L.; Huang, J. Neurofilament light chain as a biological marker for multiple sclerosis: A meta-analysis study. *Neuropsychiatr. Dis. Treat.* **2018**, *14*, 2241–2254. [CrossRef]
72. Vavasour, I.M.; Becquart, P.; Gill, J.; Zhao, G.; Yik, J.T.; Traboulsee, A.; Carruthers, R.L.; Kolind, S.H.; Schabas, A.J.; Sayao, A.L.; et al. Diffusely abnormal white matter in clinically isolated syndrome is associated with parenchymal loss and elevated neurofilament levels. *Mult. Scler. Relat. Disord.* **2021**, *57*, 103422. [CrossRef]
73. Maggi, P.; Kuhle, J.; Schädelin, S.; van der Meer, F.; Weigel, M.; Galbusera, R.; Mathias, A.; Lu, P.J.; Rahmanzadeh, R.; Benkert, P.; et al. Chronic White Matter Inflammation and Serum Neurofilament Levels in Multiple Sclerosis. *Neurology* **2021**, *97*, e543–e553. [CrossRef]
74. Puentes, F.; Benkert, P.; Amor, S.; Kuhle, J.; Giovannoni, G. Antibodies to neurofilament light as potential biomarkers in multiple sclerosis. *BMJ Neurol. Open* **2021**, *3*, e000192. [CrossRef]
75. Calabresi, P.A.; Arnold, D.L.; Sangurdekar, D.; Singh, C.M.; Altincatal, A.; de Moor, C.; Engle, B.; Goyal, J.; Deykin, A.; Szak, S.; et al. Temporal profile of serum neurofilament light in multiple sclerosis: Implications for patient monitoring. *Mult. Scler. J.* **2021**, *27*, 1497–1505. [CrossRef]
76. Jakimovski, D.; Dwyer, M.G.; Bergsland, N.; Weinstock-Guttman, B.; Zivadinov, R. Disease biomarkers in multiple sclerosis: Current serum neurofilament light chain perspectives. *Neurodegener. Dis. Manag.* **2021**, *11*, 329–340. [CrossRef]
77. Bergman, J.; Dring, A.; Zetterberg, H.; Blennow, K.; Norgren, N.; Gilthorpe, J.; Bergenheim, T.; Svenningsson, A. Neurofilament light in CSF and serum is a sensitive marker for axonal white matter injury in MS. *Neurol. Neuroimmunol. Neuroinflamm.* **2016**, *3*, e271. [CrossRef]
78. Bridel, C.; Leurs, C.E.; van Lierop, Z.; van Kempen, Z.; Dekker, I.; Twaalfhoven, H.; Moraal, B.; Barkhof, F.; Uitdehaag, B.; Killestein, J.; et al. Serum Neurofilament Light Association with Progression in Natalizumab-Treated Patients With Relapsing-Remitting Multiple Sclerosis. *Neurology* **2021**, *97*, e1898–e1905. [CrossRef]

79. Kuhle, J.; Daizadeh, N.; Benkert, P.; Maceski, A.; Barro, C.; Michalak, Z.; Sormani, M.P.; Godin, J.; Shankara, S.; Samad, T.A.; et al. Sustained reduction of serum neurofilament light chain over 7 years by alemtuzumab in early relapsing-remitting MS. *Mult. Scler. J.* **2021**, *28*, 13524585211032348. [CrossRef]
80. Cantó, E.; Barro, C.; Zhao, C.; Caillier, S.J.; Michalak, Z.; Bove, R.; Tomic, D.; Santaniello, A.; Häring, D.A.; Hollenbach, J.; et al. Association Between Serum Neurofilament Light Chain Levels and Long-term Disease Course Among Patients With Multiple Sclerosis Followed up for 12 Years. *JAMA Neurol.* **2019**, *76*, 1359–1366. [CrossRef]
81. Kuhle, J.; Plavina, T.; Barro, C.; Disanto, G.; Sangurdekar, D.; Singh, C.M.; de Moor, C.; Engle, B.; Kieseier, B.C.; Fisher, E.; et al. Neurofilament light levels are associated with long-term outcomes in multiple sclerosis. *Mult. Scler. J.* **2020**, *26*, 1691–1699. [CrossRef]
82. Disanto, G.; Adiutori, R.; Dobson, R.; Martinelli, V.; Dalla Costa, G.; Runia, T.; Evdoshenko, E.; Thouvenot, E.; Trojano, M.; Norgren, N.; et al. Serum neurofilament light chain levels are increased in patients with a clinically isolated syndrome. *J. Neurol. Neurosurg. Psychiatry* **2016**, *87*, 126–129. [CrossRef]
83. Dalla Costa, G.; Martinelli, V.; Sangalli, F.; Moiola, L.; Colombo, B.; Radaelli, M.; Letizia, L.; Roberto, F.; Comi, G. Prognostic value of serum neurofilaments in patients with clinically isolated syndromes. *Neurology* **2019**, *92*, e733–e741. [CrossRef]
84. Jakimovski, D.; Kuhle, J.; Ramanathan, M.; Barro, C.; Tomic, D.; Hagemeier, J.; Kropshofer, H.; Bergsland, N.; Leppert, D.; Dwyer, M.G. Serum neurofilament light chain levels associations with gray matter pathology: A 5-year longitudinal study. *Ann. Clin. Transl. Neurol.* **2019**, *6*, 1757–1770. [CrossRef]
85. Bjornevik, K.; Munger, K.L.; Cortese, M.; Barro, C.; Healy, B.C.; Niebuhr, D.W.; Scher, A.I.; Kuhle, J.; Ascherio, A. Serum Neurofilament Light Chain Levels in Patients With Presymptomatic Multiple Sclerosis. *JAMA Neurol.* **2020**, *77*, 58–64. [CrossRef]
86. Bittner, S.; Steffen, F.; Uphaus, T.; Muthuraman, M.; Fleischer, V.; Salmen, A.; Luessi, F.; Berthele, A.; Klotz, L.; Meuth, S.G.; et al. Clinical implications of serum neurofilament in newly diagnosed MS patients: A longitudinal multicentre cohort study. *EBioMedicine* **2020**, *56*, 102807. [CrossRef]
87. Novakova, L.; Axelsson, M.; Khademi, M.; Zetterberg, H.; Blennow, K.; Malmeström, C.; Piehl, F.; Olsson, T.; Lycke, J. Cerebrospinal fluid biomarkers as a measure of disease activity and treatment efficacy in relapsing-remitting multiple sclerosis. *J. Neurochem.* **2017**, *141*, 296–304. [CrossRef]
88. Håkansson, I.; Tisell, A.; Cassel, P.; Blennow, K.; Zetterberg, H.; Lundberg, P.; Dahle, C.; Vrethem, M.; Ernerudh, J. Neurofil ament light chain in cerebrospinal fluid and prediction of disease activity in clinically isolated syndrome and relapsing-remitting multiple sclerosis. *Eur. J. Neurol.* **2017**, *24*, 703–712. [CrossRef]
89. Zhang, Y.; Li, X.; Qiao, J. Neurofilament protein light in multiple sclerosis. *Zhonghua Yi Xue Za Zhi* **2007**, *87*, 2745–2749.
90. Haghighi, S.; Andersen, O.; Odén, A.; Rosengren, L. Cerebrospinal fluid markers in MS patients and their healthy siblings. *Acta Neurol. Scand.* **2004**, *109*, 97–99. [CrossRef]
91. Norgren, N.; Rosengren, L.; Stigbrand, T. Elevated neurofilament levels in neurological diseases. *Brain Res.* **2003**, *987*, 25–31. [CrossRef]
92. Gil-Perotin, S.; Castillo-Villalba, J.; Cubas-Nuñez, L.; Gasque, R.; Hervas, D.; Gomez-Mateu, J.; Alcala, C.; Perez-Miralles, F.; Gascon, F.; Dominguez, J.A.; et al. Combined cerebrospinal fluid neurofilament light chain protein and chitinase-3 like-1 levels in defining disease course and prognosis in multiple sclerosis. *Front. Neurol.* **2019**, *10*, 1008. [CrossRef]
93. Gaetani, L.; Salvadori, N.; Lisetti, V.; Eusebi, P.; Mancini, A.; Gentili, L.; Borrelli, A.; Portaccio, E.; Sarchielli, P.; Blennow, K.; et al. Cerebrospinal fluid neurofilament light chain tracks cognitive impairment in multiple sclerosis. *J. Neurol.* **2019**, *266*, 2157–2163. [CrossRef]
94. Gaetani, L.; Eusebi, P.; Mancini, A.; Gentili, L.; Borrelli, A.; Parnetti, L.; Calabresi, P.; Sarchielli, P.; Blennow, K.; Zetterberg, H.; et al. Cerebrospinal fluid neurofilament light chain predicts disease activity after the first demyelinating event suggestive of multiple sclerosis. *Mult. Scler. Relat. Disord.* **2019**, *35*, 228–232. [CrossRef]
95. Olesen, M.N.; Soelberg, K.; Debrabant, B.; Nilsson, A.C.; Lillevang, S.T.; Grauslund, J.; Brandslund, I.; Madsen, J.S.; Paul, F.; Smith, T.J.; et al. Cerebrospinal fluid biomarkers for predicting development of multiple sclerosis in acute optic neuritis: A population-based prospective cohort study. *J. Neuroinflamm.* **2019**, *16*, 59. [CrossRef]
96. Bhan, A.; Jacobsen, C.; Myhr, K.M.; Dalen, I.; Lode, K.; Farbu, E. Neurofilaments and 10-year follow-up in multiple sclerosis. *Mult. Scler. J.* **2018**, *24*, 1301–1307. [CrossRef]
97. Quintana, E.; Coll, C.; Salavedra-Pont, J.; Muñoz-San Martín, M.; Robles-Cedeño, R.; Tomàs-Roig, J.; Buxó, M.; Matute-Blanch, C.; Villar, L.M.; Montalban, X.; et al. Cognitive impairment in early stages of multiple sclerosis is associated with high cerebrospinal fluid levels of chitinase 3-like 1 and neurofilament light chain. *Eur. J. Neurol.* **2018**, *25*, 1189–1191. [CrossRef]
98. Van der Vuurst de Vries, R.M.; Wong, Y.Y.M.; Mescheriakova, J.Y.; van Pelt, E.D.; Runia, T.F.; Jafari, N.; Siepman, T.A.; Melief, M.J.; Wierenga-Wolf, A.F.; van Luijn, M.M.; et al. High neurofilament levels are associated with clinically definite multiple sclerosis in children and adults with clinically isolated syndrome. *Mult. Scler. J.* **2019**, *25*, 958–967. [CrossRef]
99. Novakova, L.; Axelsson, M.; Malmeström, C.; Imberg, H.; Elias, O.; Zetterberg, H.; Nerman, O.; Lycke, J. Searching for neurodegeneration in multiple sclerosis at clinical onset:Diagnostic value of biomarkers. *PLoS ONE* **2018**, *13*, e0194828. [CrossRef]
100. Tortorella, C.; Direnzo, V.; Ruggieri, M.; Zoccolella, S.; Mastrapasqua, M.; D'onghia, M.; Paolicelli, D.; Cuonzo, F.D.; Gasperini, C.; Trojano, M. Cerebrospinal fluid neurofilament light levels mark grey matter volume in clinically isolated syndrome suggestive of multiple sclerosis. *Mult. Scler. J.* **2018**, *241*, 039–1045. [CrossRef]

101. Arrambide, G.; Espejo, C.; Eixarch, H.; Villar, L.M.; Alvarez-Cermeño, J.C.; Picón, C.; Kuhle, J.; Disanto, G.; Kappos, L.; Sastre-Garriga, J.; et al. Neurofilament light chain level is a weak risk factor for the development of MS. *Neurology* **2016**, *87*, 1076–1084. [CrossRef]
102. Reyes, S.; Smets, I.; Holden, D.; Carrillo-Loza, K.; Christmas, T.; Bianchi, L.; Ammoscato, F.; Turner, B.; Marta, M.; Schmierer, K.; et al. CSF neurofilament light chain testing as an aid to determine treatment strategies in MS. *Neurol. Neuroimmunol. Neuroinflamm.* **2020**, *7*, e880. [CrossRef]
103. Modvig, S.; Degn, M.; Roed, H.; Sørensen, T.L.; Larsson, H.B.; Langkilde, A.R.; Frederiksen, J.L.; Sellebjerg, F. Cerebrospinal fluid levels of chitinase 3-like 1 and neurofilament light chain predict multiple sclerosis development and disability after optic neuritis. *Mult. Scler. J.* **2015**, *21*, 1761–1770. [CrossRef]
104. Manouchehrinia, A.; Stridh, P.; Khademi, M.; Leppert, D.; Barro, C.; Michalak, Z.; Benkert, P.; Lycke, J.; Alfredsson, L.; Kappos, L.; et al. Plasma neurofilament light levels are associated with risk of disability in multiple sclerosis. *Neurology* **2020**, *94*, e2457–e2467. [CrossRef]
105. Novakova, L.; Zetterberg, H.; Sundström, P.; Axelsson, M.; Khademi, M.; Gunnarsson, M.; Malmeström, C.; Svenningsson, A.; Olsson, T.; Piehl, F.; et al. Monitoring disease activity in multiple sclerosis using serum neurofilament light protein. *Neurology* **2017**, *89*, 2230–2237. [CrossRef]
106. Engel, S.; Friedrich, M.; Muthuraman, M.; Steffen, F.; Poplawski, A.; Groppa, S.; Bittner, S.; Zipp, F.; Luessi, F. Intrathecal B-cell accumulation and axonal damage distinguish MRI-based benign from aggressive onset in MS. *Neurol. Neuroimmunol. Neuroinflamm.* **2019**, *6*, e595. [CrossRef]
107. Kuhle, J.; Barro, C.; Disanto, G.; Mathias, A.; Soneson, C.; Bonnier, G.; Yaldizli, Ö.; Regeniter, A.; Derfuss, T.; Canales, M.; et al. Serum neurofilament light chain in early relapsing remitting MS is increased and correlates with CSF levels and with MRI measures of disease severity. *Mult. Scler. J.* **2016**, *22*, 1550–1559. [CrossRef]
108. Piehl, F.; Kockum, I.; Khademi, M.; Blennow, K.; Lycke, J.; Zetterberg, H.; Olsson, T. Plasma neurofilament light chain levels in patients with MS switching from injectable therapies to fingolimod. *Mult. Scler.* **2018**, *24*, 1046–1054. [CrossRef]
109. Ayrignac, X.; Le Bars, E.; Duflos, C.; Hirtz, C.; Maleska Maceski, A.; Carra-Dallière, C.; Charif, M.; Pinna, F.; Prin, P.; de Champfleur, N.M.; et al. Serum GFAP in multiple sclerosis: Correlation with disease type and MRI markers of disease severity. *Sci. Rep.* **2020**, *10*, 10923. [CrossRef]
110. Watanabe, M.; Nakamura, Y.; Michalak, Z.; Isobe, N.; Barro, C.; Leppert, D.; Matsushita, T.; Hayashi, F.; Yamasaki, R.; Kuhle, J.; et al. Serum GFAP and neurofilament light as biomarkers of disease activity and disability in NMOSD. *Neurology* **2019**, *93*, e1299–e1311. [CrossRef]
111. Wong, Y.Y.M.; Bruijstens, A.L.; Barro, C.; Michalak, Z.; Melief, M.J.; Wierenga, A.F.; van Pelt, E.D.; Neuteboom, R.F.; Kuhle, J.; Hintzen, R.Q. Serum neurofilament light chain in pediatric MS and other acquired demyelinating syndromes. *Neurology* **2019**, *93*, e968–e974. [CrossRef] [PubMed]
112. Håkansson, I.; Tisell, A.; Cassel, P.; Blennow, K.; Zetterberg, H.; Lundberg, P.; Dahle, C.; Vrethem, M.; Ernerudh, J. Neurofilament levels, disease activity and brain volume during follow-up in multiple sclerosis. *J. Neuroinflamm.* **2018**, *15*, 209. [CrossRef] [PubMed]
113. Kouchaki, E.; Dashti, F.; Mirazimi, S.; Alirezaei, Z.; Jafari, S.H.; Hamblin, M.R.; Mirzaei, H. Neurofilament light chain as a biomarker for diagnosis of multiple sclerosis. *EXCLI J.* **2021**, *20*, 1308–1325. [CrossRef]
114. Binder, L.I.; Frankfurter, A.; Rebhun, L.I. The distribution of tau in the mammalian central nervous system. *J. Cell Biol.* **1985**, *101*, 1371–1378. [CrossRef]
115. LoPresti, P.; Szuchet, S.; Papasozomenos, S.C.; Zinkowski, R.P.; Binder, L.I. Functional implications for the microtubule-associated protein tau: Localization in oligodendrocytes. *Proc. Natl. Acad. Sci. USA* **1995**, *92*, 1036973. [CrossRef]
116. LoPresti, P. Inducible Expression of a Truncated Form of Tau in Oligodendrocytes Elicits Gait Abnormalities and a Decrease in Myelin: Implications for Selective CNS Degenerative Diseases. *Neurochem. Res.* **2015**, *40*, 2188–2199. [CrossRef]
117. LoPresti, P. Tau in Oligodendrocytes Takes Neurons in Sickness and in Health. *Int. J. Mol. Sci.* **2018**, *19*, 2408. [CrossRef]
118. Anderson, J.M.; Hampton, D.W.; Patani, R.; Pryce, G.; Crowther, R.A.; Reynolds, R.; Franklin, R.J.; Giovannoni, G.; Compston, D.A.; Baker, D.; et al. Abnormally phosphorylated tau is associated with neuronal and axonal loss in experimental autoimmune encephalomyelitis and multiple sclerosis. *Brain* **2008**, *131*, 1736–1748. [CrossRef]
119. Anderson, J.M.; Patani, R.; Reynolds, R.; Nicholas, R.; Compston, A.; Spillantini, M.G.; Chandran, S. Evidence for abnormal tau phosphorylation in early aggressive multiple sclerosis. *Acta Neuropathol.* **2009**, *117*, 583–589. [CrossRef]
120. Ballatore, C.; Lee, V.M.; Trojanowski, J.Q. Tau-mediated neurodegeneration in Alzheimer's disease and related disorders. Nature reviews. *Neuroscience* **2007**, *8*, 663–672.
121. Mandelkow, E.M.; Mandelkow, E. Biochemistry and cell biology of tau protein in neurofibrillary degeneration. *Cold Spring Harbor Perspect. Med.* **2012**, *2*, a006247. [CrossRef] [PubMed]
122. Bartosik-Psujek, H.; Stelmasiak, Z. The CSF levels of total-tau and phosphotau in patients with relapsing-remitting multiple sclerosis. *J. Neural Transm.* **2006**, *113*, 339–345. [CrossRef] [PubMed]
123. Schneider, A.; Araújo, G.W.; Trajkovic, K.; Herrmann, M.M.; Merkler, D.; Mandelkow, E.M.; Weissert, R.; Simons, M. Hyperphosphorylation and aggregation of tau in experimental autoimmune encephalomyelitis. *J. Biol. Chem.* **2004**, *279*, 55833–55839. [CrossRef] [PubMed]

124. Rojas, J.C.; Bang, J.; Lobach, I.V.; Tsai, R.M.; Rabinovici, G.D.; Miller, B.L.; Boxer, A.L.; AL-108-231 Investigators. CSF neurofilament light chain and phosphorylated tau 181 predict disease progression in PSP. *Neurology* **2018**, *90*, e273–e281. [CrossRef] [PubMed]
125. Momtazmanesh, S.; Shobeiri, P.; Saghazadeh, A.; Teunissen, C.E.; Burman, J.; Szalardy, L.; Klivenyi, P.; Bartos, A.; Fernandes, A.; Rezaei, N. Neuronal and glial CSF biomarkers in multiple sclerosis: A systematic review and meta-analysis. *Rev. Neurosci.* **2021**, *32*, 573–595. [CrossRef]
126. Gehrmann, J.; Banati, R.B.; Cuzner, M.L.; Kreutzberg, G.W.; Newcombe, J. Amyloid precursor protein (APP) expression in multiple sclerosis lesions. *Glia* **1995**, *15*, 141–151. [CrossRef]
127. Mattsson, N.; Axelsson, M.; Haghighi, S.; Malmeström, C.; Wu, G.; Anckarsäter, R.; Sankaranarayanan, S.; Andreasson, U.; Fredrikson, S.; Gundersen, A.; et al. Reduced cerebrospinal fluid BACE1 activity in multiple sclerosis. *Multiple Sclerosis* **2009**, *15*, 448–454. [CrossRef]
128. Mathur, D.; Mishra, B.K.; Rout, S.; Lopez-Iranzo, F.J.; Lopez-Rodas, G.; Vallamkondu, J.; Kandimalla, R.; Casanova, B. Potential Biomarkers Associated with Multiple Sclerosis Pathology. *Int. J. Mol. Sci.* **2021**, *22*, 10323. [CrossRef]
129. Fagan, A.M.; Mintun, M.A.; Shah, A.R.; Aldea, P.; Roe, C.M.; Mach, R.H.; Marcus, D.; Morris, J.C.; Holtzman, D.M. Cerebrospinal fluid tau and ptau (181) increase with cortical amyloid deposition in cognitively normal individuals: Implications for future clinical trials of Alzheimer's disease. *EMBO Mol. Med.* **2009**, *1*, 371–380. [CrossRef]
130. Bos, I.; Vos, S.; Verhey, F.; Scheltens, P.; Teunissen, C.; Engelborghs, S.; Sleegers, K.; Frisoni, G.; Blin, O.; Richardson, J.C.; et al. Cerebrospinal fluid biomarkers of neurodegeneration, synaptic integrity, and astroglial activation across the clinical Alzheimer's disease spectrum. *Alzheimers Dement.* **2019**. [CrossRef]
131. Tarawneh, R. Biomarkers: Our Path Towards a Cure for Alzheimer Disease. *Biomarker Insights* **2020**, *15*, 1177271920976367. [CrossRef]
132. Li, X.; Li, T.Q.; Andreasen, N.; Wiberg, M.K.; Westman, E.; Wahlund, L.O. Ratio of Aβ42/P-tau181p in CSF is associated with aberrant default mode network in AD. *Sci. Rep.* **2013**, *3*, 1339. [CrossRef] [PubMed]
133. Janelidze, S.; Stomrud, E.; Smith, R.; Palmqvist, S.; Mattsson, N.; Airey, D.C.; Proctor, N.K.; Chai, X.; Shcherbinin, S.; Sims, J.R.; et al. Cerebrospinal fluid p-tau217 performs better than p-tau181 as a biomarker of Alzheimer's disease. *Nat. Commun.* **2020**, *11*, 1683. [CrossRef] [PubMed]
134. Telser, J.; Risch, L.; Saely, C.H.; Grossmann, K.; Werner, P. P-tau217 in Alzheimer's disease. *Clin. Chim. Acta* **2022**, *531*, 100–111. [CrossRef] [PubMed]
135. Moffett, J.R.; Ross, B.; Arun, P.; Madhavarao, C.N.; Namboodiri, A.M.A. N-Acetylaspartate in the CNS: From neurodiagnostics to neurobiology. *Prog. Neurobiol.* **2007**, *81*, 89–131. [CrossRef] [PubMed]
136. Khan, O.; Shen, Y.; Caon, C.; Bao, F.; Ching, W.; Reznar, M.; Buccheister, A.; Hu, J.; Latif, Z.; Tselis, A.; et al. Axonal metabolic recovery and potential neuroprotective effect of Glatiramer acetate in relapsing-remitting multiple sclerosis. *Multiple Sclerosis* **2005**, *11*, 646–651. [CrossRef]
137. Narayanan, S.; De Stefano, N.; Francis, G.S.; Arnaoutelis, R.; Caramanos, Z.; Collins, D.L.; Pelletier, D.; Arnason, B.G.W.; Antel, J.P.; Arnold, D.L. Axonal metabolic recovery in multiple sclerosis patients treated with interferon beta-1b. *J. Neurol.* **2001**, *248*, 979–986. [CrossRef]
138. Solanky, B.S.; John, N.A.; DeAngelis, F.; Stutters, J.; Prados, F.; Schneider, T.; Parker, R.A.; Weir, C.J.; Monteverdi, A.; Plantone, D.; et al. NAA is a Marker of Disability in Secondary-Progressive MS: A Proton MR Spectroscopic Imaging Study. *Am. J. Neuroradiol.* **2020**, *41*, 2209–2218. [CrossRef]
139. Giovannoni, G. Multiple sclerosis cerebrospinal fluid biomarkers. *Dis. Markers* **2006**, *22*, 187–196. [CrossRef]
140. Martínez-Yélamos, A.; Saiz, A.; Sanchez-Valle, R.; Casado, V.; Ramón, J.M.; Graus, F.; Arbizu, T. 14-3-3 Protein in the CSF as prognostic marker in early multiple sclerosis. *Neurology* **2001**, *57*, 722–724. [CrossRef]
141. Martínez-Yélamos, A.; Rovira, A.; Sánchez-Valle, R.; Martínez-Yélamos, S.; Tintoré, M.; Blanco, Y.; Graus, F.; Montalban, X.; Arbizu, T.; Saiz, A. CSF 14-3-3 protein assay and MRI as prognostic markers in patients with a clinically isolated syndrome suggestive of MS. *J. Neurol.* **2004**, *251*, 1278–1279. [CrossRef] [PubMed]
142. Fan, X.; Cui, L.; Zeng, Y.; Song, W.; Gaur, U.; Yang, M. 14-3-3 Proteins Are on the Crossroads of Cancer, Aging, and Age-Related Neurodegenerative Disease. *Int. J. Mol. Sci.* **2019**, *20*, 3518. [CrossRef] [PubMed]
143. Chatterjee, M.; Koel-Simmelink, M.J.; Verberk, I.M.; Killestein, J.; Vrenken, H.; Enzinger, C.; Ropele, S.; Fazekas, F.; Khalil, M.; Teunissen, C.E. Contactin-1 and contactin-2 in cerebrospinal fluid as potential biomarkers for axonal domain dysfunction in multiple sclerosis. *Mult. Scler. J.* **2018**, *4*, 2055217318819535. [CrossRef] [PubMed]
144. van Lierop, Z.Y.; Wieske, L.; Koel-Simmelink, M.J.; Chatterjee, M.; Dekker, I.; Leurs, C.E.; Willemse, E.A.; Moraal, B.; Barkhof, F.; Eftimov, F.; et al. Serum contactin-1 as a biomarker of long-term disease progression in natalizumab-treated multiple sclerosis. *Mult. Scler. J.* **2022**, *28*, 102–110. [CrossRef] [PubMed]
145. Chen, D.H.; Yu, J.W.; Wu, J.G.; Wang, S.L.; Jiang, B.J. Significances of contactin-1 expression in human gastric cancer and knockdown of contactin-1 expression inhibits invasion and metastasis of MKN45 gastric cancer cells. *J. Cancer Res. Clin. Oncol.* **2015**, *141*, 2109–2120. [CrossRef]
146. Pallante, B.A.; Giovannone, S.; Fang-Yu, L.; Zhang, J.; Liu, N.; Kang, G.; Dun, W.; Boyden, P.A.; Fishman, G.I. Contactin-2 expression in the cardiac Purkinje fiber network. Circulation. *Arrhythmia Electrophysiol.* **2010**, *3*, 186–194. [CrossRef]

147. De Vito, F.; Musella, A.; Fresegna, D.; Rizzo, F.R.; Gentile, A.; Stampanoni Bassi, M.; Gilio, L.; Buttari, F.; Procaccini, C.; Colamatteo, A.; et al. MiR-142-3p regulates synaptopathy-driven disease progression in multiple sclerosis. *Neuropathol. Appl. Neurobiol.* **2021**, *48*, e12765. [CrossRef]
148. Axelsson, M.; Malmeström, C.; Nilsson, S.; Haghighi, S.; Rosengren, L.; Lycke, J. Glial fibrillary acidic protein: A potential biomarker for progression in multiple sclerosis. *J. Neurol.* **2011**, *258*, 882–888. [CrossRef]
149. Abdelhak, A.; Hottenrott, T.; Morenas-Rodríguez, E.; Suárez-Calvet, M.; Zettl, U.K.; Haass, C.; Meuth, S.G.; Rauer, S.; Otto, M.; Tumani, H.; et al. Glial Activation Markers in CSF and Serum from Patients With Primary Progressive Multiple Sclerosis: Potential of Serum GFAP as Disease Severity Marker? *Front. Neurol.* **2019**, *10*, 280. [CrossRef]
150. Tanaka, M.; Vécsei, L. Monitoring the Redox Status in Multiple Sclerosis. *Biomedicines* **2020**, *8*, 406. [CrossRef]
151. Arslan, B.; Arslan, G.A.; Tuncer, A.; Karabudak, R.; Dinçel, A.S. Evaluation of Thiol Homeostasis in Multiple Sclerosis and Neuromyelitis Optica Spectrum Disorders. *Front. Neurol.* **2021**, *12*, 716195. [CrossRef] [PubMed]
152. Bivona, G.; Gambino, C.M.; Lo Sasso, B.; Scazzone, C.; Giglio, R.V.; Agnello, L.; Ciaccio, M. Serum Vitamin D as a Biomarker in Autoimmune, Psychiatric and Neurodegenerative Diseases. *Diagnostics* **2022**, *12*, 130. [CrossRef] [PubMed]
153. Börnsen, L.; Khademi, M.; Olsson, T.; Sørensen, P.S.; Sellebjerg, F. Osteopontin concentrations are increased in cerebrospinal fluid during attacks of multiple sclerosis. *Mult. Scler. J.* **2011**, *17*, 32–42. [CrossRef] [PubMed]
154. Jakovac, H.; Grubić Kezele, T.; Šućurović, S.; Mulac-Jeričević, B.; Radošević-Stašić, B. Osteopontin-metallothionein I/II interactions in experimental autoimmune encephalomyelitis. *Neuroscience* **2017**, *350*, 133–145. [CrossRef]
155. LoPresti, P. HDAC6 in Diseases of Cognition and of Neurons. *Cells* **2020**, *10*, 12. [CrossRef]
156. Strebl, M.G.; Campbell, A.J.; Zhao, W.N.; Schroeder, F.A.; Riley, M.M.; Chindavong, P.S.; Morin, T.M.; Haggarty, S.J.; Wagner, F.F.; Ritter, T.; et al. HDAC6 Brain Mapping with [$^{18}$F] Bavarostat Enabled by a Ru-Mediated Deoxyfluorination. *ACS Central Sci.* **2017**, *3*, 1006–1014. [CrossRef]
157. Joilin, G.; Gray, E.; Thompson, A.G.; Bobeva, Y.; Talbot, K.; Weishaupt, J.; Ludolph, A.; Malaspina, A.; Leigh, P.N.; Newbury, S.F.; et al. Identification of a potential non-coding RNA biomarker signature for amyotrophic lateral sclerosis. *Brain Commun.* **2020**, *2*, fcaa053. [CrossRef]

MDPI
St. Alban-Anlage 66
4052 Basel
Switzerland
Tel. +41 61 683 77 34
Fax +41 61 302 89 18
www.mdpi.com

*Biomedicines* Editorial Office
E-mail: biomedicines@mdpi.com
www.mdpi.com/journal/biomedicines

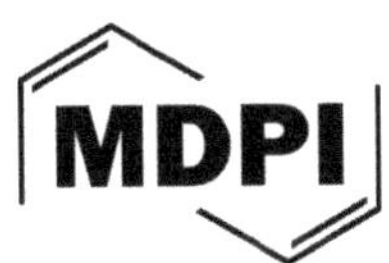

www.ingramcontent.com/pod-product-compliance
Lightning Source LLC
LaVergne TN
LVHW071008170726
843515LV00006B/1106

* 9 7 8 3 0 3 6 5 5 7 3 1 1 *